T0311640

'A CHEAP, SAFE AND NATURAL MEDICINE'

RELIGION, MEDICINE AND CULTURE IN JOHN WESLEY'S *PRIMITIVE PHYSIC*

THE WELLCOME SERIES
IN THE HISTORY OF MEDICINE

Forthcoming :

Attending Madness:
A History of Work in the Victorian Asylum

Lee-Ann Monk

The Wellcome Series in the History of Medicine series editors are
V. Nutton, M. Neve and R. Cooter.
Please send all queries regarding the series to Michael Laycock,
The Wellcome Trust Centre for the History of Medicine at UCL,
183 Euston Road, London NW1 2BE, UK.

'A CHEAP, SAFE AND NATURAL MEDICINE'

RELIGION, MEDICINE AND CULTURE IN JOHN WESLEY'S *PRIMITIVE PHYSIC*

Deborah Madden

Amsterdam – New York, NY 2007

First published in 2007
by Editions Rodopi B. V., Amsterdam – New York, NY 2007.

Editions Rodopi B.V. © 2007

Design and Typesetting by Michael Laycock,
The Wellcome Trust Centre for the History of Medicine at UCL.
Printed and bound in The Netherlands by Editions Rodopi B.V.,
Amsterdam – New York, NY 2007.

Index by Rosemary Anderson.

All rights reserved. No part of this book may be reprinted or reproduced or
utilised in any form or by any electronic, mechanical, or other means, now
known or hereafter invented, including photocopying and recording, or in
any information storage or retrieval system, without permission in writing
from The Wellcome Trust Centre for the History of Medicine at UCL.

British Library Cataloguing in Publication Data
A catalogue record for this book is available from the British Library

ISBN 978-90-420-2274-4

'"A Cheap, Safe and Natural Medicine"
Religion, Medicine and Culture in John Wesley's *Primitive Physic* –
Amsterdam – New York, NY:
Rodopi. – ill.
(Clio Medica 83 / ISSN 0045-7183;
The Wellcome Series in the History of Medicine)

Front cover:
John Wesley. Mezzotint by J. Faber, junior, 1743, after J. Williams.
Courtesy: Wellcome Library, London. Digitally coloured, 2007.

© Editions Rodopi B. V., Amsterdam – New York, NY 2007
Printed in The Netherlands

All titles in the Clio Medica series (from 1999 onwards) are available to
download from the IngentaConnect website: http://www.ingentaconnect.co.uk

Contents

*This book is dedicated
to the memory of K. Madden*

Preface

Key editions of John Wesley's *Primitive Physic: or, An Easy and Natural Method of Curing Most Diseases*, between 1747 (1st) and 1792 (24th), have been used to permit greater cross-textual analysis between this text and his other 'scientific' works written at a later date – *The Desideratum: Or, Electricity Made Plain and Useful* (1759) and *A Survey of the Wisdom of God in the Creation Or, A Compendium of Natural Philosophy* (1763). All editions of *Primitive Physic* following that of the first were corrected and enlarged by Wesley in the light of other medical and scientific discoveries. In 1755 (5th edition) he added footnotes as well as 'tried and tested remedies'. He also omitted or reduced the use of those 'extremely dangerous' 'Herculean' medicines, which included opium, bark, steel and quicksilver. In 1760 (1761, 9th edition) a postscript alerts the reader to the fact that electrical therapy was included, and in 1772 (15th edition) Wesley marked his favourite prescriptions with an asterisk. In 1781 (20th edition) a further postscript (written in 1780) contained an explanation of how particular omissions and alterations to the text had taken place as a result of contemporary medical criticism. The 23rd edition (1791) is important because it was the last written during his lifetime – this edition was re-published by Epworth Press with an editor's introduction by A. Wesley Hill in 1960. The text used and referred to here, however, is the 24th edition (London: G. Paramore, 1792). This edition is the last 'authentic' copy of *Primitive Physic* – the language and text of the 23rd edition was modernised by its editor.

The 1871 reprint of the 1st edition of *The Desideratum: Or, Electricity Made Plain and Useful* (London: Bailliere, Tindal and Cox, 1759) has been particularly useful, though there were five editions of this text in Wesley's lifetime. For *A Survey of the Wisdom of God in the Creation: Or, A Compendium of Natural Philosophy* (1763), I have drawn on the 3rd edition in five volumes (London: J. Fry, 1777). The sermons have been cited from *The Bicentennial Edition of the Works of John Wesley*, edited by Albert C. Outler, four volumes (Abingdon Press: Nashville, 1984) and, unless otherwise stated, extracts from Wesley's *Journal* have been taken from N. Curnock's eigth-volume edition (London: n.p., 1909–16). Citations from

3

Wesley's letters are drawn from J. Telford's eight-volume edited collection, *The Letters of the Revd. John Wesley, A.M.* (London: Epworth Press, 1931).

Acknowledgements

Examining the centrality of medicine and healing to John Wesley's theology has meant that I have necessarily needed to draw on the expertise of academics who inhabit very different worlds. In this, I have been extremely fortunate in being able to utilise a range of knowledge from leading scholars in the disciplines of eighteenth-century medicine, theology, literary criticism and cultural studies.

I owe an enormous debt of gratitude to Dr Brian Young, who not only read this work in its Doctoral thesis form, but who provided the initial inspiration for my chosen topic as an undergraduate at the University of Sussex. Dr Young put research and teaching opportunities my way as a postgraduate and, indeed, this book has developed and grown out of a Masters dissertation completed in 1998 at the University of Sussex. It was Dr Young who introduced my work to Dr John Walsh – a terrifying prospect, which, by turns, proved to be rewarding and vital. Dr Walsh's penetrating and thorough reading of my work, combined with his incisive common sense and valuable 'bibliographical jottings', have benefited this study considerably and for this I am deeply honoured.

I would very much like to express thanks to Revd Dr Jane Shaw, my DPhil supervisor, who steered a steady path between intellectual comment and practical assistance. Dr Shaw also presented me with ample research opportunities that helped to cast fresh perspectives on work relating to Wesley. The advice and comments given by thesis examiners, Dr Jeremy Gregory and Dr Perry Gauci, as well as suggestions made by journal editors and reviewers, have been gratefully received and are now fully incorporated into this book. I want also to acknowledge here the editors of *Clio Medica* and to thank Michael Laycock for his diligence.

Many thanks to Professor Norman Vance whose learned wit and refreshing candour still illuminates the margins of a very rough first draft thesis chapter. He might be glad to know that those diligent annotations were subsequently followed up and carefully integrated into the work. The tremendous generosity of Professor Randy Maddox must also be acknowledged here. In what can only be described as an act of sheer benevolence, Randy Maddox provided me with a bibliography of John Wesley's medical references – a compilation on which he had been working.

As is often the case with parallel research projects, Maddox's findings arrived too late for me to utilise in my doctoral thesis. I am, however, very grateful to Randy Maddox for his encouragement and can, at least, acknowledge here his forthcoming chapter that shares so many common interests and concerns.[1] There are a number of other academics too, whom I wish to thank at Lincoln College. The kind support of Rector Paul Langford, my College Advisor, and Dr Anne Marie Drummond who offered much needed practical help at a critical time while writing my thesis.

The primary texts used for research into this topic were obtained from a range of libraries, including the Bodleian Library, Radcliffe Science Library, British Library, John Rylands University Library and the Wellcome Trust Centres for the History of Medicine (both in London and Oxford). Smaller college libraries included those of Regent's Park, Lincoln and Corpus Christi. I am extremely grateful for all the assistance given to me by the staff working in those libraries. At this juncture, I wish to state that research for this work would not have been possible without the financial assistance of both the Arts and Humanities Research Board and the Wellcome Trust Centre for the History of Medicine. Concerning the latter, I would like to acknowledge the late Professor Roy Porter. When first embarking on the unpredictable journey that is academia, Roy Porter was kind enough to offer invaluable insights into an array of matters that were of concern to me at that time but which also included advice on funding. The immense contribution Porter has made to the history of medicine and his subsequent influence over my work will quickly become apparent to any reader of this book.

Finally, I wish to make one or two personal acknowledgements. Thanks to Graham Collis for the extensive bibliographies he compiled for me while engaging in (non-academic) research – these bibliographies were purely a by-product of his own consuming passion for early-modern history. Louise Payne-Madden's clarity and focus on a methodological point served to remind me of the direction my work needed to go, while the invigorating and inspiring cross-channel telephone conversations I have had with Alison Faiers provided much needed distraction as well as motivation. My deepest thanks and gratitude must go to Dr David Towsey, whose formidable intelligence, combined with tireless patience and unruffled demeanour, safeguarded me against complete insanity. This work was written for Kitty and Zac Towsey whose very existence brought it urgently to fruition. Any infelicities that remain here are, of course, my own.

Note

1. R.L. Maddox, 'A Heritage Reclaimed: John Wesley on Holistic Health and Healing' in M.E.M. Moore (ed.), *A Living Tradition* (Nashville, TN: Kingswood Books, forthcoming).

PRIMITIVE PHYSIC:

OR,

An EASY and NATURAL METHOD

OF

CURING

MOST

DISEASES.

By *JOHN WESLEY*, M.A.

Homo sam; humani nihil a me alienum puto.

THE TWENTY-FOURTH EDITION.

LONDON:

Printed by G. PARAMORE, *North-Green, Worship-Street;*
And sold by G. WHITFIELD, at the Chapel, City-Road,
and at all the Methodist Preaching-Houses in Town and
Country. 1792.

Frontispiece to Primitive Physic.
Courtesy: Wellcome Library, London.

PART I

**THE MEDICAL HOLISM
OF *PRIMITIVE PHYSIC***

1

Introduction:
Primitive Physic Explain'd in an Easy and Natural Method

> Without any concern about the obliging or disobliging any man living, a mean
> hand has made here some little attempt, towards a plain and easy way of curing
> most diseases. I have only consulted herein, Experience, common sense, and the
> common Interest of Mankind.
>
> John Wesley, 'The Preface', *Primitive Physic* (1747)[1]

John Wesley's medical manual, *Primitive Physic: Or, An Easy and Natural
Method of Curing Most Diseases*, was one of the most popular medical
volumes published in eighteenth-century England – twenty-three editions
went to press in his lifetime; the last and thirty-seventh edition was
published in 1859.[2] No one was more surprised at the public's response to
Primitive Physic than Wesley himself, as is apparent in the 'Postscript' to the
fifth edition of 1755:

> It was a great surprise to the Editor of the following Collection, that there
> was so swift and large a demand for it; that three impressions were called for
> in four or five years; and that it was not only re-published by the Booksellers
> of a neighbouring nation; but also inserted by parts in their public papers,
> and so propagated through the whole kingdom. This encouraged him
> carefully to revise the whole, and to publish it again with several alterations,
> which it is hoped may make it of greater use to those who love common
> sense and common honesty.[3]

Primitive Physic was certainly in great demand, but to categorise this text
as simply 'populist', as most historians continue to do, is to obscure its rich
cultural meanings and discursive contexts. This interpretation conceals the
extensive range of authoritative references drawn from a variety of European
sources that are brought to bear by Wesley in *Primitive Physic*.

On the face of it, *Primitive Physic* is a manual which seems to contain a
strange combination of common sense and religion. There is no doubt that
emphasis on the populist strains of *Primitive Physic* can largely be attributed
to the effective nature of Wesley's rhetoric, of which the passage previously
quoted is a good example. Here, Wesley seeks to convince, comfort and

reassure his reader that *Primitive Physic* is concerned to steer an empiricist course between the Scylla of abstruse medical theory and the Charybdis of speculative philosophy. 'Plain', 'easy', 'experience' and 'common sense' are words used specifically to make explicit the practical orientation of his text. Historians, particularly historians of medicine, could be forgiven for failing to see beyond the distortions of polemical discourse in Wesley's medical and scientific work. Yet the widespread appeal of *Primitive Physic*, what Wesley regarded as its very strength, came to be caricatured in twentieth-century historiography as evidence of an 'absurd, fantastic compilation of uncritical folklore'.[4]

Criticism on this basis was often strangely reminiscent of that levelled at Wesley by those anxious to guard their status as 'professional' physicians, and whose reaction now appears to be oddly disproportionate. If the Methodist movement as a whole raised serious objections, Wesley's medical manual seems to have rubbed salt into the wounds of its detractors. Arrows of stinging criticism flew from every quarter, and feverish accusations of 'quackery' gushed from the quills of physicians, satirists and clergymen alike.

Part of this reaction can be attributed to the shock waves felt by Georgian society in response to an ardent Evangelical revival – one that appeared to wield an unhealthy influence over the lower orders. The emotional 'convulsions' of those 'enthusiastic' elements within the Methodist movement, combined with its leader's penchant for dispensing medical advice, offended good taste, moderation and polite cultural standards. Critics thus sought recourse to satire, frequently the best remedy for religious distemper, in the form of garish caricatures, which depicted Wesley as a religious and medical quack.[5]

It was only a matter of time before eighteenth-century presses groaned under the sheer volume of pamphlets, articles and tracts which sought to establish a connection between Methodism and religious madness, be it the 'old fanaticism' of seventeenth-century Puritanism, or the authoritarian tyranny of Rome. The potency of this argument can be seen most clearly in Bishop Lavington's classic discussion of the subject, *The Enthusiasm of Methodists and Papists Compared*, written in three parts between 1749 and 1754. Lavington cited as his main source and authority Henry More's *Enthusiasmus Triumphatus* (1656), which had set out to reveal a link between religious inspiration and madness. Interestingly, More's text was abridged and published as *Enthusiasm Explained* in 1739, largely as a result of the growth of Methodism. Following on from where More had left off, Lavington argued that zeal and enthusiasm were fevers and diseases of the mind, both of which were intimately connected to Catholicism and Methodism.[6]

Figure 1.1

John Wesley preaching outside a church.
Wellcome Library, London.

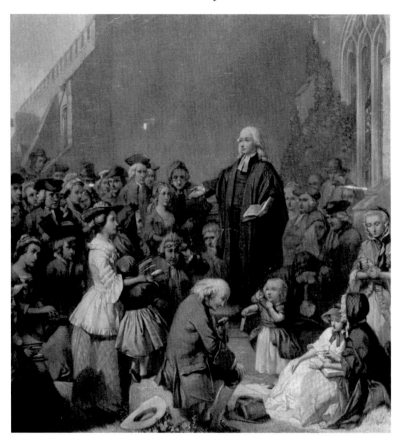

Contemporary anxiety over letting the genie of enthusiasm out of the bottle is only part of a multi-faceted and complicated story. In many instances, the gleeful dismemberment of *Primitive Physic* by critics was unjustified and unwarranted. An examination of how this reaction fits into a complex web of attitudes must also bear in mind that where criticism was unnecessarily cruel, or even irrational, its motivation remains a mystery, which proves impossible to unravel. The opprobrium heaped upon *Primitive Physic* is not suggestive of any actual quackery committed by Wesley, and a close reading of his medical manual reveals a surprising array of sources as well as opening up his relationship to medicine, 'science' and theology. Here, the now freighted word 'science' in its early-modern context is used in a deliberately anachronistic way: like the philosopher John Ray and the philosopher-divine William Derham, Wesley understood 'science' to mean natural philosophy, which of course carried its own distinctive theological bias. This bias was concerned, primarily, with using natural philosophy to undercut the worst deistic excesses of mechanical or speculative philosophies. Just as few scholars have detected the scientific and philosophical perspectives that underpin Wesley's theology,[7] it has also been the case that many have ignored the theological context in which Wesley wrote his scientific work.[8] Demonstrating the powerful interplay between science, medicine and theology that takes place in *Primitive Physic* is one of the main concerns of this book.

This is not to suggest that Wesley's medical remedies were underpinned by a view of healing that relied purely upon faith. An explicit aim here is an avoidance of a lengthy consideration of Wesley's interest in faith healing and the miraculous. I have examined instead the way in which Wesley deploys religious, scientific and medical discourses on their own terms in *Primitive Physic*. For example, 'The Preface' to *Primitive Physic* points to how man and nature are conditioned by God, but the remedies contained in the main body of the text rely entirely upon empirical and rational claims for their efficacy. Here, the connection between 'The Preface' and 'Collection of Receipts' shows the trajectory of Wesley's work in general: it transforms a divinely-ordered universe into an explanation of how that order works itself out in ways that are rationally verifiable and probable. Wesley endeavoured to do this by way of ensuring medical credibility whilst protecting his integrity as a Christian.

Primitive Physic exemplifies Wesley's role as what Henry D. Rack has called a 'cultural mediator'.[9] The mediation of complex material to the literate and semi-literate in eighteenth-century England was intimately linked to Wesley's rhetoric of 'plain' language, which also contained a deep theological imperative connected to his missionary zeal for practical piety. 'Plain style' belies the full complexity and multiple layers constructed in Wesley's prose, where he made a conscious move to reject ornate style in favour of the Horatian rule to make 'concise your diction, let your sense be clear, not with weight your words fatigue the ear'.[10] Certainly, he makes this move explicit in the other 'scientific' works: *The Desideratum: Or, Electricity Made Plain and Useful*, published anonymously in 1759, and *A Survey of the Wisdom of God in the Creation: Or, A Compendium of Natural Philosophy* – the latter of which was heavily amended, re-worked and enlarged with footnotes. Originally a Latin work entitled *Elementa Philosophiae Practicae et Theoreticae* (1703), this text was written by John Francis Buddaeus of Jena University.[11]

Wesley's scientific work was motivated, not merely from a popularising impulse – which, for some of Wesley's modern-day critics, seems to imply a downgrading of intellectual material – but also fed into a much broader religious and social aim. Some time ago, Robert. E. Schofield commented that the three major scientific works written by Wesley could be broken down into three simple categories: practical (*Primitive Physic*), 'scientific' (*Desideratum*) and religious (*Compendium*).[12] This, I think, is partially true, though in writing *Primitive Physic*, Wesley twinned the roles of pastor and physician to combine simple, traditional methods of healing with the new scientific and medical discoveries of his day. Exposing this symbiotic relationship can help to undermine the still all too common misrepresentation of John Wesley as unthinking 'enthusiast', anti-theoretical 'empirick' responding to Enlightenment rationalism, principally Newtonian science.[13]

Drawing on the seminal work of J.D. Walsh, scholars such as A.C. Outler, R.E. Brantley, Henry D. Rack, Isabel Rivers, Brian W. Young and Phyllis Mack have focused on the eclectic and complex nature of Wesley's theology. These scholars have raised important questions and challenged some of the caricatures of both John Wesley and Methodism in general.[14] Though engaged in very different projects, a common theme shared by this academic work is an acute sensitivity to language. By identifying the language of religion current during the early-modern period, the work of Isabel Rivers has managed to unpack, even deconstruct, terms such as 'reason', 'enthusiast' and 'orthodox'. By contrast, but by no means contrary to this work, the way in which Wesley used the language of empiricism and 'rationalism' when appealing to men of reason *and* religion are themes covered by A.C. Outler, Henry D. Rack and Phyllis Mack.

These scholars have shown us the difficulty of imposing a uniformity to the language of the period under discussion. Using this aspect of their work has helped to question that type of Foucauldian analysis which privileges 'discursive constructions' to ascribe a unifying theme to variegated human experiences over long periods of time. Such an analysis denies historical contingency and ignores points of division and contact between very different groups. With regard to the period and topic under discussion here, social and cultural historians of medicine have long pointed to both the shared and contested knowledge between lay medics, apothecaries, physicians and patients. Here, no uniformity can be ascribed to the 'medicalisation' of language or, indeed, practice, nor did any one dominant discourse subsume the other. Instead, it was the case, as Phyllis Mack suggests, that a wide range of epistemologies of disease and pain co-existed.[15]

On the subject of Wesley's interest in philosophy, science and medicine, vital contributions have been made by Henry D. Rack, W.J. Turrell, John C.

English, R.E. Schofield, J. Cule, J.W. Haas, G.S. Rousseau and Phillip W. Ott. Collectively, this work has done a great deal to break down traditional dichotomies by teasing out the 'rational' elements of Wesley's thought.[16] English and Haas have shown how Wesley's ambivalent attitude to the anti-Newtonian writings of religious thinker, John Hutchinson, means that he continues to be cast as an anti-intellectual with unorthodox scientific leanings. Phillip W. Ott and Randy Maddox are scholars who have written illuminating articles and lectures on particular features of Wesley's medical holism. Ott has produced several engaging and pithy articles on the way in which Wesley used medical imagery and metaphor to describe the pursuit of health (spiritual and physical) as 'therapy' for the soul.[17] More recently, Maddox has felt the need to identify Wesley's 'serious interest in health and healing' because this aspect of his ministry has been consistently ignored. Few in Wesleyan traditions today, he argues, 'are aware that Wesley published a collection of advice for preserving health and treating diseases….'[18] Even when they are aware, many still believe that *Primitive Physic* represents an embarrassing collection of folk remedies and old wives' tales.[19] Both Ott and Maddox focus on the theological mainsprings of Wesley's interest in medicine, but an analysis covering the rich context of his engagement with medicine has not yet been undertaken in a sustained way.

The central place of medicine and healing to both Wesley and the Methodist movement continues to be overlooked by historians generally, whilst historians of medicine still regard *Primitive Physic* as a populist text to be downplayed on this basis. A serious consideration of *Primitive Physic* in all of its contextual complexity has yet to take place by an historian. G.S. Rousseau's article, 'John Wesley's "Primitive Physick" (1747)', written for the *Harvard Library Bulletin* in 1968, briefly summarised and contextualised the significance of this important work.[20] Rousseau opened the way for a lengthier and more detailed investigation into the actual methods deployed by Wesley. This article thus serves here as a useful starting point to locate *Primitive Physic* in its intellectual, religious, social and cultural context. Moving on from Rousseau's article, this book will investigate Wesley's dialogue with a broad sweep of medical practitioners while tracking the course of those treatments arranged in *Primitive Physic*. In so doing, the full extent of this text's typicality can be uncovered and revealed.

Wesley's life-long passion for science and medicine attests to the fact that he cannot easily be ascribed to any anti-rationalist or 'Counter-Enlightenment' camp. Furthermore, detailed evidence can show how his physic compares favourably to that of other pious medical men – not only those with an empiricist cast of mind, such as John Locke and Thomas Sydenham, but also practitioners like Dr George Cheyne and Dr Richard Mead who were thoroughly Newtonian in their outlook. Breaking down the categories of empirical and speculative approaches, but also of 'professional' and 'lay knowledge', will provide a more complex picture of a man who was coming to terms with changes in medical theory, language and practice.

For Wesley, social and personal development did not depend exclusively on enlightened thinking or religious faith, but on rationalism (head) and religion (heart) working together within an overall framework of holism or 'wholeness' – working together whilst demonstrating their own strengths. *Primitive Physic* provides its reader with an interpretation of the universe that is organised (though not pre-ordained) by God, and this cosmography prefaces a series of individual medical remedies. Significantly, the remedies listed in *Primitive Physic* are required to stand or fall on empirical efficacy and are judged, therefore, according to rationalistic standards. The success of those remedies was used by Wesley to serve his vocation of practical piety, which was motivated by a holistic view of nature – a view inspired by the spiritualism of Primitive Christianity. Exploring the hermeneutics of Wesley's Primitive Christianity in Chapter 2 does not simply offer the reader a theological detour, but provides us with the best way of assessing the considerable medical achievement that *Primitive Physic* represents.

The providential organisation of man and nature means that the promotion of bodily health becomes an act of spiritual vindication. Yet the two domains of this discourse – religion (spiritual health) and medicine (bodily health) – are kept distinct by Wesley. As already noted, it was essential to keep each domain distinct in order to maintain intellectual credibility – theologically and medically. Wesley makes this manoeuvre on the one hand, but on the other sees no contradiction in bringing those discourses together to serve his mission: a mission to improve the world in which he lived.

Wesley's medical remedies did not need to rely on faith, but an acknowledgement of his epistemology of spirit need not, as Susan Juster has argued, become a 'quirky if entertaining journey down an atavistic path'. Rather, it should lead directly 'to some of the most pressing intellectual and political changes facing early modern Britons'.[21] In this context, it is apparent that John Wesley personifies those very tensions and contradictions which lie at the heart of English enlightened thinking. Individuals like Wesley, a learned, classical scholar who was deeply committed to practical piety, confound simplistic polarities. Contextualising a figure who continues to be regarded as anti-Enlightenment allows one to make this point, whilst simultaneously undercutting interpretations that pit 'orthodox' against 'unorthodox', 'Reason' against 'Enthusiasm'.

As is now sufficiently well known, 'reason' contained multiple meanings in the period under analysis and its role was frequently open to question. Dr Johnson identified a great fear faced by his contemporaries when he suggested that the most alarming threat to society was the uncertain continuance of reason. David Hume wryly noted that the ratio of folly to reason in his age had not significantly changed from that of ages past. Often, reason became a field on which duels instigated by diverse parties were fought.[22] While most enlightened thinkers were keen to demonstrate the reasonableness of Christianity, it was also the case that just as many were eager to show that reason itself retained its theological principle.[23] Wesley makes this explicit in his *An Earnest Appeal to Men of Reason and Religion* (1743) and his awareness of the complex nature of reason, combined with a serious commitment to science and medicine, proves that the act of pairing oppositions such as 'reason' and 'unreason' is illusory. The lines of Enlightenment thinking are less sharp and more fluid, whilst each antithesis is more complex and less consistent than historians once imagined.[24]

The virtue of recent Enlightenment historiography lies in the fact that it has shown us the limitations of seeing the 'Enlightenment project' of modernity as being predominantly rationalist and thus secular. As a critique, this has now reached a point of self-dissolution, and the arguments surrounding it are stale. In recent years, Enlightenment scholarship has steered a *via media* between triumphant grand narrative and a pessimistic analysis that sees the Enlightenment as bestowing the legacy of its dark side onto the twentieth century in the form of exclusivity, religious intolerance and ethnic cleansing.[25] Starting with Kant's idea of Enlightenment as a continuing, rather than completed, process of human understanding, this scholarship has done much to restore the contradictory tensions, self-doubt and self-questioning that preoccupied many philosophers, theologians and writers.[26] Those studies that have been concerned to draw out common European Enlightenment themes whilst respecting national and local experiences have provided a variegated geography of the Enlightenment, which has successfully managed to recapture a sense of the period as a whole.[27]

Concomitant to this development is the fact that medical and scientific historiography has reorientated itself towards forging an interesting relationship with histories of Enlightenment, but more specifically, social, cultural and religious histories. These links have led to many transformations taking place within the history of medicine, with a number of scholars amply demonstrating the fluidity of Enlightenment medical practice.[28] Roy Porter and other well-known historians of medicine, such as William F. Bynum, Christopher Lawrence, Anita Guerrini and Joan Lane, amongst others, have identified the crucial role played by religion and piety in the practice of medicine. The significant contribution made by these scholars lies in the fact that they have done much to blur the lines of demarcation between 'professional' and 'quack', secular and religious, to provide a more dynamic picture of the connections between medicine, religion and 'superstition'.

In addition to this, under the influence of Jürgen Habermas's classic text, *Strukturwandel der Öffentlichkeit* (1962), translated in 1989 as *The Structural Transformation of the Public Sphere. An Enquiry into a Category of Bourgeois Society*, medicine and science have come to be regarded as part of a 'public realm', characterised by 'polite' standards and the commodification of a robust print culture.[29] This text has been crucial to the development of the historiography of medicine and science, and its influence can be seen most clearly in the works of Roy Porter, Jan Golinski, Simon Schaffer and Stephen Shapin. With commercial and consumer-led imperatives becoming a major driving force behind medical practice, and the medical needs of the wealthy shaping orthodox medicine – a development that Wesley bitterly denounced in 'The Preface' to *Primitive Physic* – the boundary between doctor, non-medical practitioner and patient in Georgian England is now recognised as having been sufficiently unclear.[30]

Re-figuring the Enlightenment to reveal its nervous solidarity in this way has greatly benefited Wesley, who becomes less of an anomaly and begins to resemble someone typical of a vibrant European print culture which was rich in a variety of intellectual and theological traditions. Even the most radical of sceptics, those amongst the *philosophes*, who wished to escape established traditions, canons and orthodoxies, did so, not by providing a 'secular' critique in contradistinction with, or absolutely external to Christian tradition, but via an internal questioning, which owed a debt to the very object of its critique. It is now well known that the clerical nature of English enlightened philosophy, science and medicine flourished within a context of piety, so that interpretations of illness, for example, continued to be imbued with religious meanings.[31] Although it remains the case that history of medicine scholars continue to downplay John Wesley's contribution to the medical scene, it is also fair to say that some have significantly modified their views and are more willing to acknowledge the rational, empirical elements of his work.[32] Utilising the methodology set down by those scholars concerned to show the fluidity of eighteenth-century medical practice, a fully contextualised *Primitive Physic* can give us great insight into the ideological mix of Wesleyan thought. This insight necessarily involves a critique of the misconceptions that have grown out of what is usually regarded as Wesley's 'opposing' tendencies of rationalism and 'enthusiasm'.

Examining the centrality of medicine and healing in Wesley's theology provides greater scope for what in modern academic parlance is termed 'inter-disciplinarity'. It is certainly the case that Wesley's practice of medicine has been traditionally neglected by historians because it falls between disciplines. Methodologically, this study wishes as its starting point to avoid both rigid subject boundaries and modern 'inter-disciplinariness', working instead, back to an original insight – an insight that can bring a range of traditions under consideration. Finally, the fact that John Wesley, founder and leader of the Methodist movement, continues to be more revered than read, more eulogised than understood, means that a critical approach to *Primitive Physic* is still needed. The objective here is to conduct an exploration of Wesley's medical holism before demonstrating how *Primitive Physic* represents an enlightened empirical approach to medicine. *Primitive Physic* was not simply bounded by the immediate practical needs of its readership, but participated in several significant and interconnected intellectual debates. An assessment of Wesley's contribution to medicine must make two important observations; the first involves looking at how the reciprocal relationship between theology and Enlightened philosophy was expressed in his written work. Attention to this is crucial because various opponents evoked different responses. Various motivations and factors need to be taken into account, even when analysing a single, seemingly straightforward, text. The motivating force behind Wesley's explication of man's post-lapsarian condition in the first paragraph of 'The Preface' to *Primitive Physic* is distinct from the practical remedies suggested in Wesley's collection of receipts. Yet it is also vital to see how these very different manoeuvres cannot be separated from Wesley's holistic conception of medicine. This latter point leads on to my second observation. It is essential to understand how Wesley translated his intellectual endeavours into a pragmatic and workable practical piety – a practical piety that drew on the tradition of Primitive Christianity to meet the physical and spiritual needs of the poor in eighteenth-century England.

This process reveals the teleology of Wesley's thinking and praxis. He combined simple traditional medicine with the best scientific discoveries of his day because healing was central to his theology. Sickness of the flesh implied sickness of the spirit, but if allusions were made to the divine in 'The Preface', Wesley's medical practice was thoroughly empirical and duly recorded as such in the main body of *Primitive Physic.* Contemporary critics and subsequent scholars who claimed that Wesley spiritualised illness by attributing madness to demonic possession must not have read the prescriptions for lunacy, madness and nervous disorders in *Primitive Physic,* all of which tie in with eighteenth-century medical practice. Before launching into an exploration of Wesley's conception of healing and assessing his contribution to the world of Georgian medicine, it will be necessary first to say a word or two about the methodological approach taken here.

As far as Wesley was concerned, the greatest benefit to mankind could be found in making available an 'easy' and 'natural' method for curing most diseases. The success of this method lay, not simply in its popularising impulse, but in the fact that this seemingly 'simple' manual contained a hermeneutics of enormous versatility and power – one that has been overlooked or missed by many historians. Wesley's determination to convey complex material in 'plain' language amounted to a rhetoric that was multi-layered. *Primitive Physic* is a manual that is focused towards very specific problems – this even includes setting out practical solutions for man in his post-lapsarian fallen state. Specifying its focus in this way allowed Wesley to articulate otherwise diverse, complex and unmanageable bodies of knowledge to *useful effect*. In this sense, his advice was not merely practical in its basis but contained a hermeneutic for theoretical knowledge.

Identifying this removes one barrier, but leaves behind an obvious methodological problem, which involves the arrangement and articulation of diverse and complex material. When unpicking the fabric of Wesley's texts to demonstrate the myriad of allusions made, how is one to avoid falling back into the complexity and confusion that he successfully controlled? One way of managing the manifold themes that are brought to light is to respect those boundaries and limitations put in place by Wesley himself. It therefore becomes necessary to articulate the various bodies of knowledge according to the sequence of specific, practical applications with which Wesley gave them life. This refers back to my earlier point about the necessity of observing how Wesley's intellectual pre-occupations came to be translated practically in the public realm; how he makes distinct the practical and physical, whilst theoretically reconciling his (spiritual) conception of healing with eighteenth-century medical practice. Wesley's solution was to adopt a pragmatic empirical approach that was practical in its effects, while also taking a stance that treated together body, mind and spirit – although this latter pietistic, holistic stance very much depended on the receptivity of the person being treated.

In order to control, arrange and articulate the endlessly intricate themes that are unearthed by Wesley's medical manual, the structure of this book has needed to loosely follow that of *Primitive Physic*. Part One of this volume thus examines 'The Preface' to Wesley's text in its broadest possible context. Tracing the contours of the first three sections of 'The Preface' in Chapter 2, draws out particular overarching theological themes that shaped Wesley's thinking and praxis, Primitive Christianity and practical piety. These themes are analysed by way of providing a hermeneutical key to his medical practice. Wesley's sermons are also a useful general source for reiterating the centrality of healing to his theology, seen most vividly in the recurrence of medical language and imagery in this rather unexpected context. Attention has also been paid to the correlation between Primitive Christianity, practical piety and the tradition of natural philosophy and empirical medicine, which

Wesley adopted from, amongst others, Francis Bacon, Robert Boyle, Thomas Sydenham and John Locke. Related to, but also bridging these themes, is the theological imperative behind Wesley's 'plain' style where a brief explication is offered.

Sections Four to Fifteen of 'The Preface' form the basis of a discussion in Chapter 3 about the eighteenth-century medical scene. The complex position *Primitive Physic* adopts in the quarrel between the modern and ancients – physic as an art or science – is extrapolated from the historiography Wesley formulates to criticise some aspects of Georgian medical practice. An opportunity to compare Wesley's criticism with actual contemporary medical practice naturally presents itself here, which in turn gives rise to an analysis of those contemporary medical writers whom Wesley esteems and cites in *Primitive Physic*. It also seemed appropriate, when looking at Wesley's critique of Georgian medical practice, to include an investigation into some of the criticisms levelled back at *Primitive Physic*, thereby making plain the dialogical nature of the text. A detailed inquiry into the validity of Dr William Hawes's *An Examination of the Rev Mr John Wesley's Primitive Physic* (1776), in relation to observations made by other physicians about Wesley's text, highlights the concerns and preoccupations of an established 'professional' physician and founder of the Royal Humane Society.

Section Sixteen of 'The Preface' shifts its focus onto regimen, and here Wesley presents his reader with a 'few Plain, easy Rules [added to, but] chiefly transcribed from Dr. *Cheyne*'.[33] Wesley breaks this section down into sub-sections I-VI, placing them under the following headings that make up the 'non-naturals': air, diet, sleep, exercise, evacuations and the passions. The series of rules that are listed under each of the headings are examined in Chapter 4 to indicate the way in which Wesley sees a symbiotic relationship between science, regimen, health, temperance, morality and purity. This chapter is notable for identifying the importance Wesley attached to the primary role played by regimen in the area of preventative medicine. Regimen, though powerfully connected to morality and virtue in Wesley's mind, was a practical concern; it provided a safe and cost-effective way of ensuring the health of those poorer members of society.

Part II, or Chapter 5, turns its attention to the main body of *Primitive Physic* and its collection of receipts. Certain key diseases that dominated eighteenth-century life have been assembled and brought under consideration. Rousseau has suggested that the reason why historians have failed to analyse Wesley's text is due to *Primitive Physic* being 'a difficult book for anyone other than a medical historian to evaluate'.[34] One of the main problems with reading *Primitive Physic* is the apparent opacity of the enumerative style of its receipts. These receipts do not merely represent the sum total of their individual remedies, but constitute substantive meaning and argument in their articulation. Chapter 5 thus hopes to bring to light these complex bodies of knowledge and attendant medical debates current in eighteenth-century England. The enumerative style of *Primitive Physic* was a mechanism used by Wesley to assemble complex bodies of knowledge. It was also his way of rooting *Primitive Physic* in that tradition of medical empiricism espoused by Robert Boyle – though, as will become clear, Wesley drew on a variety of other eighteenth-century medical sources. This makes it difficult to simply regard *Primitive Physic* as belonging to that class of 'kitchen-physic' prevalent in late-seventeenth century England.

The remedies suggested by Wesley are subjected to a two-fold analysis. This involves looking at exactly how Wesley's remedies compare to those of other contemporary medical practitioners and noting the way in which articles change over time in various editions of *Primitive Physic*. Particular notice has been taken of the incorporation of new scientific and medical discoveries, such as electrical therapy. Attendant to this are the omissions made in later editions, which take into account new medical findings or current debates. An examination of this process is aided by checking the 'Postscript' to relevant editions of *Primitive Physic*. This goes some way to providing an explanation for some omissions – though not all. Where this has failed, cross-textual analysis of Wesley's other scientific work, and extracts from his *Journal* and *Letters*, are important for gleaning insights into the omissions, as well as casting light on how he practised medicine generally.

Enough now has been said about the arrangement of Wesley's text here. What then, of other sources? It should be clear that a wide variety of other printed primary sources have been brought together; sources ranging from scientific tracts expounding upon electricity and the chemical composition of mineral water, to medical manuals theorising about the role of 'obstructions' in febrile diseases. Other sources have included an extensive range of theological writings, pietistic works and patristic studies that wielded influence over, or were of interest to, Wesley. Examining such a wealth and diversity of material has proved, in itself, to be a useful exercise in methodology, as it has enabled a modern academic historian to examine heterogeneous texts in a manner akin to an eighteenth-century scholar.

It could be said that intellectual and cultural history, or at any rate, an inter-disciplinary approach, is the way in which modern scholarship characterises a type of intellectual activity that did not need to be justified by eighteenth-century scholars. Wesley, and other scholars like him, sought to create some boundaries whilst erasing others in a series of conceptual shifts and re-alignments which brought entire traditions under consideration. Methodologically, this study wishes to work back to this original insight – though necessarily working back from disciplinary structures and divisions that have accumulated in the intervening period.

Paradoxically, by focusing sharply on his medical manual, Wesley's entire intellectual field of vision is brought vibrantly to life. In working through the local concerns and interests articulated in *Primitive Physic*, one can clearly see the way in which Wesley engaged in the larger context of eighteenth-century intellectual life. Following the contours of Wesley's thinking, through all of its contradictory twists and turns, and over vastly contrasting areas of interest, has helped to create more meaningful connections. This in turn has helped to produce a greater understanding of the interplay between theology, medicine and enlightened empiricism, which is at work in *Primitive Physic*. Finally, by questioning those distinctions usually drawn between Wesley's 'popular' medical work and other 'orthodox' volumes, this study seeks to veer away from traditional medical histories and triumphant or Whiggish Enlightenment historiography.

That Wesley managed to reconcile such diverse elements so seamlessly, without worrying about compromising his religious convictions or threatening the integrity of his medical practice, is a remarkable achievement in itself. This manoeuvre was critically important to him and fed into a deeper sense of intellectual pride, seen in the obvious pleasure he gained from meeting the curate, turned physiologist, inventor and member of the Royal Society, Stephen Hales. Hales successfully combined his passion for science and medicine with active priestly duties in Teddington, Middlesex, and it is clear that Wesley felt a great affinity with this man. In the course of a conversation in 1753, Hales had shown Wesley several experiments, and the remarks recorded in his *Journal* are illustrative of the impression Hales made: 'How well do philosophy and religion agree in a man of sound understanding'.[35] Immediately, Wesley recognised in Hales his own desire to put an active religion and experimental philosophy to useful effect. It is this motivation, and John Wesley's hermeneutics of Primitive Christianity, to which we now turn in following chapter.

Notes

1. J. Wesley, *Primitive Physic: Or, An Easy and Natural Method of Curing Most Diseases,* 24th edn (London, 1792), ix.
2. A later edition (38th) was also published in London but the date for this is uncertain. Another 'popular' medical volume was William Buchan's *Domestic Medicine* (1769). Buchan's volume was aimed at a higher income group; it sold for six shillings, as compared to Wesley's *Primitive Physic*, which sold for one shilling. I treat some of the arguments contained in this first section of the Introduction elsewhere. See, D. Madden, 'Experience and the Common

Interest of Mankind: The Enlightened Empiricism of John Wesley's *Primitive Physic*', *British Journal for Eighteenth-Century Studies*, 26, 1 (2003), 41–53.

3. Wesley, *op. cit.* (note 1), xv. The 'neighbouring nation' referred to is Ireland, but *Primitive Physic* was also printed in Wales and France.

4. J.H. Plumb, *England in the Eighteenth Century* (London: Penguin, 1950), 95–6. There are numerous references to Wesley's populist and 'unorthodox' scientific leanings – too many to cite. Here, I will refer only to those key works where this argumentation is made explicit. Roy Porter's early work, significantly perhaps, follows a similar trajectory to that of his mentor and old supervisor J.H. Plumb. See R. Porter, *Mind Forg'd Manacles: A History of Madness in England from the Restoration to the Regency* (London: Penguin, 1987), *Health For Sale: Quackery in England 1660–1850* (Manchester: Manchester University Press, 1989); R. Porter (ed.), *Patients and Practitioners* (Cambridge: Cambridge University Press, 1985). See also A. Suzuki, 'Anti-Lockean Enlightenment? Mind and Body in Early Eighteenth-Century English Medicine', in R. Porter (ed.), *Medicine in the Enlightenment* (Amsterdam: Rodopi, 1995), 336–59. Suzuki argues that *Primitive Physic* is an 'aggressively anti-intellectual, anti-theoretical and populist medical advice manual intended explicitly for the poor' (349). In contra-distinction to this, however, an earlier work by L.S. King, *The Medical World of the Eighteenth Century* (Chicago: University of Chicago Press, 1958), summarised Wesley's contribution to medicine. King argued that Wesley represented the best of the empiric tradition in medicine (39).

5. A.M. Lyles, *Methodism Mocked: The Satiric Reaction to Methodism in the Eighteenth Century* (London: Epworth Press, 1960).

6. G. Lavington, *The Enthusiasm of Methodists and Papists Compared*, 2nd edn (London, 1754), H. More, *Enthusiasmus Triumphatus* (1656), with an introduction by M.V. Deporte (California: University of California Press, 1966). The connection between religious inspiration and madness had been established by Meric Casaubon, whose *Treatise Concerning Enthusiasm, As it is an Effect of Nature* (London, 1655), Henry More had drawn upon. As is indicated by the title, Casaubon sought to demonstrate that, not only was enthusiasm an effect of nature, but it was mistaken by man for divine inspiration. See P.J. Korshin (ed.), *Casaubon's 'Treatise'* (Florida: Scholars Facsimiles and Reprints, 1970). After the publication of Henry More's work it became commonplace to speak of enthusiasm as the force of 'fancy' causing the individual to lose contact with reality. This 'distemper', though false, could be cured and John Locke also dealt with the issue of enthusiasm in a manner reminiscent of More when he argued in Book IV of his *Essay*, that the fancies in man's brain are sometimes mistaken for revelation. See Locke, *Essay Concerning Human Understanding*, John Yolton (ed.), (1690; London: Everyman, 1994). I do not wish to engage here in a full analysis of

25

how religious inspiration came to be valorised in terms of 'enthusiasm', which involved a medical language that described it primarily as a physical disorder or madness. There are already a large number of excellent works on this subject. See, for example, M. Heyd, *'Be Sober and Reasonable': The Critique of Enthusiasm in the Seventeenth and Early Eighteenth Centuries* (New York: E.J. Brill, 1995). Also, M. De Porte, *Nightmares and Hobbyhorses: Swift, Sterne and Augustan Ideas of Madness* (San Marino, CA: The Huntington Library, 1974) and the introductory chapter by Ole Peter Grell and Roy Porter in which they see how Enlightenment physicians allude to the affinity between sectaries and lunatics: 'In individuals such aberrations had long been blamed on demonic possession; now it was the turn of entire religious sects to be "demonized" on medico–philosophical authority...' (5). O.P. Grell and R. Porter, 'Introduction', in *idem* (eds), *Toleration in Enlightenment Europe* (Cambridge: Cambridge University Press, 2000), 1–22.

7. An obvious, though rare exception, is R.E. Brantley's *Locke, Wesley and the Method of English Romanticism* (Gainesville: University of Florida Press, 1984).

8. J.W. Haas, 'John Wesley's Views on Science and Christianity: An Examination of the Charge of Anti-Science', *American Society of Church History*, 63 (1994), 378–92.

9. H.D. Rack, *Reasonable Enthusiast: John Wesley and the Rise of Methodism* (London: Epworth Press, 1992).

10. Quoted by E.B. Bardell, 'Primitive Physick: John Wesley's Receipts', *Pharmacy in History*, 21 (1979), 111–21: 116.

11. Hereafter referred to as the *Compendium*. John Francis Buddaeus, a pietist who was Professor of Philosophy and Religion, had been recommended to Wesley when he visited Jena in 1738–9. See R.E. Schofield, 'John Wesley and Science in 18th Century England', *Isis*, 44 (1953), 331–40. The first two-volume edition was an abridged version of the Latin work by Buddaeus, but included notes from William Derham's *Physico–Theology: Or A Demonstration of the Being and Attributes of God from his Works of Creation* (1713), John Ray's *The Wisdom of God Manifested in the Works of the Creation* (1691). The 1777 edition was extended to five volumes and included extracts from Charles Bonnet's *The Contemplation of Nature* (1764). Haas, *op. cit.* (note 8), 383.

12. Schofield, *op. cit.* (note 11).

13. Haas, *op. cit.* (note 8), 379.

14. J. Walsh, 'Origins of the Evangelical Revival', in G.V. Bennett and J.D. Walsh (eds), *Essays in Modern Church History in Memory of Norman Sykes* (Oxford: Oxford University Press, 1966), 132–62; J. Walsh, 'John Wesley and the Community of Goods', in K. Robbins (ed.), *Protestant*

Evangelicalism: Britain, Ireland, Germany and America, c.1750–c.1950: Essays in Honour of W.R. Ward (Oxford: Oxford University Press, 1990), 22–50; A.C. Outler, 'Introduction', in *idem* (ed.), *The Bicentennial Edition of The Works of John Wesley*, (Nashville: Abingdon Press, 1985), Vol. I, *Sermons*, 1–100; Rack, *op. cit.* (note 9); I. Rivers, *Reason, Grace and Sentiment: A Study of the Language of Religion and Ethics in England, 1660–1780*, 2 vols (Cambridge: Cambridge University Press, 1991); B.W. Young, *Religion and Enlightenment in Eighteenth-Century England* (Oxford: Clarendon Press, 1998); P. Mack, 'Religious Dissenters in Enlightenment England', *History Workshop Journal*, 49 (2000), 1–23.

15. See H. Aarsleff, *From Locke to Saussure: Essays on the Study of Language and Intellectual History* (London: Athlone, 1982); Mack, *op. cit.* (note 14).

16. W.J. Turrell, *John Wesley: Physician and Electrotherapist* (Blackwell: Oxford, 1938); Schofield, *op. cit.* (note 11); J.C. English, 'John Wesley and Isaac Newton's "System of the World"', *Proceedings of the Wesley Historical Society*, 48/3 (1991) 69–86; J. Cule, 'The Rev. John Wesley, M.A. (Oxon.), 1703–1791: "The Naked Empiricist" and Orthodox Medicine', *The Journal of the History of Medicine*, 45 (1990), 41–63; Haas, *op. cit.* (note 8); G.S. Rousseau, 'John Wesley's "Primitive Physick" (1747)', *Harvard Library Bulletin*, 16 (1968), 242–56; P.W. Ott, 'John Wesley on Health: A Word for Sensible Regimen', *Methodist History*, 18 (1979–80), 193–204; P.W. Ott, 'John Wesley on Health as Wholeness', *Journal of Religion and Health*, 30 (1991), 43–57; P.W. Ott, 'Medicine as Metaphor: John Wesley on Therapy of the Soul', *Methodist History*, 33 (1995), 178–91. My thanks to Amanda Porterfield for drawing attention to an earlier essay written by H.Y. Vanderpool while this work was being revised for book publication. Vanderpool's essay considers Wesley's medical practice in the context of later Wesleyan–Methodist healing traditions. See H.Y. Vanderpool, 'The Wesleyan–Methodist Tradition', in R.L. Numbers and D.W. Amundsen (eds), *Caring and Curing: Health and Medicine in the Western Religious Traditions* (New York: Macmillan, 1986), 317–53.

17. Ott, 'John Wesley on Health as Wholeness', *ibid.*; Ott, 'Medicine as Metaphor', *ibid*; R.L. Maddox, 'A Heritage Reclaimed: John Wesley on Holistic Health and Healing' in M.E.M. Moore (ed.), A Living Tradition (Nashville, TN: Kingswood Books, forthcoming).

18. Maddox, *ibid.*

19. Maddox, *ibid.* Maddox cites recent examples, R.H. Stone, *John Wesley's Life and Ethics* (Nashville: Abingdon Press, 2001) and J. Munsey Turner, *John Wesley: The Evangelical Revival and the Rise of Methodism in England* (Peterborough: Epworth Press, 2002).

20. Rousseau, *op. cit.* (note 16). To some extent Rousseau's article follows a similar trajectory to A. Wesley Hill's *John Wesley Among the Physicians: A*

Study of Eighteenth-Century Medicine (London: Epworth Press, 1958) in that it provides a brief overview of Wesley's medical practice. Rack's article, 'Doctors, Demons and Early Methodist Healing', in W.J. Sheils (ed.), *Studies in Church History*, Vol. 19, *The Church and Healing* (Oxford: Oxford University Press, 1982), also provides a brief explication of Wesley's 'amateur' medicine in the context of Methodist spiritual healing. Earlier articles include those written by B.G. Thomas, 'John Wesley and the Art of Healing', *American Physician*, 32 (1906), 295–8, W.R. Riddell, 'Wesley's System of Medicine', *New York Medical Journal*, 99 (1914), 64–8 and G. Dock, 'The Primitive Physick of Revd John Wesley: A Picture of Eighteenth-Century Medicine', *The Journal of the American Medical Association*, 64 (1915), 629–38.

21. S. Juster, 'Mystical Pregnancy and Holy Bleeding: Visionary Experiences in Early Modern Britain and America', *William and Mary Quarterly*, 57 (2000), 249–88: 253.

22. G. Kelly Armstrong, 'Irrationalism and Politics in the Eighteenth Century', *Studies in Eighteenth-Century Culture*, 2 (1972), 239–53.

23. M. Hagner, 'Enlightened Monsters', in W. Clark, J. Golinski and S. Schaffer (eds), *The Sciences in Enlightened Europe* (Chicago: University of Chicago Press, 1999), 175–217.

24. Rivers, *op. cit.* (note 14).

25. For a classic account of this pessimistic view, see M. Horkheimer and T. Adorno, *Dialectic of Enlightenment*, trans J. Cumming (London: Allen Lane, 1973).

26. I. Kant, 'An Answer to the Question: "What is Enlightenment"', in Hans Reiss (ed.) *Kant's Political Writings* (Cambridge: Cambridge University Press, 1970), 54–60.

27. This recent scholarship includes Grell and Porter (eds), *op. cit* (note 6), and Clark, Golinski and Schaffer (eds), *op. cit* (note 23). The introduction to the latter provides an excellent historiography because of the complete, yet succinct, synthesis of the existing material. Clark, Golinski and Schaffer (eds), 'Introduction', *op. cit* (note 23), 3–31: 20.

28. J. Lane, *A Social History of Medicine: Health, Healing and Disease in England, 1750–1950* (London: Routledge, 2001); A. Guerrini, *Obesity and Depression in the Enlightenment: The Life and Times of George Cheyne* (Oklahoma: University of Oklahoma Press, 2000); Clark, Golinski and Schaffer (eds), *op. cit.* (note 23); S.C. Lawrence, *Charitable Knowledge: Hospital Pupils and Practitioners in Eighteenth-Century London* (Cambridge: Cambridge University Press, 1996). L.I. Conrad *et al.* (eds), *The Western Medical Tradition* (Cambridge: Cambridge University Press, 1995); R. Porter (ed.), *Medicine in the Enlightenment* (Amsterdam: Clio Medica, 1995); C.J. Lawrence, *Medicine in the Making of Modern Britain, 1700–1920* (London:

Routledge, 1994); J. Barry and C. Jones (eds), *Medicine and Charity Before the Welfare State* (London: Routledge, 1991).

29. J. Habermas, *The Structural Transformation of the Public Sphere: An Enquiry into a Category of Bourgeois Society*, trans T. Burger (Cambridge, MA: MIT Press, 1989). The influence of Habermas over the history of Enlightenment science and medicine has been noted by Dorinda Outram. She argues that the way in which historians like Roy Porter have used his work is problematic due to the fact that Habermas did not assign science a specific place in the public realm: 'Historians who follow Habermas can find no way from within that theory to explain why, or whether, science could be assigned this centrality'. Neither does this approach provide a solution to the relationship between history of science and cultural history. Whilst Habermas's theory releases historians from the dark view of science and technology put forward by Horkheimer and Adorno, the description of an Enlightenment which sees it as an 'innocent creation' of reading, writing, conversation and amateur science is one divested from the 'consideration of power'. Outram's latter point regarding the consideration of power is particularly relevant to this study in as much as Wesley's cultural mediation of medical and scientific ideas to a 'popular' audience was an attempt to alter the distribution of the power carried by that knowledge. See D. Outram, 'The Enlightenment Our Contemporary', in Clark, Golinski and Schaffer (eds), *op. cit* (note 23), 32–40.

30. N.D. Jewson, 'Medical Knowledge and the Patronage System in Eighteenth-Century England', *Sociology,* 8 (1974), 369–85; R. Porter and D. Porter, *In Sickness and in Health* (New York: Blackwell, 1989); C.J. Lawrence, *op. cit.* (note 28); J. Brewer and Roy Porter (eds), *Consumption and the World of Goods* (London: Routledge, 1993). These scholars have identified the diversity of medical practitioners operating in a non-regulated marketplace.

31. Lawrence, *ibid.*, 12; R.D. Lund (ed.), *The Margins of Orthodoxy: Heterodox Writing and Cultural Response* (Cambridge: Cambridge University Press, 1995); J.D. Walsh, C. Haydon and S. Taylor (eds), *The Church of England. c.1689–c.1833: From Toleration to Tractarianism* (Cambridge: Cambridge University Press, 1993); Young, *op. cit.* (note 14); R. Porter (ed.), *The Enlightenment in National Context* (Cambridge: Cambridge University Press, 1981).

32. The analysis Roy Porter offers in his earlier works (see note 4 above) concerning Wesley's contribution to medicine differs significantly to that given in his later work, which is more explicit in its identification of Wesley's empiricism. This can be seen particularly in R. Porter and G.S. Rousseau, *Gout: The Patrician Malady* (London: Yale University Press, 2000).

33. Wesley, *op. cit.* (note 1), xi

34. Rousseau, *op cit.* (note 16), 245.

35. Wesley, N. Curnock, (ed.), *The Journal of the Revd John Wesley, A.M.,* 8 vols (London: n.p., 1909–1916), Vol. IV, 73.

2

John Wesley's Hermeneutics of Primitive Christianity and Practical Piety

One grand preventative of pain and sickness of various kinds, seems intimated by the grand Author of Nature in the very sentence that intails death upon us: 'In the sweat of thy face shalt thou eat bread, till thou return to the ground'.

John Wesley, 'The Preface', *Primitive Physic*

Hereby the great physician of souls applies medicine to heal this sickness; to restore human nature, totally corrupted in all its faculties... 'in Adam ye all died;' in the second Adam, 'in Christ, ye all are made alive' now 'go on' from 'faith to faith', until your whole sickness be healed...

John Wesley, *Sermon on Original Sin* (1759)[1]

Primitive Christianity

Primitivism provided a holistic framework for Wesley's thinking and praxis, both generally and in *Primitive Physic*. This was his *modus operandi* and the ideals of Primitivism, whether it applied to the Apostolic age or an ancient standard in physic, are intricately woven into 'The Preface' of Wesley's medical volume. The theme of wholeness was central to his theology and structured all of his work, in its written, oral and practical forms.[2] The motif of Primitive Christianity was deeply personal. From an early age Wesley inherited the traditions of both Puritan and Anglican practical piety directly from his parents, Samuel and Susannah Wesley, who taught him to revere the Apostolic age, that first and golden period of the Christian Church.[3] Born on 17 June 1703, at the family home of Epworth Rectory in Lincolnshire, Wesley's parents, however, were originally of dissenting stock, but conformed to the Church of England.

He was born into an era in which Christian antiquity and patristic studies had been a focal point for theological, ecclesiastical and moral discourse for more than a century.[4] Patristics involved making a theological study of the Church Fathers, usually between the first and eighth centuries, though sometimes extending its reach to encompass thirteenth-century theologians. It was primarily concerned with the emergence of Christianity and the early Church. During the seventeenth century, the University of Oxford played a prominent role in this debate, while providing a stronghold for High Church Anglicanism, with numerous Anglican leaders and writers expressing their approbation of Primitive Christianity.[5] Writings from the patristic revival were readily available to Wesley as a scholar at Oxford and he made a point of studying a great number of them, including William Cave's *Primitive Christianity* (1672) and Anthony Horneck's *The Happy Ascetick* (1681).[6] Bishop Jeremy Taylor's *The Whole Duty of Man* (1657) and *Ductor Dubitantium* (1660) also served to teach Wesley the Christian life of *devotio* and provided guidance on inward holiness.

After attending Charterhouse school, Wesley was elected scholar of Christ Church, Oxford, in 1720, graduating in 1724 before becoming a fellow of Lincoln College in 1726. His reading of patristic texts, combined with his involvement in the Holy Club at Oxford, helped to compound the reverence for Primitive Christianity that had been instilled into him as a child. Like an historian, Wesley sensed that he had discovered something precious that had hitherto been lost, and felt compelled to make ancient texts intelligible through his writings and sermons.[7] He esteemed those writings closest to The Acts, over and above second- and third-century texts, and believed that exceptional purity existed in this period; the most authentic commentators on Scripture were those nearest the fountain, which were also eminently imbued with that Spirit. He articulated this in *An Address to the Clergy* (1756), a reworking of a sermon written by his father, and again in 1777 when giving his sermon *On Laying the Foundation of the New Chapel*.[8]

During his time at Oxford, Wesley had a voracious appetite for patristic writings and A.C. Outler has suggested that one of the bonuses of an Oxford education was a living sense of history.[9] The Holy Club, initially intended as a fellowship for the study of classical literature and the New Testament, soon shifted its attention towards patrology and the cultivation of practical piety.[10] In tandem with this development, the Holy Club came to regard itself as an experiment in early Christianity and, reminiscing late in life, Wesley emphasised its performative nature by claiming that the movement sought to practice the community of goods modelled in The Acts.[11]

There was, however, nothing programmatic about Wesley's use of Primitive Christianity and his conception of the early Church altered significantly over time. During his missionary trip to Georgia (1735–7) Wesley came into contact with the evangelical primitivism of the Moravian Brethren, and this association deepened his understanding of the spirit of early Christianity. The simplicity and discipline of this group led him to question the idealised, static and conservative view of Primitive Christianity that he inherited from his father. Another indication of Wesley's non-programmatic use of Primitive Christianity is evidenced by his avoidance of writing an explicitly prescriptive treatise or essay on the subject.[12]

Wesley internalised patristic texts to such an extent that the act of weaving together intricate and complex sources became second nature to him. He allowed no authority to approach that of Scripture, but patristic evidence pointed to Scriptural truth and could be used to illuminate or allude to esoteric and obscure passages in the Bible. There are no citations of patristic authors in 'The Preface' to *Primitive Physic* where Scriptural citation and 'plain' style is the preferred method. Yet Wesley's interpretation of the Genesis story given in the opening three sections to 'The Preface' is heavily laden with patristic influences, including St Clement of Rome's *First Epistle*, St Clement of Alexandria's *Paedagogus* and the *Spiritual Homilies* of St Pseudo-Macarius.

Genesis is the beginning of the story and so 'The Preface' opens with a Miltonian cosmography, a belief that in the beginning there was no need for medicine because Adam knew no sin, no pain, sickness nor bodily disorder:

> The habitation wherein the angelic mind, the Divinae Particula Aura abode, although originally formed out of the dust of the earth, was liable to no decay. It had no seeds of corruption or dissolution within itself. And there was nothing without to injure it: heaven and earth and all the hosts of them were mild, benign and friendly to human nature.[13]

Now, since man had 'rebelled against the Sovereign', the seeds of weakness, sickness and death are 'lodged in our inmost substance; whence a thousand disorders continually spring, even without the aid of external violence'.[14] Man's fall from grace means that nature conspires against him: the sun sheds unwholesome influences, the earth exhales poisonous damps and the air is replete with shafts of death. The environment is loaded with lethal micro-organisms and Wesley's conception of original sin here is fused with the experimental philosophy of Robert Boyle, which sought to explain the relationship between hostile environment and disease in purely physical terms.

Man's distempered nature, the result of original sin, is vividly described in terms of sickness and disease in Wesley's sermon, *The One Thing Needful* (1734):

> Our nature is distempered as well as enslaved; the whole head is faint and the whole heart is sick. Our body, soul and spirit, are infected, overspread, consumed, with the most fatal leprosy. We are all over, within and without, in the eye of God, full of diseases, and wounds, and putrifying sores. Every one of our brutal passions and diabolical tempers, every kind of pride,

sensuality, selfishness, is one of those deadly wounds, of those loathsome sores, full of corruption, and of all uncleanness.[15]

The Earth had become 'one great infirmary', full of sick people waiting to be healed.[16] Wesley was inspired by Augustine's holistic view of nature, but disease was not merely divine punishment in terms of human bondage. As the passages cited from *Primitive Physic* at the beginning of this chapter show, Wesley believed that a merciful God provided the antidotes to nature's poisons. Illness and death, the result of man's fall, are unavoidable, but Christ, the ultimate physician, healed the sick and bore the sins of man *bodily* on the cross: 'By nature ye are wholly corrupted, by grace ye shall be wholly renewed'.[17] God had provided salvation through Christ so that the tension between corruption and renewal could be resolved.[18] Salvation, in this sense, was physically and spiritually healing.[19] Christ the physician, healer of body and soul, served to link the material and spiritual worlds, hence the Latin word for health, but also salvation – *saluus* – powerfully connects physic and religion together.[20] Yet nowhere does Wesley suggest that health of the body and soul is one and the same: 'faith does not overturn the course of nature: natural causes still produce natural effects'.[21] In 'The Preface' he evokes the divine physician, but by no means is his belief in providential medicine articulated in the main text of *Primitive Physic*. As Maddox points out, while it was the case that man was made perfectly complete in his resurrected state, Wesley 'resisted the tendency to minimise the physical dimension of God's healing work in the present world'.[22]

The *spiritual* world could not affect *physical* organs and the Incarnation gave tremendous significance to the body as something holding intrinsic value in its own right. The tangible nature of Christ's resurrection, asserted in The Acts, was a doctrine held dear in the early Church: resurrection involved the whole person, as opposed to the Greek-inspired inner 'pneumatic' personality or the alienated soul of Judaism.[23] The body was on loan to man, and in I Corinthians, St Paul states that man's body was a 'temple of the Holy Spirit': it belonged to God.[24] As the locus of ordered limits, its transgression was sacrilegious: 'Do you not know that your bodies are members of Christ?'[25] The body was a gift and as such, Wesley states in his sermon, *The Good Steward* (1768), one had to take care of that 'exquisitely wrought machine' – here he deliberately alluded to Cartesian mechanistic language to make a basic, but fundamental, theological point.[26]

The language that Wesley deploys in many of his sermons is repeatedly shot-through with mechanistic, physiological and medical themes, further pointing to his understanding of health in terms of a well-ordered machine.[27] This vision of man in his pristine, pre-lapsed state is given in *The Fall of Man* (1782):

But how fearfully and wonderfully wrought into innumerable fibres, nerves, membranes, muscles, arteries, veins, vessels of various kinds! And how amazing is this dust connected with water, with enclosed, circulating fluids, diversifies a thousand ways by a thousand tubes and strainers! Yea, and how wonderfully is air impacted into every part, solid or fluid, of the animal machine; air, not elastic, which would tear the machine in pieces, but as fixed as water under the pole! But all this would not avail, were not ethereal fire intimately mixed both with this earth, air and water. And all these elements are mingled together in the most exact proportion; so that while the body is in health, no one of them predominates, in the least degree, over the others.[28]

Wesley's grasp of iatromechanical philosophy is clear, particularly when one contrasts it with the following extract taken from Dr George Cheyne's *The English Malady: Or, A Treatise of Nervous Diseases of all Kinds* (1733):

[T]he human body is a Machine of an infinite Number and Variety of different Channels and Pipes, filled with various and different liquors and Fluids, perpetually running, glideing, or creeping forward, or returning backward, in a constant Circle, and sending out little Branches and Outlets, to moisten, nourish, and repair the Expenses of Living.[29]

Pristine purity is Wesley's overriding theological concern in his sermon on the Fall and the primal elements are used to illustrate the holistic character of nature. An extension of this principle can be seen in *Primitive Physic* where Wesley seeks to reconcile man with the primal elements. Wesley's sermon, however, also seeks to explicate Genesis in eighteenth-century medical language: man's body is a system of 'fibres' and 'nerves', through which 'fluids' can circulate unhindered. In its medico–theological imagery, his sermon echoes Stephen Hales's *A Sermon Preached before the Royal College of Physicians* (1751). Hales was eager to point out to his medical colleagues that man's body was a beautiful symmetrical structure that reflected the 'brightness' of his soul:

What a vast variety of parts differing from each other, are nourished by the same blood, whereby *we are cloathed with skin and flesh and fenced with bones and sinews*, and all those parts are, not only in themselves of an admirable texture, but also justly adapted to be useful to each other? With what excellent art is that curious hydraulick engine the *heart* framed, forcibly to impell the blood with rapidity through the minute channels, and meanders of the body?[30]

Wesley's first 'University sermon', *The Image of God*, which he preached at St Mary's in 1730, made frequent use of contemporary medical language, borrowing phrases such as 'open' and 'obstructed' vessels to explain man's state before and after the Fall. In this sermon, Wesley admitted that he could only offer a 'probable' account of Genesis, based on conjecture rather than Scripture. Before the Fall, he argues, the original 'particles' of man's body were 'incorruptible', which meant that no external 'substance' ever 'adhered to any part of it':

> By this means both the juices contained must have been still of the same consistence, and the vessels containing them have kept the same spring, and remained ever clear and open.[31]

Again, we can see how Wesley adapted the mechanistic vocabulary of Cheyne to describe the pre-lapsarian body, one in which 'juices' could move around unobstructed through 'open' vessels. In its pristine state, man's body was designed to function indefinitely; disorder only ensued as a result of corruption via an external noxious agent.[32] This noxious agent came in the form of forbidden fruit, which contained a deadly juice:

> [T]he particles of which were apt to cleave to whatever they touched. Some of these, being received into the human body, might adhere to the inner coats of the finer vessels; to which again other particles that before floated loose in the blood, continually joining, would naturally lay a foundation for numberless disorders in all parts of the machine... the solid parts of the body would every day lose something of their spring, and so be less able to contribute their necessary assistance to the circulation of the fluids.[33]

Notwithstanding the fact that Adam masticated and ingested death with this fruit, an antidote was available. Had he taken fruit from the Tree of Life, Adam could have restored his body to immortality. This would have remedied Adam's slow, languid death by its 'thin, abstersive nature, particularly fitted to counteract the other, to wipe off its particles, wheresoever adhering....'[34] An 'abstersive', such as linseed oil, was a 'cleansing' remedy, that could draw away ill-humours or obstructions, and Wesley's use of medical language and imagery helped to create contemporary resonances by way of elucidating and making Genesis more meaningful.

As a clergyman, Wesley regarded it as permissible to move between the providential and physical worlds. His approach to medicine in *Primitive Physic* is thoroughly empirical, but his conception of healing was holistic. He saw brute existence as only one part of man's being, and in this he shared much in common with pietist medics, such as Herman Boerhaave and Cheyne. Cheyne, in fact, cited I Corinthians on the title page of 'Discourse I' to his *An Essay on Regimen* (1740): 'There is a natural body, and there is a spiritual body'. This citation was intended to complement the title of 'Discourse I' which was: 'Philosophical Conjectures about the nature and qualities of the original Animal Body'.[35] Man's nature and health were inextricably linked; he was a unity of body, mind and soul and this is what Wesley meant when he referred to 'inward and outward' health.[36] This sentiment was expressed by the second-century Christian theologian, Clement of Alexandria, whose works, amongst an impressive range of other patristic writings, Wesley esteemed and revered. Clement stated that the:

> [G]ood Instructor, the Wisdom, the Word of the Father, who made man, cares for the whole nature of His creature; the all-sufficient Physician of humanity, the Saviour, heals both body and soul.[37]

For Wesley, healing the 'whole' man consisted of using all the means that 'reason and experience can dictate', but this was contained within the definite theological framework of Scripture, interpreted by reason and confirmed by experience.[38] His theme of 'wholeness', closely related to perfection and holiness, was extracted from the Eastern Christian liturgical works of Pseudo-Macarius.[39] It is constructed in all of his work, but the perspective in *Primitive Physic* is quite clear. Dying is inevitable, yet God has planted in man a strong desire to live. If man is plagued with a thousand disorders, the human goal involves actively recovering the sense of wholeness, purity and perfection (through grace) which characterised the original order. The promise of physical *and spiritual* perfection was something that Hales wanted to remind his listeners of the Royal College of Physicians:

> God, who has thus curiously wrought our wonderful frame out of the dust, knowing how prone we are to disorder it, by irregularities, of his tender fatherly care for us, has not only implanted in us a strong desire of life, and self preservation; but has also strictly enjoined us of all destructive irregularities and vices; and the practice of those virtues, which are so well adapted to our nature; that they have a natural tendency, not only to keep the body in order, but also *to give health to the soul* as well as marrow to the bones.[40]

Before any attempt could be made to recover that happy state of grace, man had to begin by accepting that he lived in the grip of a mighty power, that of the flesh. Here an important distinction needed to be made between the 'body' and 'flesh'. St Paul's anthropology involved a threefold conception of *soma* (body), *sarx* (flesh) and *pneuma* (spirit).[41] The body does not merely represent an undisciplined entity with attendant physical needs; bodily weakness points to a state of helplessness, but *flesh* signifies man's rebellion against God – this is what Wesley is referring to in 'The Preface' when he describes the seeds of death being in our 'inmost substance'. Wesley is keen to restate this in his *Compendium*:

> How admirably has God secured the execution of his original sentence, upon every child of man, *Dust thou art, and unto dust shalt thou return?* From the moment we live, we prepare for Death, by the adhesion of dust, mixt with all our aliments, to our nature dust; so that whatever we eat or drink, to prolong life, must sap the foundation of it. Thus in spite of all the wisdom of Man, and all the precautions which can be used, every morsel we take poisons while it feeds and brings us nearer to the Dust from whence we came.[42]

We see here how he used a type of medical language to suggest that a 'rationalised' mode of regimen is insufficient to make man 'whole' again.

This 'fleshly' rebellion, which encompasses the body, signifies something far greater than man's mortal coil. The fleshly was, in the words of St Paul, the dark counter law of 'sin which dwells in my members'.[43] Man is a being not simply torn between body and soul, but also between flesh and spirit. Life lived in the flesh is subject to this dark power reared in rebellion, but a life lived in Christ is freedom: 'the Spirit of Him, who raised Jesus from the dead dwells in you, he will… give life to your mortal bodies also.[44] St Paul connects the concept of *pneuma* here with the Hebraic tradition of *ruach*, 'breath of God', to insist that our *mortal bodies* can be given life.[45]

Spirit conveyed the divine element in man, which could be directed by God's grace to good conduct in opposition to the flesh. To live a holy and pious life, in Jesus, is to live eternally. Schism and dissension divided the flesh and spirit, body and soul, man and God, but Jesus was manifest in man's flesh. Hence Wesley's sermon, *The Trouble and Rest of Good Men* (1735), suggests that 'the Great Physician of souls is continually present' in man.[46] The sacrament affects man's body as it receives in it the seed of an immortal nature and the Eucharist is the immortal medicine for every *spiritual* malady.

The Incarnation made it possible for man, potentially at least, to repair the violence of original sin and lead a happy (holy) life. A life of simplicity and sensible regimen seeks to imitate Christ and replace the fruit taken from the Tree of Knowledge. Pursuit of perfection to combat the disorder of original sin was exemplified by the Primitive Christians, and this was outlined by the patristic scholar Anthony Horneck in *The Happy Ascetick*. Horneck's work made a lasting impression on Wesley when he read it in Oxford in 1729:

> What advantages the soul can be supposed to give the body, the same did the first Christians afford to the benighted world; and whatever inconveniences

the body puts the soul to, the same did the bespotted world bring upon the first Christians.[47]

Through God's grace, the early Christian community blossomed under the *ruach*, 'breath' or Spirit of God and so Wesley believed that Primitive Christianity was the 'vital breath' of the Church.[48] In imitation of Christ, the early Christians become emblematic of resistance to the 'fleshly' world while simultaneously, and paradoxically, becoming symbols of an acceptance of humility.[49]

A disciplined, well-ordered holy life did not involve the rejection of bodily health, or medicine to cure disease.[50] Nor did it imply unnecessary physical suffering. D.J. Melling points out that early Christianity had a profound respect for the medical profession as long as doctors exercised their role in a humble unmercenary spirit. In this context the doctor's healing function provided a theologically illuminative image of the salvic role of Christ.[51] Sickness and disease, in fact, could pose a threat to spiritual life: illness could induce febrile imaginings, thereby creating self-indulgence, anger or blasphemy.[52] Where possible, sickness should be avoided and doctors during the patristic period had a variety of medical resources at their disposal that could offer relief and healing.[53] Where suffering was unavoidable, Christians were challenged to find meaning in this suffering by way of spiritual growth.[54] In this sense, Melling argues, the Christian spiritual tradition enabled suffering to be accepted as a gift, 'a transforming gift that temporarily reshapes the sufferer's life....'[55] This is something quite distinct from those individuals, groups or sects who practised extreme asceticism and held the body in contempt.[56] Providence had endowed nature with remedies for human experimentation which could aid the development of medicine and mitigate physical pain. Diadochos, Bishop of Photike in the late-fifth century, believed that the Creation provided man with a rich source of natural cures.[57] A belief in the providential and healing power of nature continued to be firmly extolled in the seventeenth and eighteenth century, even amongst 'professional' physicians. Thomas Sydenham, the so-called 'English Hippocrates', described by Wesley in *Primitive Physic* as 'the great and good Dr Sydenham',[58] argued that although nature determined disease, it was also the case that nature could provide the appropriate cure:

> The Supreme Deity, by whose power all things are produced, and upon whose nod they depend, hath in his infinite wisdom, so disposed all things, that they betake themselves to their appointed works after a certain order and method; they do nothing in vain; they execute only that which is the most excellent and which is best fitted for the universal fabric and for their own

proper natures. They are engines that are moved not by any skill of their own, but by that of a higher artificer.[59]

'The Preface' to *Primitive Physic* reinforced the sentiments expressed by Sydenham: 'one grand preventative of pain and sickness of various kinds, seems intimated by the grand Author of Nature'.[60] The 'Bread or herb of the field' can restore man to health and strength.[61]

Health was a positive value to be promoted, and Clement of Alexandria decreed that the 'harmonious mechanism of the body contributes to the understanding which leads to goodness of nature'.[62] Clement advocated a moderate diet, combined with physical exercise. Lack of exercise, he stated, led to an excess of perspiration and faeces – the latter of which brought about a secondary undesirable consequence, that is, excessive lust.[63] For Clement of Alexandria, bodily health promoted mental agility, which in turn increased the capacity for self-control and moral rectitude. A frugal lifestyle, with controlled fasting as a remedy for excess, instilled physical self-restraint and clarity of thought.[64] Gluttony, on the other hand, produced physical slothfulness and led to an uncontrolled lifestyle, which resulted in dullness of mind.[65]

Fasting not only imitated the Primitive Christians, it subdued the body, which preserved physical and spiritual health. Furthermore, as had been made clear in the *Epistles* written by St Cyprian, third-century Bishop of Carthage, self-control of the body was emblematic of the Church: one could not allow the polluted waters of heresy to infect its body.[66] This important connection was made by St Ignatius, first-century Bishop of Antioch, in his *Epistle to the Trallians*. St Ignatius cautioned his reader to:

> Partake of Christian food exclusively; abstain from plants of alien growth, that is, heresy.... Heretics weave Jesus Christ into their web – to win our confidence, just like persons who administer a deadly drug, mixed with honeyed wine, which the unsuspecting gladly take – and with baneful relish they swallow death.[67]

Counsels of poverty, chastity, obedience and self-discipline were an attempt to recover Christ's pure body – the body of the Church.

William Cave, the Anglican scholar of the patristic revival, wrote in glowing terms about the virtue of early Christians, who practised fasting, 'singular continence and charity', piety and humility, obedience and honesty, and whose laws were 'so just and rational, in all its designs so divine and heavenly'.[68] Primitive Christianity demonstrates that holiness was the only ornament of early Christians who managed to achieve the closest thing to earthly perfection. Wesley also taught that bodily health was inextricably linked to salvation and 'true' faith, qualities that should not be separated from the good, holy life. He drew on Horneck, but sought inspiration from the seventeenth-century bishop and writer of devotional works, Jeremy Taylor.

On the issue of fasting, Taylor had insisted that health should be borne in mind and was not in favour of strict asceticism or unnecessary suffering. Wesley's moderate stance on asceticism concurred with that of Taylor, and at Oxford he put to use Taylor's *The Rule and Exercises of Holy Living* (1650).[69] He resolved to begin and end each day with thoughts of God; to be moderate in sleeping, eating and drinking; to be diligent in work and to moderate the passions and self-examination. This work, combined with Cheyne's *An Essay of Health and Long Life* (1724), meant that well before *Primitive Physic* was conceived, Wesley had developed 'a rationalised mode of life' that was conscious of being directed by the will of God.[70]

Horneck's text also set out a comprehensive list of exercises, the application of which could lead to Godliness. The exercises laid out in *The Happy Ascetick*, he argued, would keep the soul awake and strengthen it in the same manner that meat gave vigour to the body. It was vital for Christians to look after their souls: 'till we learn to exercise ourselves into Godliness, we are slaves....'[71] By contrast, the souls of Primitive Christians were 'nourished' by the Holy Spirit, which helped them to achieve 'high degrees of piety'. Horneck cites the New Testament on fasting, whilst advising his reader to recoil from extreme asceticism:

> It would be vain, and next to ridiculous to desire any of my readers to tread in the steps of [those] giants in fasting, yet I must with great seriousness exhort you to make abstinence your frequent exercise... by fasting I mean total abstinence from meat and drink, or where nature is not able to bear it, an abstinence from all pleasant food.[72]

As indicated by the title, *The Happy Ascetick* did not advocate extreme mortification but provided examples of when fasting was appropriate. Horneck implied that extreme acts of fasting led only to self-gratification and warned his readers to guard against this allegedly Catholic trait.

In common with Horneck and Taylor, Wesley adopted a moderate stance towards asceticism and fasting, though he regarded self-denial as an essential part of Christian living. He extols the virtues of fasting in 'The Preface' to *Primitive Physic*, where it features as one of his 'easy' rules in Section Sixteen (sub-section II), placed under the 'non-natural' heading of 'Eating and Drinking': 'Nothing conduces more to health, than abstinence and plain food, with due labour'.[73] The 'rational' elements of this rule and how it pertained to physical welfare will be examined later, but Wesley was keen to identify its theological significance. The history of this practice, from the

Old Testament through to the early Christian Church, and its appearance in the Anglican Homily on Fasting, is outlined in his *Sermon on the Mount.*[74] An explicit statement on the subject is given in his *Thoughts Upon Self Denial* – the writing of which was an act of practical piety in and of itself:

> If so much has been said… on the subject already, what need is there to say or write any more? I answer: there are considerable numbers, even of people fearing God, who have not had the opportunity either of hearing what has been spoken or reading what has been written.[75]

Wesley criticised the obscure and inaccessible style of other clergymen and theologians who had written on the subject:

> [They] speak of it in so dark, so perplexed, so intricate, so mystical a manner, as if they designed to conceal it from the vulgar, rather than explain it to common readers.[76]

He set out to explain exactly what self-denial should mean to the 'common' reader, which was linked, he argued, to taking up the cross for Jesus. Here, Wesley made clear his casuist concern with missionary activity. Fasting, he suggests, is a valuable aid to prayer: to obey God is to glorify him with body and soul.

Conversely, gluttony and self-indulgence are sins that readily lend themselves to other types of intemperate behaviour. On this, Wesley followed the logical thinking set down by Pseudo-Macarius, Taylor and Horneck, by stating that self-denial does not merely refer to eating and drinking. Though it is stated as such in *Primitive Physic*, self-denial pertained to all of the senses: 'Control the appetite and you will more easily control all bodily desires' (Ephesians, 6:2).[77] Drawing on the fifteenth-century ascetical writings of Thomas à Kempis, Wesley taught that the holy life forbade man to crave luxuries: such craving was an indication that the body (flesh) was rebelling against the spirit.[78] Man naturally inclined towards greed and lust, and so the passions needed to be bridled. Fasting was one way of achieving this.

Contrary to the criticism and controversy evoked by Holy Club members, Wesley did not endorse extreme asceticism. Methodists, however, did observe feast and fast days in imitation of the early Church.[79] Robert Nelson, Non-juror and close friend of the Wesley family, wrote *A Companion for the Festivals and Fasts of the Church of England* (1704), taking note of how meticulous the ancient Christians had been in their weekly and annual fasts. After reading this, Wesley resolved to abstain from food on Wednesdays and Fridays – the Primitive Christians chose these days because Christ had been betrayed on the former and crucified on the latter – and from 1732 Wesley observed all of the fast days appointed by the Church.[80] He also gave up meat and wine in preference for vegetables and rice – an eating pattern that was to be repeated four years later in Georgia, when he lived for several days on one type of food only.

Wesley did not think it necessary to take Scripture literally on the issue of fasting or self-denial; clearly, it would be inappropriate for eighteenth-century Christians to give up their houses, land, wives and children to live an ascetic life. Methodists were called upon to make self-denial meaningful to their own situation, and Wesley's advice was therefore practically orientated. He was nonetheless concerned to draw comparisons between the virtue, temperance and abstinence of early Christians, and the indolence, luxury and idleness of his own age, a recurring theme in many of his sermons. Christian sobriety and temperance could provide the perfect remedy to counter this whilst curbing passions of the flesh. Drawing on the first-century convert, St Clement of Rome, Wesley insisted that self-control was within the reach of most Christians: the Incarnation made it possible for every *body* to undergo transformation, a transformation that could lead to holiness (wholeness) and perfection.[81]

Wesley's fascination with Eastern Christian liturgy, specifically that of the fourth-century Christian thinker Pseudo-Macarius, and that of his contemporary, the Biblical exegete, Ephraem Syrus, lay in their description of perfection (wholeness) being the goal of Christian life. The early source of this influence undoubtedly came to Wesley via his father, but according to a diary entry for July 1736, he 'read Macarius and sang'.[82] Christian perfection (wholeness) came to hold a central place in Wesley's theology, and here he attempted to fuse together eastern and Anglican traditions. He made particular use of Macarius' rhetoric of the heart, which is most evident in the sermons where Wesley envisages the stages of perfection as an experience of the heart. First, man's heart is possessed by evil. He then progresses to having a heart indwelt by sin *and* grace. Finally, he owns a heart that is full of God. Heavily influenced by Macarius, Wesley understood Christianity as an awakening of the spiritual senses – one whereby man could attain a direct and palpable spiritual awareness of God dwelling in his heart.[83] This spiritual awareness was akin to a physical sensation.

Macarius expressed a holistic, rather than dualistic, anthropology, which was inspired by St Paul's rhetoric of the heart. Wesley borrowed extensively from this interpretation, not only to explicate Christian perfection, but also to explain faith in terms of a circumcision of the heart. It is the 'medicine' of faith, Wesley argues in his sermon, *The Circumcision of the Heart* (1733), which can make man 'whole'.[84] Macarius' rhetoric of the heart is pivotal to Wesley's holistic conception of healing. In the *Fifty Spiritual Homilies*, man's heart has multiple meanings. Physically, it controls the body: 'the heart directs and governs all the other organs of the body' and if the heart stops, then the human body dies.[85] But the depth of man's heart is infinite, and for this reason it has symbolic importance: it is the moral and spiritual centre of the whole person.[86] It is from the heart that 'grace penetrates throughout all parts of the body'.[87] For Wesley, the heart was moral centre, where Christ lives, and he describes it as 'the fountain of life'.[88] Man's heart was all-embracing, and if the heart lies at the centre of Macarius' theology, then it is the *Fifty Spiritual Homilies* that are central to Wesley's thinking, praxis and rhetoric.

The doctrine of Christian perfection, which is so strongly emphasised in the *Homilies*, is not intended to be blandly optimistic, and Wesley's use of Macarius to expound his distinct version of Christian perfection does not, in any way, chime with Shaftsburian Enlightenment ideas of perfectibility. Like Macarius, Wesley believed that Christians could expect to face spiritual and physical suffering right until the end of their lives. *Imitatio Christi* involved a constant struggle for perfection with a resignation to God's will.[89] Wesley's emphasis on the struggle involved here was closely allied to his complex and sophisticated historical analysis of Primitive Christianity. This was a dynamic, as opposed to an idealised, static interpretation, of the early Church – the latter of which had been provided by many seventeenth-century Anglican writers. By contrast, Wesley believed that the 'mystery of iniquity', closely related to original sin, troubled even the golden age.[90] This is conveyed in the Pauline epistles and existed in the New Testament era, tarnishing the image of the Jerusalem Church – Wesley's supreme model of Primitive Christianity. J.D. Walsh points out that Wesley's:

> [H]istorical realism, combined with his consciousness of the potency of original sin, led him to stress the fragility of this primal state. Even in the Acts the worm was in the bud.[91]

Those defects within the Church increased throughout the second and third centuries, despite periodic revivals and isolated pockets of piety, until the fall of Constantine.[92]

The 'mystery of iniquity' posed a threat to even the best of Churches. Its remedy could be found in an active faith: in missionary activity and practical piety. Anglican texts, like those of Cave and Horneck, could be utilised for prescriptive and missionary purposes, and Wesley's inclusion of these works in his *Christian Library* (1749–55) attests to this. The following passage from Horneck's *Happy Ascetick* is worth quoting at length because there is no doubt its rhetoric would have appealed to Wesley:

> The light they came attended withall filled the world, as the sun doth the universe, which comes from its Eastern conclave, and presently diffuses and

spreads its light over all the surface of our hemisphere. So soon did the world feel the influences and operations of those new stars and were forced to acknowledge their divine power and virtue; for they pressed through the chaos mankind lay in, as souls do pierce through bodies and the life, sense and understanding they taught was wholly new, so different from what was in the world before, that man gazed at the spectacle and lost themselves in admiration... with this kind of life, the first Christians amazed an unbelieving world... some who may chance to read these lives will look upon the account I have given you as a spiritual romance, an emblem rather of what men might be, rather of what they generally are.[93]

Horneck indicates that the 'spiritual romance' of his prose is intended to have a profound effect on the reader. Its prescriptive nature is made all the more evident by the fact that Horneck closes his work by directing his reader to a list of patristic writings. This prescriptive element had its desired effect; having read the work of those early Christians, Wesley came to regard their example as being emblematic of his own Methodist mission.

The light of the New Testament did, indeed, contrast vividly with that of the Old, and Primitive Christians were called upon to carry the torch into the darkest corners of the world: Christ's redemptive radiance would enlighten those who wanted to see. For Wesley, the brilliance of this light cast many dramatic shadows, shadows that reached down to his own so-called 'enlightened' age. He thus deliberately likened his mission to that of the Primitive Christians, who had tirelessly sought to transform a 'deluded' world into one of holiness and perfection. For Christians like Wesley this was necessarily going to involve a struggle. As Horneck argued, the 'body seems to long for nothing as much as the ruin of the soul....'[94] Yet Horneck also put his finger on what was vitally important by presenting Primitive Christianity as being emblematic of what men *might* be, as opposed to what they generally are. This paradox lies too at the heart of Wesley's holistic theology and is represented in his tract, *The Character of a Methodist* (1742), where he outlines the ideal to which Methodists should and could aspire.[95] Significantly, the inscription beneath the title, taken from St Paul (Philippians, 3:12–14), states 'not as though I had already attained'.[96] Many years later, Wesley acknowledged that the source of inspiration for this sermon came from the Christian character, drawn by Clement of Alexandria, in the seventh book of *Stromateis* – though the theme of Christian struggle is prominent and recurring in much patrology, not least Macarius' *Fifty Spiritual Homilies*.

Given Wesley's rich theological background, in which the traditions of Puritanism and Anglicanism came together, it is hardly surprising perhaps, that his conception of Primitive Christianity should have developed in complex and interesting ways. At Oxford, Wesley espoused a more conservative, establishmentarian and High Church interpretation of Primitive Christianity, though even here he tentatively pushed the limits of this inherited view of primitivism.[97] This primitivism developed under the spiritual guidance of German pietists, but Wesley never completely aligned himself with that form of Primitive Christianity, mainly because of its rejection of ecclesiology. He worried too much about denying Church authority and his ambivalence on the issue of where authority should ultimately rest shows how difficult it was for him to resolve this complication. This difficulty troubled Wesley a great deal throughout his career as Methodist leader.

Contact with the Moravian Brethren, combined with his Aldersgate conversion experience, helped Wesley to orientate himself to the task of reviving ancient Christian morality and spirituality. He may not have agreed entirely with the Moravians on every theological point, but German pietism served to deepen Wesley's Anglican conception of *devotio* and practical piety by its insistence that every Christian should look out for the spiritual welfare of his fellow men. This responsibility should not be confined exclusively to office holders, and Wesley sought to revive the full significance of the word *diakonos* (in The Acts) for 'servant'. In this sense every Christian should serve as the best representative of God.

Eamon Duffy has argued that Wesley's Aldersgate conversion experience put an end to primitivistic notions that had preoccupied him in Oxford and Georgia.[98] While it was certainly true that he allowed no authority to touch that of Scripture after his conversion experience, Wesley continued to study and use early Christian texts, which he believed could complement God's own story.[99] In this, he approached ancient scripts in the manner of an English liberal scholar. After Aldersgate, there was no significant change in Wesley's preoccupation with Primitive Christianity and L.L. Keefer has suggested that 1738 was, in fact, crucial to his development of it: Aldersgate re-focused Wesley's primitivism away from a heavy emphasis upon ecclesiastical institutions to a theology that was more soteriologically based.[100]

The Primitive Christians of the 'purest ages' inspired Wesley's preaching and encouraged him to create a movement based on his vision of the ancient Church. He was convinced that Methodist doctrine, discipline and depth of piety came nearer to the Primitive Church than any other group. Methodism, he argued in *Laying the Foundation of the New Chapel* in 1777, was the 'old religion, the religion of the Bible, the religion of the Primitive Church'.[101] Visiting the sick, and providing medical advice to poorer members of society, was justified as meeting pressing needs, but it is also clear that Wesley derived pleasure from comparing this act of piety to earlier examples in Christian history.[102] 'Justification by Faith' never allowed Wesley to become self-satisfied or complacent and he worried incessantly about Methodism 'falling away' like the early Church. A huge threat to the efficiency of Christianity was increasing wealth and riches, which inured Methodists from feeling a sense of charity to those less fortunate members of society.[103] To safeguard against this, Methodists needed constantly to engage in acts of charity: charity was the fruit of faith. Utilising those cardinal virtues identified by Macarius (prayer, temperance and alms giving), Wesley saw that the good and holy life, *imitatio Christi*, demanded an active faith, combined with a duty to God and one's neighbour.

Wesley's medical manual, *Primitive Physic*, fitted into a wider context and was characteristic of a movement that placed a premium on social action. This social action was an active faith, undertaken in Christ's name, but informed by those shining examples of early Christians who attempted to achieve pristine purity in the form of physical and spiritual health. The Methodist movement was a 'socially concerned Christianity',[104] and now that the theological context of Wesley's holism has been explored, the following section wishes to examine in more detail the impetus behind Wesley's emphasis on active faith and practical piety.

Practical piety

The deep-rooted significance of Primitivism and its motif for providing a holistic framework from which Wesley worked is explained by Keefer, who suggests that it provides the hermeneutic key for understanding his life. Indeed, it runs through every stage of Wesley's life, providing a unifying theme, which can explicate his soteriology, the existential core of his theology: 'Primitivism explains the comprehensive nature of Wesley's Methodism, an eclectic breadth that defies labels, and it provides the background to his social concern.'[105] It should now be clear exactly how Primitivism fed into Wesley's concept of healing. An active faith or practical piety that was linked to Primitivism provided a backdrop to Wesley's social concern, and was of particular relevance in the realm of medicine and welfare. Central to this social concern was the principle of duty: to God, oneself and one's neighbour.

The compulsion to heal was closely bound up with Wesley's passionate commitment to Primitive Christianity, but the tradition of clerical medicine was also very strong. Like many other clergymen, Wesley felt a *duty* and obligation to practise physic. There is an abundance of evidence to show that English clergymen were encouraged to practise medicine by way of pastoral care, indicated in the Church's willingness to dispense medical licenscs.[106] In the 'Preface' to his *Medicinal Experiments: Or, A Collection of Choice and Safe Remedies For the Most Part Simple and Easily Prepared* (1692), Robert Boyle noted that Anglican bishops had authorised his book in order to encourage clergymen to use it in their dioceses.[107] According to the 'dictates of philanthropy and Christianity', Boyle stated that the receipts set out in his manual were intended for those poor living 'in places where physicians are scarce, if at all to be had… by poor people [who] cannot find a fee or surgeon, or a doctor.'[108]

Many rural areas relied on clergymen as a valuable source of medical advice[109] and Henry D. Rack has seen how priests were often required to be 'benevolent' amateurs, dispensing simple remedies as 'fathers' of their community – this, he suggests, continued well into the nineteenth century.[110] Evidence of this can be seen in an anonymously published text, *The Family Guide to Health* (1767), which sought to supply a physician where one could not be obtained. The existence of this text, and many others like it, shows that clerical medicine continued well into the Enlightenment period. *The Family Guide*, dedicated to the 'parochial clergy', makes the following important observations:

> The affluent has ever at command the best advice which the world can minister. But upon you principally the eyes of the poor are fixed for counsel and instruction. To give it throughout your several charges is the business of your profession… [this] would add greatly to your office and the relief of those committed to your care. The world has been long since admonished of the expediency of having recourse in sickness to a physician in Holy orders. To call a clergyman who has studied physic, is just equivalent.[111]

In common with Dr Samuel Tissot's *L'Avis au Peuple sur sa Santé* (1762), and to a lesser extent *Primitive Physic*, *The Family Guide* was not merely intended to be a popular medical manual. The medical knowledge drawn from the 'most eminent physicians' was to be mediated through the clergy in the form of pastoral care.[112]

Bishop Gilbert Burnet's *Discourse of the Pastoral Care* (1692), a work well known to Wesley, recommended that clergymen study physic so that they might engage in acts of charity.[113] The principle of pastoral care was strong in both the Puritan and Anglican traditions, as seen in Richard Baxter's *The Reformed Pastor* (1656) and George Herbert's *The Country Parson* (1671), both of which were texts known and loved by Wesley. In the latter work, Herbert states that the country parson regards the day as lost when not engaged in acts of charity: 'the country parson is full of charity; it is his predominant element'.[114] Wesley's mixed theological background, glimpsed in his appreciation of both Puritan and Anglican texts, is worth noting briefly for its relationship to medical practice.

The close proximity between Non-conformity and medicine is not a subject that will be explored here but, as is now well known, a large number of Non-conformist ministers were forced to rely on their work as physicians after the Ejection in 1662. Wesley's great grandfather, Bartholomew Westley, Rector of Catherston in Dorset, found himself in this very position. An interesting subsidiary point here is that, although Wesley's father conformed to the Anglican Church, his uncle, Matthew Wesley, remained a Non-conformist and practised medicine as an apothecary in London – a trade noted for its association with dissenting religion. John Wesley's family background epitomises the complex religious and medical interconnections that were characteristic of the Restoration period and continued to influence eighteenth-century life.

Wesley's background is a good example of the changing religious alliances that took place during the seventeenth century: Samuel Wesley broke with the Puritanism of his own family background, but retained a belief in the importance of repentance, conversion and rebirth. He married into the Annesley family, a family that was Non-conformist and heavily Puritan in its outlook, and although Samuel Wesley was keen to demonstrate the continuity between Primitive Christianity and Anglicanism to his own children, he greatly esteemed Puritan leaders, such as Stephen Charnock and John Bunyan.[115] In fact, Samuel Wesley had difficulty in making a complete and decisive break with the Puritan traditions that were inherited from his father, John Wesley. This complicated and rich heritage filtered down through the generations, and L. Tyerman has noted a striking similarity between the ministry of John Wesley (snr) and that of the Methodist leaders:

> Indeed, we find in John Wesley's history an epitome of the Methodism which sprang up, through the instrumentality of his grandsons John and Charles; his mode of preaching, matter, manner and success, bear a striking resemblance to theirs and their co-adjutors.[116]

Given the tenacity of practical piety as a principle in both the Non-conformist and Anglican faiths, combined with a strong tradition of clerical medicine within his family, it seems wholly appropriate that John Wesley (jnr) should want to dispense physic to his extended parish.[117]

It was this concoction of practical piety and Christian enlightened thinking, typified by Wesley's family, which gave rise to the Anglican philanthropic and reformation movements prevalent in the late-seventeenth-century period. In terms of providing an example of active faith, the Society for the Reformation of Manners (SRM), which was founded in 1677, and the Society for Promoting Christian Knowledge (SPCK), instituted in 1698, were powerful sources of influence over Wesley and Methodism as a whole.

Anglicans had been at the forefront of initiatives to establish health care and hospitals during the Restoration period, as part of a bigger campaign to reform manners and morality.[118] Wesley's older brother, Samuel, played a crucial role in this, and the Charitable Society, to which he belonged, was responsible for opening the first voluntary hospital in London.

The Westminster Infirmary had its origins in the Charitable Society, but the opening of Westminster paved the way for a number of other voluntary hospitals, which was ironic given that the initial aim of the Charitable Society was to relieve the sick and needy in their homes.[119] The Society minutes of 1719 are particularly informative here.[120] They show how the Society set out to provide free medical advice to the sick–poor and to: 'procure them the advice of physicians or assistance of surgeons and nurses....'[121] Of primary concern was to care for the *souls* as well as the bodies of those sick–poor: 'the Society designs to reclaim the souls of the sick....'[122]

The Charitable Society was based on a specific model: the Society for Promoting Christian Knowledge (SPCK). As members of the SPCK, Samuel Wesley (jnr) and Henry Hoare provided the connecting link between both societies. Samuel Wesley was also a board member of the most famous and successful charity school, the Grey Coat School, which had opened in 1698. Like the Infirmary, the school was located in the parish of Westminster. Adrian Wilson sees how the Charitable Society, which created Westminster Infirmary, was designed to extend into the care of the sick–poor a form of charitable provision that sought to educate poor children: 'it drew on the same personnel, the same methods and the same religious motive: the care of the sick was linked with their eternal salvation....'[123] Physical and spiritual health were inextricably linked, but the giving of alms, a central precept of Christianity, meant that philanthropy, if undertaken in the right spirit, constituted a religious act of piety, which was a duty to God: such an act could bring about personal salvation.[124]

Duty and personal salvation were principles uppermost in John Wesley's mind shortly before undertaking his Georgian mission – an extended act of piety. In a letter to Dr Burton dated 10 October 1735, Wesley makes plain his reasons for going to America:

> My chief motive is the hope of saving my own soul. I hope to learn the true sense of the gospel of Christ by preaching it to the heathen. They have no comments to construe away the text; no vain philosophy to corrupt it; no luxurious, sensual covetous, ambitious expounders to soften its unpleasing truths. They have no party, no interest to serve, and are therefore fit to receive the gospel in its simplicity. They are as little children, humble, willing to learn, and eager to do, the will of God.... I then hope to know what it is to love my neigbour as myself, and to feel the powers of that second motive

to visit the heathens, even the desire to impart to them what I have received – a saving knowledge of the gospel of Christ.[125]

Duty (to God, oneself and one's neighbour) is the motivating force here. Unfortunately, Wesley's idealistic attitude was to bring bitter disappointment; the Native Americans were not the docile, simple or unspoiled children that he had imagined and hoped for. Nor was this 'heathen' naturally inclined towards receiving the Gospel. Wesley's missionary attempt in Georgia proved to be an unmitigated failure.

This trip to America, however, was inspired and motivated by SPCK ideals of practical piety. He regarded it as an opportunity to instigate Primitive Christianity in an environment and context that closely resembled the ancient Church of apostolic times.[126] Here, the alliance of Primitive Christianity and practical piety would bear fruit, though this feature of Methodism had long-since been espoused by Anglican philanthropic societies like the SRM and the SPCK. Methodism used this example to utilise the ideals of Primitive Christianity while strongly emphasising the value of charity. Tyerman has also noted the similarities:

> [C]onverted young men soon found the benefit of their weekly conferences with each other. Each person related his religious experience to the rest, and thus they became the means of building themselves up in the faith of Christ. The reader will at once perceive that John Wesley's United Societies of Methodists, with their weekly class meetings, instituted sixty-two years afterwards, were almost, if not altogether, an exact revival of these weekly meetings, begun in 1677.[127]

Wesley understood that there was an intimate relationship between the growth of practical piety and the revival of interest in patristic ancient texts during this period: the former was a direct outworking of the latter, and this was personified in the Anglican patristic scholar, Anthony Horneck.

The way in which Horneck's text, *The Happy Ascetick*, exerted its influence in terms of Primitivism over Wesley has been outlined already. But Horneck wielded significant influence over the Methodist movement in unexpected and various ways. He brought together a number of traditions, including German piety and Anglican devotion. A native of Bacharach in Germany, Horneck travelled to England early in life and, after an education at The Queen's College, Oxford, he became a leading figure in the Anglican reformation societies in London.[128] He aimed to renew spiritual life in the Church and, along with Bishop William Beveridge, was actively involved in collecting funds for the poor; in fact, Bishop Gilbert Burnet noted that it was Anthony Horneck and William Beveridge who chiefly conducted the reformation societies.[129] Tyerman observes that their fund-raising relieved many poor families. Debtors and 'sundry prisoners' were set at liberty, some went into a trade, and orphans were also maintained. Poor scholars also received assistance to go to university.[130]

Each member of the society made a weekly contribution to the public stock for pious and charitable ends.[131] Tyerman sees in this an unbroken line between those religious societies instituted by Horneck and Beveridge and the Methodist societies later set up by John and Charles Wesley. Beveridge and Horneck were, he argues:

> [P]ioneers of the Methodist societies, and prepared their way. Their origin and number indicate the existence of a large amount of experimental and earnest piety… they were instrumental in beginning and establishing about one hundred schools in London and its suburbs, in which thousands of poor children were taught gratuitously, and were carefully educated in good manners.[132]

The Methodist 'welfare' programme of establishing schools, encouraging literacy, visiting hospitals, opening medical dispensaries and campaigning for better conditions in gaols, corresponded with the experimental pious works undertaken by Anglican reformation societies. Wesley's commitment to healthcare was motivated by the active duty of practical piety, and *Primitive Physic* quite literally represents what he tried to achieve. Methodist social, educative and health-care initiatives, in tandem with lending services and anti-slavery campaigns, also fitted in with English enlightened values – values that grew out of a Christian culture.

Those involved in this type of initiative were actively seeking to Christianise the communities that they helped. Thomas Bray, founder of the SPCK, argued that the purpose of the Society was to undertake missionary work as a means of extending the Church's influence at home and abroad. To engage in active faith was a way of reinvigorating Anglicanism, thereby promoting 'the pure and primitive Christianity which we profess'.[133] Primitive Christianity was fostered institutionally through the SPCK and this, combined with practical piety, was a way in which Anglicanism could counter the threat of dissent, Socinianism and deism.[134] Wilson argues that Anglicanism wielded very little power in the metropolis, with dissent flourishing in areas like Westminster in the wake of the Toleration Act (1689). Organisations like the SPCK grew up, therefore, in response to this political climate. Wilson's analysis is acute, though he overplays the High Church orientation of the SPCK and pays less attention to the *eirenic* Anglicanism of these societies.[135]

Practical piety involved much more than political rhetoric, which seems to imply that an automatic unity existed between various faiths brought together by societies like the SPCK. Groups and individuals gathered together under the SPCK banner to orientate themselves towards specific goals to 'improve' society, but it was also true that a considerable amount of tension and disunity existed within philanthropic movements. Potential controversial, political and religious issues, however, tended to be by-passed or glossed-over by recourse to a heavy emphasis on practical holiness – a point made by Samuel Wesley (snr) in *A Letter Concerning the Religious Societies* (1699). The design of these societies, he argued, was not to create religious schism and division. It was to show every Christian that glory to God involved the welfare and salvation of themselves and their neighbours.[136] Samuel Wesley's *Letter* expressed a desire to see these societies formed in every major town and in it he is also keen to point out that this type of initiative was not novel; significantly, the Church of Rome was indebted to its progress as a result of such endeavours. An example of this, he argued, could be seen in France, where the Marquis de Renty had founded similar groups in 1640. These societies consisted of devout persons, meeting on a weekly basis, to discuss ways in which to provide relief to the poor, sick and needy.[137] Reference to this example was his way of providing a cautionary reminder to his Anglican peers.

Given Samuel Wesley's gentle reminder of the ever-present threat of Roman Catholicism means that there is no doubt that religion and politics came together in complex ways. But debate continues in earnest amongst scholars about the motivation behind the philanthropic initiatives undertaken during the seventeenth and eighteenth centuries.[138] Deborah Valenze has identified a pietistic component and seen how the eighteenth century fine-tuned charitable works undertaken during the Restoration period – evidenced by the number of hospitals and asylums that opened in Georgian England. In a society that was professedly and uniformly Christian, she argues, such gestures were often outwardly related to religious belief. Recent scholarship has done much to correct an analysis that not only regarded philanthropic charitable initiatives and welfare reforms as separate entities, but one in which the 'rational' nature of both was over-emphasised. Enlightenment scholars of history and medicine are now far more willing to acknowledge the vitally important role that pietistic Christianity played in health and welfare reform. As Samuel Johnson observed in 1758, 'Charity, or tenderness for the poor' was considered to be 'inseparable from piety.'[139]

Valenze argues that eighteenth-century charity was closely connected to the 'manifestation of monetary or material generosity towards the less fortunate by beneficiaries of the new commercial age'.[140] She makes use of Felicity Heal's paradigm shift, occurring between the sixteenth and seventeenth centuries, from individual and household acts of charity to a type of benevolence organised through institutions and state-administered poor laws, to argue that the meaning of 'benevolence' came to be specialised in the Georgian period. This took the form of organised charity, such as the founding of hospitals, dispensaries and asylums and was linked, not directly to increased wealth, but to contemporary anxiety about growing affluence and the distribution of wealth. It is also important to include the Dispensary Movement as part of this type of organised benevolence. Bronwyn Croxson argues that this movement has received very little attention from historians who, she says, have advanced two explanations for the post-1770 Dispensary Movement in London:

> Firstly, dispensaries were institutions designed to advance the interests of a particular group of physicians who were 'outsiders' in the London medical market and therefore unable to gain hospital positions; and secondly, dispensaries were founded because hospitals were unable to meet the needs of the sick poor.

Croxson believes that both of these explanations are incomplete. She suggests that the benefactors who supported dispensaries were motivated by social status, fashion, and a desire for contact with subordinate recipients of charity:

> The elite figureheads associated with a particular dispensary also contributed to its image, not least because their political affiliation could be used to attract like-minded benefactors... these private and political ends provide a clear explanation for the support forthcoming for dispensaries that [did] not rely on benefactors having an altruistic concern for the needs of the poor.[141]

This 'altruistic' concern was the 'public' face of such initiatives and presented in terms of providing humanitarian relief to the poor. Croxson's analysis, though cynical, is certainly worth some serious consideration, but Wesley, who opened dispensaries in London and Bristol in 1746, should not be construed in this political and economic context. However, while Wilson has emphasised the 'politics of medical improvement' in early-Hanoverian London, a recent article written by Paola Bertucci sees how this might also be applied to Wesley's involvement with the Dispensary Movement, which, she says, is 'indicative of his attempts to gain the trust of the sick poor in competition with Dissenters' philanthropy'. In addressing the poor, Wesley was reaching people who would not be cared for by the medical establishment, while offering a High Church alternative to Dissenters' philanthropy. This is most marked, she argues, in Wesley's practice as an 'electric healer', which was driven by a political theology that sought to instil the 'principles of obedience and subordination to religious and political authority'.[142] She believes that Wesley's 'medical philanthropic activities', which also included visits to the sick by Methodists, formed part of a High Church campaign to counter the threat of dissent and deism, 'associated with the diffusion of a political theology which had passive obedience and social subordination among its main tenets and the maintenance of social order as one of its main concerns'.[143] For Bertucci this is evidenced by *Primitive Physic*, which 'emphasised the necessity for proper behaviour and prescribed moderation as the most effective preventative medicine: temperance of the passions, prayer and regimen were the recommended remedies to prevent sickness, just as passive obedience to the king was necessary to prevent political turmoil'.[144]

Bertucci is the latest in a long line of scholars who have stressed social and political discipline as being the main motivation behind organisations like the SRM, the SPCK and indeed, the Methodist movement.[145] It is easy to trace the source of 'social discipline' or 'social control' arguments, particularly when organisations like the SRM enforced an active policy whereby magistrates were informed of the behaviour of particular sabbath-breakers, drunkards and adulterers. 'Reformation' societies were so called, precisely because they sought to promote Christianity by repressing 'vice' and reforming what was regarded as socially unacceptable behaviour. Samuel Wesley (snr) stated as much in his *Sermon Preached Before the Society for the Reformation of Manners* at St James's Church, Westminster, in 1698. He described the immoral nature of the metropolis and, drawing on themes of Primitive Christianity, observed that:

> Our infamous theatres seem to have done more mischief to the faith and morals of the nation than Hobbes... with as much reason we may exclaim against our plays and interludes as did the zealous fathers against the pagan spectacles, and justly rank those, as they did the others, among those pomps and vanities which our baptism obliges us to renounce and abhor....[146]

Sixty-five years later, John Wesley preached before the same Society, from the same text, in West Street Chapel, Seven Dials.[147]

Acts of charity carried multiple motives and Susan C. Lawrence points to the diverse nature of philanthropic initiatives, some of which could also include genuine sincerity. She argues that finding economic, political and social interests, no matter how manipulative and mean-spirited they appear to be, fails to wipe out the sincerity and generosity with which 'men and women gave of their time and money'.[148] Philanthropic endeavours, such as the opening of infirmaries and dispensaries, were intended to heal the sick, but Roy Porter also sees how they functioned as a 'social balm'.[149] The infirmary was frequently the ideal vehicle for *practical* benevolence.[150] Those who espoused the cause of charity stressed the 'pole star of duty – duty to

God, duty to humanity' – which did not necessarily preclude an egotistical element.[151] Ego may have dictated a need for increased 'professional' status or cash benefits on the part of the giver. Moreover, charitable acts bore the mark of civilised, polite and gentlemanly behaviour:

> Duty and pleasure, but also prudence. As the future Archbishop Secker – himself a trained doctor – put that trinity: 'Religion, humanity, common Prudence, loudly require us to rescue' the sick poor.[152]

As Bernard Mandeville noted in his *Essay on Charity and Charity Schools* (1724), it might have been the case that 'pride and vanity' built 'more hospitals than all the virtues together'.[153]

Mandeville, in fact, stunned his contemporaries by pointing out in his *Fable of the Bees* (1723 and 1728) that what appeared to be virtuous acts were by no means motivated by Christian piety. Philanthropic acts were usually met with widespread public approval and so it could just as easily be the case that men were simply miming the conventional signs of Christian piety. This made it impossible to distinguish between genuine acts of charity and those that were driven by selfish motives. E.J. Hundert sees how Mandeville thereby 'redescribed the scene of moral activity' in Augustan England – a point that was picked up by Wesley when he suggested that Mandeville 'cordially recommends vice of every kind'; not only as useful now and then, but as absolutely necessary at all times….'[154] The *Fable*'s notorious maxim, 'Private Vices, Publick Benefits', epitomised Mandeville's view that society was bounded together, not by Christian commitment, but by competition, exploitation and vice. In this context, Hundert argues, a person's character is nothing more than 'an artefact crafted by role-players within theatrical forms of social exchange'.[155]

It was certainly the case that many of his contemporaries suspected Wesley of miming the signs of practical piety. Frequently, Wesley's character became garishly theatrical as he was cast in the role of French effete or cunning rake, usually with a Catholic [sic] proclivity for 'drunkenness', sexual perversion, corruption and licentiousness. Theophilus Evans, author of *The History of Modern Enthusiasm from the Reformation to the Present Times* (1752), noted that: 'the neighbouring kingdom of France has been no less pestered with wild and extravagant opinions, and sometimes under the specious pretence of spiritual devotion'.[156] Evans informs his readers that Wesley bewitches his flock at nocturnal meetings, after which there follow extraordinary 'scenes of debauchery', where 'bastards' are brought into the world by young female 'devotees'.[157] Wesley's motives were continually called into question and subjected to intense scrutiny – despite the fact that his concern for the physical and spiritual welfare of the poor was genuine.

Genuine concern for the spiritual welfare of the sick–poor continued well into the eighteenth century, proof of which can be seen in the fact that hospitals held regular prayer services. Lawrence has shown that many hospital governors thought that regular Christian instruction could produce a reformation in the morals and manners of patients.[158] Patients' minds would be particularly susceptible to Christian instruction when their bodies were weighed down by physical pain and suffering. She looks to the minutes of governors' meetings to show how hospitals had strict rules against swearing, gambling, excessive drinking and indecencies. This was combined with directions to see that a hospital's chaplain did his duty, to purchase the spiritual readings for the wards, and to encourage visiting governors to instil submission to divine authority.[159] Hospitals were provided with bibles and common prayer books, as well as other 'improving' literature such as the devotional works of Jeremy Taylor.[160] Methodists frequently preached in hospitals, and Wesley's *Journal* shows that he made a point of touring and inspecting the hospitals of every major town he visited.

The motivations behind philanthropic and charitable acts were manifold, but crucial to note is the way in which religion provided the language for social change. It was only through religious reformation that seventeenth- and eighteenth-century philanthropists could envision instituting social reformation: religious belief, charity, welfare and social organisation were tightly bonded together.[161] Key to this reformation was the concept of duty, an example of which can be seen, argues L. Haakonssen, in the fact that Enlightenment medical ethics grew out of this Christian precept – albeit a precept that had been elaborated from the material of Stoic and Roman Law. In common with the clergyman, an eighteenth-century physician's duties were divided into those he owed God, himself and the benefit of mankind. Central to this system of practical ethics was the idea that the public imposed a set of duties, which constituted an office or role for life.[162]

Evidence of this can be seen in a wealth of medical, clerical–medical and scientific tracts, which are prefaced with statements referring to this three-fold duty. Citing Tissot's *L'Avis au Peuple sur sa Santé* as the main source of inspiration, William Buchan argues in the 'Preface' to *Domestic Medicine* (1769) that:

> There certainly cannot be a more necessary, a more noble, more Godlike action than to administer to the wants of our fellow men in distress… to assist… the endeavours of the humane and benevolent in relieving distress; to eradicate dangerous and hurtful prejudices; to guard the ignorant and credulous against the frauds and impositions of quacks and impostors; and

to show men what is in their power, both with regard to the prevention and cure of diseases, are certainly worthy of the physician's attention.[163]

The sentiments expressed here were repeated in a large number of medical and scientific works. Hence Bishop Berkeley felt 'indispensably obliged, by the Duty every Man owes Mankind' to write and publish *The Medicinal Virtues of Tar Water* (1744).[164] To provide 'cheap' and 'natural' remedies in an 'easy' method was Wesley's duty to 'Mankind', as indicated in the title to his medical manual: *Primitive Physic: Or, An Easy and Natural Method of Curing Most Diseases*:

> Who would not wish to have a physician always in his house, and one that attends without fee or reward? To be able (unless in some complicated cases) to prescribe to his family as well as himself? If it be said, but what need is there of such attempt? I answer, the greatest that can possibly be conceived. Is it not needful in the highest degree, to rescue men from the jaws of destruction... from pining away in sickness and pain, either through ignorance or dishonesty of physicians?[165]

The title and tenor of *Primitive Physic* is more than a little reminiscent of Boyle's *Medicinal Experiments: Or, A Collection of Choice and Safe Remedies, For the Most Part Simple, and Easily Prepared*, and it was Boyle's intention also to make accessible cheap remedies:

> [F]or medicines so simple, and for the most part so cheap, I have found all of them to be good of their kind: and though I think that most of them are safer than many other medicines that are in great request, yet I do not pretend that those should play the part of medicines and physicians too; but that they may be employed by one who knows how to administer them discreetly.[166]

Boyle felt compelled to prepare physic 'by the dictates of philanthropy and Christianity' but intended his receipts to be of practical use to the poor living in the country.[167] Physicians were more difficult to come by in the country and the artisan or labourer needed to self-medicate during times of illness – primarily because his family depended upon him financially. Loss of income through illness, disease or death could render a family completely destitute. This is made clear 'to the Parochial Clergy' in the anonymously written *The Family Guide to Health*:

> How often, when called upon, to visit the sick, have you seen them perishing and hurried to an untimely grave for want of a little advice and the application of proper means; and those means, it might be easy to procure, had not the knowledge of ascertaining them, been also wanting.[168]

Medics like Buchan were keenly aware of this danger, which is hardly surprising given that so many diseases could carry away a family's sole breadwinner:

> The poor often perish in diseases for want of proper nursing… no one can imagine, who has not been witness of these situations, how much good a well disposed person may do, by only taking care to have such wants supplied.[169]

Buchan, who was originally sent to Edinburgh to study divinity, but who abandoned his calling in favour of a career in medicine, wanted to instil into the 'poor' the importance of 'proper food, fresh air, cleanliness, and other pieces of regimen necessary in diseases'.[170] Philanthropic and charitable endeavours presented a cost-effective way for those poor members of society to keep themselves in a reasonable state of health. Loss of labour through illness, Porter argues, represented 'a direct debit to the community, with the risk of further charges if they and their families fell on to the parish.'[171] Yet in terms of health and longevity, many also argued that the artisans' or country folks' 'simple' life contrasted favourably with the luxurious, indolent and urban lifestyle characteristic of polite society, of which 'gouty' conditions attested all too visibly. Tissot wrote *L'Avis au Peuple sur sa Santé* by way of tackling diseases faced by the rural poor in Lausanne. However, its sister manual, *An Essay on the Disorders of People of Fashion* (1771), sought to redress the balance of prescriptive medical works designed for the poor and aimed its fire at the urban middling classes. While the Swiss physician believed that the main causes of disease amongst the rural poor were excessive labour, insanitary conditions and drunkenness, he regarded the country labourer's diet and outdoor lifestyle as being exemplary. Cheyne expounded a similar view in as much as he believed that the 'moderate' diet generally espoused by the middling ranks was the best example to follow in tandem with a firm commitment to regimen. The connection Cheyne made between the condition of gout and a moneyed lifestyle, both of which he saw as being symptomatic of a 'civilised' age, was nevertheless sufficiently complex and ambivalent. Noted already is the fact that Wesley advocated a simple ascetic lifestyle to counter the pernicious dangers of a rich and wealthy lifestyle.

In terms of benevolence and practical piety, a variety of medics, clerical–medics and scientists sought to state their intention explicitly from the outset. Joseph Priestley in 'The Preface' to *The History and Present State of Electricity* (1767) argued that the cultivation of piety was essential to philosophers: 'true' philosophy promotes piety. Citing David Hartley as a useful guide on this point, Priestley extracts the relevant passages from *Observations on Man* (1749) to lend weight to his argument:

> Since the world is a system of benevolence, and consequently its author the
> subject of unbounded love and adoration, benevolence and piety are our
> only true guides in our inquiries... the only keys which will unlock the
> mysteries of nature... when the pursuit of truth is directed by this higher
> rule, and entered upon with a view to the Glory of God, and the good of
> mankind, there is no employment more worthy of our natures, or more
> conducive to their purification and perfection.[172]

Through Hartley, Priestley makes a direct connection between practical
piety and Christian purification. Furthermore, philosophy, if undertaken in
the right spirit and directed by the will of God, could become an act of
practical piety.

There were, of course, substantial points of difference in terms of
theoretical and methodological approach, but the principle expressed here
by Priestley echoes that of those experimental philosophers and medics
involved in the Oxford Philosophical Club and Royal Society. For Boyle,
philosophical or medical work reflected a pious commitment to improve the
condition of mankind:

> And therefore I reckon the investigation and divulging of useful truths in
> physick... among the greatest and most extensive acts of charity... by which
> a man may... oblige mankind.[173]

As a Christian philosopher, Boyle was concerned to integrate his medical
and scientific discoveries into God's divine plan. Boyle's broad-based,
eclectic, but empirical, approach was utilised by way of promoting medical
reform; knowledge gained here should not be exclusive, but disseminated
widely for the interest of mankind. This espousal of practical piety led Boyle
to encourage individual responsibility for health and welfare – welfare that
was cost-effective.[174]

All of this bears a striking resemblance to the approach taken by Wesley
in *Primitive Physic*. Like Boyle, Wesley wanted to demonstrate that an active
Christian faith was perfectly compatible with medical and scientific research,
particularly if that research could be serviceable and cost-effective to
mankind. Far from these two modes of operation being in conflict, scientific
research, if conducted in the right spirit – by marking off its inherent
limitations – could, in itself, become an act of practical piety. Moreover, the
dissemination of knowledge gained from such activity constituted a form of
active faith and this was closely allied to the principle of 'plain' language,
which also contained a theological imperative.

This latter point will be investigated later, but it will be necessary first to
examine how the experimental, empirical and pragmatic method utilised by
Boyle and other colleagues at the Oxford Philosophical Club and Royal

Society, informed Wesley's methodological approach. Wesley's identification of the theological mainsprings of natural philosophy, and its close correlation to the empirical method used by Boyle, Sydenham and Locke, was incorporated as part of an active faith, which put enlightenment to useful, practical effect. Here, Wesley followed the example set down by those Anglican practical pietists who incorporated medical and welfare reform into a much bigger vision of human and spiritual development.

Enlightened empiricism as a philosophy of nature

John Wesley may not have been a systematic 'Enlightenment' thinker, but his cast of mind fitted well with English enlightened thinking. If a philosophical empiricism meant that he was less than triumphant about the capacity of human knowledge, this did not prevent him from actively attempting to acquire the knowledge needed to comment on scientific or medical experiments. Indeed, he used this enlightened empiricism by way of encouraging men and women to relieve and improve their physical conditions.

Wesley studied, commented on and, in some cases abridged, a range of works by enlightened authors, which included Isaac Newton, Robert Boyle, John Locke, Peter Browne, René Descartes, Nicholas Malebranche and David Hartley.[175] The enlightened ideas put forward by these authors, J.W. Haas argues, were 'filtered through a pluralistic theological lens' and examined with a 'theologian's eye'.[176] Yet, contrary to accusations made by a number of nineteenth-century historians, Wesley did not subject science and philosophy to theology.[177] His adoption of the empirical tradition corresponded instead with a late-seventeenth- and early-eighteenth-century desire to reconcile Scripture and natural philosophy.[178] In this context, as the work of Andrew Cunningham and John Hedley Brooke has now established, a reconciliatory, as opposed to purely conflictual, relationship between religion and science in the form of natural philosophy could protect Christianity from the threat of deism and atheism.[179] Here, Wesley reflected a trend in Anglican theology, which 'aspired to bridge, but not obliterate, differences between theology, philosophy and science'.[180] Natural history, philosophy and science could point to the wisdom of God, and Wesley put the works of the philosopher–divines John Ray and William Derham to useful effect in his *A Survey of the Wisdom of God in the Creation: Or, A Compendium of Natural Philosophy*.[181]

Wesley followed in the English empiricist tradition, set down by Francis Bacon and taken up by members of the Philosophical Club in Oxford and the Royal Society in London.[182] The former group included, amongst many others, Boyle, Sydenham and Locke. Observed against a backdrop of seventeenth-century political strife and religious schism, empiricism was a methodological approach that attempted to arrive at a consensus over matters of fact in the realms of science, philosophy and medicine. K. Dewhurst has shown that the empirical medical works of Sydenham and Locke led to a steady progress in clinical medicine based on observation.[183] Sydenham believed that the search for ultimate causes of disease was speculative and in vain:

> I have been very careful to write nothing but what was the faithful product of observation. I neither suffered myself to be deceived by idle speculations, nor have deceived others by obtruding anything upon them but downright matters of fact... the function of a physician [is the] industrious investigation of the history of diseases, and of the effect of remedies, as shown by the only teacher, experience. True practice consists in the observations of nature: these are finer than speculations. Hence the medicine of nature is more refined than the medicine of philosophy.[184]

Physicians should concern themselves only with the 'outer husk' of things, since God had designed man's senses to perceive only this, which meant that human capacity for knowledge was necessarily limited. It was on this basis that Sydenham rejected the use of microscopes in scientific investigation, insisting that they were artificial and therefore of no practical use.[185]

Both Sydenham and Locke were opposed to *a priori* hypotheses and favoured instead an accumulated mass of observed facts; this could help to build up a more accurate clinical picture of disease and sickness. Locke makes plain his feelings on the matter in a letter addressed to Dr Thomas Molyneux in 1692:

> I perfectly agree with you concerning general Theories, that they are for the most part but a sort of waking Dream, with which, when Men have warm'd their own Heads, they pass into unquestionable Truths, and then the ignorant World must be set to right by them: Though this be, as you rightly observe, beginning at the Wrong end, when Men lay the Foundation in their own Fancies, and then endeavour to suit the Phenomena of Diseases, and the Cure of them to those Fancies....[186]

Empiricism could provide general, but more reliable, explanations – a process Boyle described as the 'interrogation of nature'.[187] Boyle's method in medicine, which, like Sydenham and Locke, he regarded as a sub-set of natural philosophy, sought to unite diverse bodies of knowledge based on facts. In *Primitive Physic* Wesley follows the same experimental, empiricist method utilised by Sydenham, Locke and Boyle by bringing together a complex range of medical approaches.

An enlightened empirical method that privileged fact over theoretical speculation was of huge significance to Wesley's scientific and medical work. As Haas points out, Wesley's writings 'bear ample witness that an empirical approach permeated both his theology and natural philosophy.'[188] Wesley greatly esteemed those English empiricists for paving the way to 'true' philosophy – a discipline that was keen to show the limitations of human knowledge even as it strove to develop it. Concerning those limits of human knowledge, critics and commentators have tended to see an anti-intellectual strain in Wesley's insistence on this point – a stance that many have interpreted as being directed specifically at Newton.[189] Wesley understood that Newton himself had repudiated *a priori* speculations, preferring an empirical approach, which set out plain facts over and above hypothesis. Newton formulated the law of gravity but did not seek to uncover divine causes. Porter thus comments: 'in Newtonianism, British scientific culture found its enduring rhetoric: humble, empirical, co-operative, pious, useful'.[190] Wesley was, however, also keenly aware from his reading of Samuel Clarke's *A Demonstration of the Being and Attributes of God* (1705) that natural philosophy – or a philosophy of nature – was at one and the same time protective of the sacred in nature whilst lending itself to deistic, if not atheistic, interpretations.[191] His antipathy was directed, not at Newton, but that brand of Newtonian or deist thinking which he believed threatened to over-play man's intellect by subordinating faith to reason, thus removing God entirely from the picture.[192]

Like Cheyne and John Hutchinson, Wesley was eager to combat the deist tendencies of Newton's philosophy. His approach to scientific, philosophic and medical inquiry was thus threefold: to retain, first, a prominent place for the Creator; second, to emphasise strongly the limitations of human knowledge, thus preserving the supernatural character of faith. This could be achieved by rejecting speculative philosophy in favour of an experimental, empirical approach based on experience. Finally, Wesley wanted to put all knowledge to useful effect for the common interest of mankind. This three-fold method can be seen in all of Wesley's scientific works where the principle is logically worked through, though not explicitly stated. It is at work in 'The Preface' to *Primitive Physic*, where, in Section One, Wesley states that the 'grand Author of Nature' can help to restore man's health. In Section Eleven, the reader is informed that some 'lovers of mankind' have attempted to 'explode' hypotheses and 'fine-spun theories' in order to make physic 'a plain intelligible thing, as it was in the beginning: having no more mystery in it than this, "such a medicine removes such a pain".' Section Thirteen is a statement of Wesley's intention to provide an 'easy way of curing most diseases' for the 'common interest of Mankind'.[193]

This method did not in any way preclude an active engagement with scientific and philosophical research. Nor did Wesley's approach seek to subvert the disciplines of philosophy, science and medicine to theology. It sought, instead, to undermine the slick certainties of 'Reason' with its proclivity for excessive rationality and system-building, the result of which could usher in a type of 'madness' akin to 'enthusiasm'. On this, Wesley had much in common with other English enlightened thinkers who regarded excessive rationalism and systematic philosophy as major irritants. In this context system-building was equated with the sin of pride, which ran contrary to the principle of practical piety. Wesley rails against this tendency in 'The Preface' to his *Compendium*:

> Does not the same survey of the Creation, which shows us the wisdom of God, show the astonishing ignorance and short-sightedness of man? For when we have finished our survey, what do we know? How conceivably little? Is not every thinking man constrained to cry out, And is this all? Do all the boasted discoveries of so enlightened an age, amount to no more than this? *Vain man would be wise!* Would know all things! But with how little success does he attempt it? How small a part do we know even of the things that encompass us on every side.[194]

The glimpsing of God's wisdom showed that man, after all his research, was stumbling in the dark.

System-building could evoke vanity and pride, but threatened to create schism or civil discord. Barbara Beigun Kaplan notes that it led people to hold differing opinions, 'thus fragmenting the quest for knowledge' by frustrating an attempt to achieve religious unity through a collaborative effort.[195] Ambivalent attitudes to *a priori* speculative systems, or distaste for the uncritical worship of reason, may have had more to do with religious ethics in Georgian England rather than a philosophical scepticism. But at the very least, discussions about the nature and limitation of knowledge were a careful balancing act between natural science or philosophy and theology: knowledge of the world and knowledge of God. Rom Harré summarises this very well when he suggests that in eighteenth-century Britain:

> Every discussion of the epistemology of natural science from this period must be understood against the presumption that its author was almost certainly scrutinising his own reasoning for its theological consequences in the knowledge that so too was everyone of his readers.[196]

An empirical strain continued to dominate eighteenth-century medical practice, in spite of the changes that took place in medical theory and discourse. This strain could even be seen in those most iatro–mechanical and 'rational' of physicians, such as Cheyne and Mead.

Wesley's *An Earnest Appeal to Men of Reason and Religion* (1743) and *A Farther Appeal to Men of Reason and Religion* (1745) spin upon the axis of rationalism and faith. The *Appeals* corroborate a Lockean definition of the 'reasonableness' of Christianity, only deftly to undercut its deist and rationalist implications with dialectical logic and skill.[197] Like Locke, Wesley insisted that any claim to revelation had to be confirmed by reason, but this did not mean that reason could obtain any degree of certainty when determining whether revelation was of divine origin. Establishing its validity was a matter of probability; reason could confirm Scripture, but it could not falsify Christianity with any degree of certainty.

Reason was central to Christian doctrine, but in terms of giving faith, hope, love or even instilling real virtue, it was utterly incapable. Reason could not explain faith in rational terms, and in spiritual matters the faculty of reason depended exclusively upon faith:

> What then will your reason do here? How will it pass from things natural to spiritual? From the things that are seen to those things that are not seen? From the visible to the invisible world? What a gulf is here! By what art will reason get over the immense chasm?

> Faith is that divine evidence whereby the spiritual man discerneth God and the things of God. It is with regard to the spiritual world what sense is regard to the natural. It is the spiritual sensation of every soul that is born of God.[198]

Not since Eden had man really known God. After the Fall, all man could rely on was religious intuition and faith. Drawing on Locke's *The Reasonableness of Christianity* (1695), but also the *An Essay Concerning Human Understanding* (1690), Wesley demarcates the limit of human knowledge in his sermon on the *Imperfection of Human Knowledge* (1784). He utilises I Corinthians (13:9), 'we know in part', to indicate that man's intellect is infallible because he is *de facto* imperfect.[199]

Using Pauline rhetoric, Wesley adopts an empiricist and distinctively Lockean tone to convey this message in a letter to Bishop William Warburton, written in 1763:

> How little does the wisest of men know of anything more than he can see with his eyes! What clouds and darkness cover the whole scene of things invisible and eternal! What does he know even of himself, as to his invisible part? What of his future manner of existence? How melancholy an account does the prying learned philosopher (perhaps the wisest and best of all heathens), the great, the venerable Marcus Antonius give of all these things!

What was the result of all his serious researches? Of his high and deep contemplation…Poor Antonius! With his wealth, his honour, his power, with all his wisdom and philosophy!

What points of knowledge did he gain?
That life is sacred all – and vain!
Sacred how high? And vain how low?
He could not tell – but died to know.[200]

Heathen philosophers had been stumbling in the dark and *died to know* the 'truth'. They depended on reason to lead them to the truth but, as Locke pointed out in *The Reasonableness*, 'some parts of that truth lie too deep for our natural powers easily to reach, and make plain to mankind, without some light from above to direct them'.[201] True knowledge was disclosed by revelation and further confirmed by reason and experience. The beautiful simplicity of Christianity lay in its balance between reason and revelation.

Paradoxically, true knowledge was revealed to man after an acknowledgement that the human intellectual faculty was imperfect and infallible. The 'office' of faith could lead man out of the darkness and give birth to a new understanding, which would reveal true knowledge. Boyle stated that scientific and medical discoveries intended for the improvement of mankind were ultimately a revelation from God. Such revelations sprang from the labour of pious research and on this both Bacon and Boyle argued that philosophy could instil great faith. God rewarded the faithful who undertook philosophical research in the spirit of practical piety by granting gradual insights into the workings of nature. This was the motivating force of those belonging to the Philosophical Club at Oxford, the legacy of which left its mark on Wesley.[202]

In spite of the limitation of human knowledge brought about by the Fall, Boyle insisted that the efforts of those who wished to understand nature could eventually arrive at a type of refined approximation of how it worked. This would encourage the philosopher and scientist to carry on with his investigations in the hope of arriving at probabilistic, though not certain, knowledge.[203] In 'The Preface' to *The Desideratum: Or, Electricity Made Plain and Useful,* Wesley is eager to let his reader know that the search for ultimate causes via speculative philosophy is fruitless:

But who can be assured of this or that hypothesis, by which he endeavours to account for those facts? Perhaps the utmost we have reason to expect here is, a high degree of probability.[204]

Wesley, like Boyle and Locke, did not deny that man could know the existence of God through nature and natural law, but the essential character of nature could only be revealed by God to man. Wesley's view on the virtue of empirical scientific research was expressed as such in the *Compendium*:

> He [God] does not impart to us the knowledge of himself immediately; that is not the plan he has chosen; but he has commanded the heavens and the earth to proclaim his existence, to make him known to us. He has endued us with facilities susceptible of this divine language, and has raised up men who explore their beauties and become their interpreters. Natural philosophy treats both of God himself and his creatures, visible and invisible....[205]

It is plain how Wesley's *Compendium* made use of John Ray's *The Wisdom of God Manifested in the Works of the Creation* (1691). In the latter work, Ray had set out 'by virtue of his function' to 'write something on Divinity' and wished to show exactly how the heavens and earth could 'proclaim' God's existence and 'make him known' to man.[206] No man, however, could find out the internal workings of nature or God, though the office of faith could supply this want.

In his letter to William Warburton, Wesley reminds his opponent of the supernatural framework of faith, while placing his argument in that Lockean tradition which strongly rejected deism. An attempt to go beyond what was humanly possible in the sphere of knowledge might produce various negative psychological conditions. These states of mind included the uncritical worship of reason, a debilitating scepticism or doubt, and the dangerous flights of mystical fancy, which could lead man into superstition, delusion or nervous disorder. With the precision of a surgeon's knife, Wesley manages to dissect the accusations of 'fanaticism' and 'enthusiasm' levelled at Methodism by Bishop Warburton. Turning Warburton's argument on its head, Wesley argued that it is excessive rationalism, not an active faith, which produced psychological distress.[207] Wesley made this very same point in the *Compendium*:

> It will be easily observed that I endeavour throughout, not to *account for* things, but only to describe them. I undertake barely to set down what *appears* in Nature, not the *cause* of those appearances. The *facts* lie within the reach of our senses and understanding; the *causes* are more remote. *That things* are so, we know with certainty: But *why they are so*, we know not. In many cases we cannot know; and the more we inquire, the more we are perplext and intangled. God *hath so done his works*, that we may admire and adore: But *we cannot search them out to perfection...* the more we labour to penetrate into the Nature of this Divine Principle, the more it seems to retire and withdraw itself from our most studious researches.[208]

He made clear that distinction between empirical knowledge and knowledge of the internal workings of nature. In *An Earnest Appeal,* Wesley claimed that 'ideas of faith differ *toto genere* from those of external sensation.[209] This was further complicated, though, by the analogy he drew between an empirical sensorium and what he referred to as a type of spiritual 'sense' or immaterial 'reality'.[210] Outler has seen how this analogy was extrapolated from a concept that had its origins in Descartes, but was further elaborated by Malebranche.[211] It is this analogy that allowed Wesley to regard man as a unity of body, mind and spirit, and determined his thinking about health in holistic terms. With perfect consistency Wesley could thus maintain a position that distinguished between a Lockean empirical knowledge of tangible reality, while making claims for a type of intuitive knowledge of God – since spiritual 'reality' does not come within the orbit of empirical or rational knowledge. Hence, as Outler wryly remarks, Wesley was both an 'avowed empiricist' and 'unembarrassed intuitist who openly claimed his heritage to Christian Platonism'.[212]

Scholars have seen how this approach was unique and particular to Wesley.[213] However, Laura Bartels Felleman has suggested that another powerful source of influence on Wesley in this regard was Cheyne, who also combined a heightened awareness of the 'spiritual senses' with an empirical approach to epistemology.[214] Maddox has also noted how Cheyne's writings played a major role in nurturing Wesley's mature emphasis on the interconnection between physical, emotional and spiritual health.[215] Cheyne criticised Locke's faulty description of the human faculties which, he argued, were incapable of giving man a proper sense of the spiritual world.[216] Cheyne's critique would certainly have struck a cord with Wesley, as seen in the following passage from *An Earnest Appeal* where empiricism is blended together with Christian Platonism or a 'spiritual sense' of an immaterial realm:

> And seeing our ideas are not innate but must originally come from our senses, it is certainly necessary that you have senses capable of discerning objects...not those only which are called 'natural senses', which in this respect profit nothing as being altogether incapable of discerning objects of a spiritual kind, but spiritual senses... it is necessary that you have the hearing ear and seeing eye, emphatically so called; that you have a new class of senses opened in your soul, not depending on organs of flesh and blood, to be the '*evidence* of things not seen' as your bodily senses are of visible things....[217]

The empirical method adopted by Wesley when approaching medicine and science, however, meant that he had no desire to present a metaphysical system for the natural world. Instead he sought, like Boyle, Locke, Ray and Derham, to harmonise nature with Scripture and the wisdom of God – hence the appropriateness of the title to his compendium: *A Survey of the Wisdom of God in the Creation: Or, A Compendium of Natural Philosophy*. He also spells this out in the affirmation of a letter received from a friend in 1748. Dr Robinson's letter was published in the February,1779, issue of the *Arminian Magazine*:

> Natural philosophers busy themselves about two things, the history of facts and the causes to its effects. No man I think can with any reason pretend to the second, til he has enriched his memory with a large flock of natural history; which alone, if we should never get further is very profitable for life and godliness, teaching us many things useful in common life; and creating in an attentive mind a high reverence for the creator, whose power, wisdom, goodness and the considerate view of the creatures very sensibly demonstrates and more feelingly than abstract reasonings.[218]

Speculative philosophy was reminiscent of that branch of knowledge espoused by the 'Schoolmen' who, in Wesley's view, had neglected natural philosophy. The English empiricists, on the other hand, understood well the defects of School philosophy and 'incited lovers of Natural philosophy' to a diligent search via 'many experiments and observations':

> After this, not single persons only, but whole societies applied themselves carefully to make experiments; that having accurately observed the structure and properties of each body, they might the more safely judge of their nature. And the advantages which have arisen from hence manifestly appear from the memoirs of the Royal Society....[219]

Medicine could teach man many 'useful' things for 'common life' and Wesley agreed with Boyle that physic should be regarded as a branch of natural philosophy, which was subject to the same empirical method of fact-finding:

> Dr Harvey improved Natural philosophy, by another no less eminent discovery: for he was the first of the moderns that shewed all animals to be generated from eggs... another remarkable discovery in the last century was that of the transfusion of blood... what pity, that so important an experiment should ever fall into disuse!

> It cannot be denied that physicians have finally improved this branch of philosophy, as they have continual opportunities of making new discoveries in the human body. In diseases themselves, the wonderful wisdom of the author of Nature appears: And by [this] means... many hidden recesses of

the human frame are unexpectedly discovered. The powers of medicine also variously exerting themselves, lay open the secrets of Nature.[220]

The second of the two above-cited passages from the *Compendium* shares many of its assumptions with the following extract taken from the 'Preface' to Cheyne's *An Essay on Regimen*:

True philosophy is the science of living the most happily... physic is one branch of this philosophy, and regards but one part of our composition... true philosophy takes in the whole extent of our Being, from its distant beginning to its most advanced stages... true physic is that only which directs how the body may be preserved the most healthful....[221]

Physic was a branch of natural philosophy, and so healing the body by recourse to empirical methods was perfectly valid. The medical works of Boyle, Sydenham and Locke were augmented by those of Cheyne and Hartley – the latter of which showed Wesley that the body was a system of nerve fibres, which transmitted sense perceptions to the brain.[222] This stance was bolstered by an avowedly empiricist belief that the essential nature of matter was impenetrable and thus unknowable. The following observations about the 'Nerve' contained in the *Compendium* clarifies this:

A *Nerve* is a whitish, round, slender body arising from the brain, which is supposed to convey the animal spirits, to all parts of the body. What these spirits are, none can show: Nay, we are not sure they have any being, whether the nerves are hollow canals, or only solid threads...

...are the nerves in general hollow canals, which contain a circulating fluid? Or are they solid threads, which being highly elastic, vibrate variously to occasion various sensations? The latter supposition is wholly overthrown by the phenomena of wounded nerves.

But what is this fluid? Who can tell? We may very probably conjecture, it consists of the same circulating fluids from which it seems to be derived, and with the nervous fibrils which we suppose it is designed to nourish and repair. But it may likewise consist, and perhaps chiefly, of some subtle fire or ether, diffused thro' the whole system of Nature, and acting by Laws unknown to us.[223]

A range of possibilities concerning the physiology of the nerve are presented here, but Wesley accepted the utility of regarding the human body as a machine and tended to use Cartesian mechanical language where appropriate.

In this he shared much in common with Boyle who did not attempt to articulate a mechanistic account of the body, but wished to use the body–machine analogy as a tool to further understand human physiological processes and demonstrate the sovereignty of God.[224] Like Boyle, Wesley found a convincing argument in the concept of the body as finely tuned machine: the human frame provided further evidence of God's handiwork. 'The wisdom of God' was, in fact, reflected in the human body and is stated as such by Wesley in the *Compendium*:

> And how eminently this is displayed first, in the *situation* of its parts and members? They are situated most conveniently for use, for ornament, and mutual assistance. 1. For use. The principal senses are placed in the head, as sentinels in a watch-tower. How could the eyes have been more commodiously fixed, for the guidance of the whole body? The ears, likewise, made for the reception of sounds, which naturally move upward, are rightly placed in the uppermost parts of the body: And, so are the nostrils, as all odours ascend.[225]

Exactly how Wesley put medical language to use in his work, specifically his sermons, has already been identified but his acute awareness of the medium of language is indicative of Wesley's methodology as a whole.

If philosophical research had the capacity to become an act of practical piety that could bring man closer to God, the dissemination of such knowledge also constituted a form of active faith. The way in which knowledge was mediated was crucially significant. Language functioned as a tool through which an understanding of complex material could be arrived at, but this was also closely allied to the principle of 'plain' language – a principle that contained a theological imperative, which was multi-layered. For Wesley, God's own story was mediated via the simple and plain language used by the Apostles and Primitive Christians. In the Gospels it carried with it a missionary purpose, which was powerfully connected to faith and the imperative of practical divinity. Acts of practical piety brought with them a heightened spiritual awareness of God and 'true' knowledge, which in turn needed to be made accessible to those seeking enlightenment. The teleology of Wesley's thinking and praxis is evident here, but the vital role played by 'plain' language in bridging Primitive Christianity, practical piety and true knowledge will be examined in the final section of this chapter.

John Wesley's rhetoric of 'plain' style

We have already identified the way in which Wesley represents the story of Genesis in the opening three paragraphs of 'The Preface' to *Primitive Physic*. This part of 'The Preface' has its 'origin' in Genesis, though an array of patristic sources was woven into the fabric of this text to demonstrate Scriptural truth. Wesley's repeated claim to be *homo unius libri* was

71

misleading and this very statement exemplifies his rhetoric of 'plain' style. The plain style characteristic of Wesley's preaching and writing owes a huge debt to his family background, which blended Non-conformist, Puritan elements with Anglicanism.[226]

The numerous unacknowledged influences in Wesley's work mean that it is easy to oversimplify and underestimate his learning. Yet Wesley's claim to be the man of one Book should not imply that he was an unthinking literalist. His dexterity with ancient languages meant that Wesley understood their flexible nature, which in turn alerted him to the danger of literal interpretation. Nor did Wesley's espousal of plain style simply stem from a popularising impulse, but had a deep moral and theological imperative. It is Wesley's veiled learning that gives all of his work a depth and originality rarely found in typical popularisers.[227]

Eighteenth-century authors and writers rarely acknowledged their sources or 'borrowings', but it is true to say that Wesley ingested his sources to such an extent that they often seemed to be refined out of existence: biblical references are left unacknowledged and citations of patristic authors are comparatively few. Wesley took to heart his father's advice to 'master' and 'digest' any given text.[228] This can be seen in 'The Preface' to *Sermons on Several Occasions*, where he stresses a deliberate intention to 'forget all that ever I have read in my life'.[229] This disavowal, Outler suggests, was Wesley's way of hiding his learning, so that he could avoid alienating his reader or listener.[230] His thorough ingestion of sources is also connected to a powerful tradition of sublimation in Christian history. This ingestion and sublimation has a number of important theological principles, including a missionary concern with practical piety which necessarily involved spreading the divine word in a simple and plain language.

The Puritan strains in Wesley's background meant that he was acutely aware of the intimate relationship between sublimation and plain style. Christian history was not simply the chronicle of institutions; it was the (divine) story of the preached word and its success or failure in different contexts.[231] Wesley's use of plain language represented more than a pragmatic approach, though this motivation was crucially important because of its relationship to practical piety. This can be seen in his following statement on the issue of plain language:

> I think it my duty to see every phrase be clear, pure, and proper. Conciseness, which is now, as it were, natural to me, brings *quantum sufficit* of strength. If, after all, I observe any stiff expression, I throw it out, neck and shoulders. Clearness, in particular, is necessary… to instruct people of the lowest understanding….[232]

The Latin tag here is illustrative of the fact that Wesley could never quite escape his classical training, though this in no way mitigates the plain style. George Lawton notes, in fact, that in the sermons, but also other works, 'Latin and Greek quotations... rub shoulders with the language of the marketplace, the tavern, and the meeting-house'.[233] Wesley believed that there was a dignity in the simplicity of plain style that could appeal to men of all ranks. Furthermore, he knew how men of all ranks discoursed and, as Lawton suggests, almost everything Wesley wrote was designed to communicate, vindicate, convince, persuade and move: 'It was essentially rhetorical... even the *Journal* is of this nature, although it is easy to forget the fact'.[234]

The 'ornate' style of English sermonising was an unnecessary distraction from God's word. Eusebius of Caesarea, the father of Church history, stressed the importance of writing God's story and *The History of the Church* sets out to record 'the lines of succession from the Holy Apostles', the 'men... who were ambassadors of the divine word'. Eusebius insisted that no language could explain the essence and nature of Christ.[235] Language could not explain the full significance and mystery of the Incarnation and must therefore point to another mode of expression to make the unknowable comprehensible. Metaphor might achieve this aim and this mode was critical to Wesley's articulation of theology and its esoteric themes. Language could not fully explain the workings of God and Wesley used medical metaphors extensively, of which he had a particular fondness.[236] Metaphor functioned as a tool, in the same way as patristic evidence, to illuminate complex, esoteric biblical themes and make clear Scriptural truth. Little attention should be drawn to the preacher or writer, who was simply the channel or mediator through which Scriptural truth could be conveyed. Thomas à Kempis thus advised the reader of *Imitatio Christi* not to be 'influenced by the importance of the writer, and whether his learning be great or small; but let the love of pure truth draw you to read.'[237]

Love of pure truth impelled Wesley to read voraciously, write prolifically and act as 'ambassador of the divine word' to his Methodist followers. In the context of Christian history as divine story – though not a predetermined one – it is clear that a moment of repetition and *kenosis* occurs in his use of the plain style of preaching and writing – just as it does in St Paul's *Epistles*. St Paul's language is imbued with that of the Septuagint to reassure his readers that he and they share a common tradition and faith, a tradition that was bigger than the Apostle, St Paul himself.[238]

Kenosis, the Greek word for 'emptying himself', is taken from St Paul's account of the Incarnation when Christ humbled himself by breaking away from divinity to become man. This breaking device is a movement of discontinuity, a break from the heavy influence of divine power. Wesley's adoption of plain style becomes a way of emptying and humbling himself to God. Here, we can see also how the principle of *kenosis* fitted into an empiricist methodology – a methodology that placed heavy emphasis on the limitation of human knowledge. For Wesley, *kenosis*, or humbling oneself towards the *imitatio Christi*, had a two-fold purpose. Firstly, it emulated the Primitive Christians for whom Wesley had so much respect. Secondly, it was a way that Wesley could place himself *fons et origo*.

On the second point, acts of charity, preaching and writing could take on a missionary purpose if undergone in a spirit of practical piety; philosophical and medical research could constitute an act of piety if conducted for the benefit of mankind. Such acts contained the potential to become imbued with a supernatural or divine power and an empirical approach could complement and confirm this belief. With its acknowledgement of human intellectual fallibility, empiricism promises to bring with it a capacity to glimpse divine revelation and 'true' knowledge. Practical piety, in the form of charitable acts, preaching, writing or research, does not, therefore, simply reproduce or emulate the origin of Primitive Christianity; it can actually become that origin. In this sense, Wesley's missionary trip to Georgia was a conscious manoeuvre on his part to go back to the origin. Convinced that the Gospel was revealed in situations akin to Apostolic times, the word of God could only be discovered in an actual repetition of the early Christians who preached to the pagans.[239] Wesley makes this patently clear when describing an experience he had while attending a Moravian service in Georgia:

> After several hours spent in conference and prayer, they proceeded to the election and ordination of a Bishop. The great simplicity, as well as solemnity, of the whole, made me forget the seventeen hundred years between, and imagine myself in one of those assemblies where form and state were not; but Paul the tent-maker, or Peter the fisherman presided; yet with the demonstration of the Spirit and Power.[240]

Wesley was struck by the 'great simplicity' of the Moravians, whom he believed to be closer to Primitive Christianity than any other religious group. This desire to place himself *fons et origo* was intimately bound up with his rhetoric of simplicity and plain style; in his written work it was the conscious adoption of the simple literary style of The Acts and the Gospels.

The New Testament is characterised by its missionary spirit and by the effective expansion of the word. In his written (and oral) work, Wesley seeks to emulate the performative structure of this plain style and its missionary purpose. Patristic writings are valuable in as much as they can create a 'living continuity' between contemporary Christians and the New Testament, but this evidence, or that of any other, should not undermine the authority of Scripture.[241] Hence, Wesley's oft-quoted method of Scripture: interpreted by Christian tradition, reviewed by reason and appropriated by experience. The lives of Primitive Christians were inspirational and Wesley insisted in *A Plain Account of the People Called Methodists* (1748) that Methodists 'generally found, in looking back, something in Christian antiquity, likewise nearly parallel' to Methodism.[242]

A Plain Account was an open letter to his close friend the Revd Vincent Perronet, Vicar of Shoreham, Kent, and its function was intended to be an apology for the Methodist movement. In it, particular features of Methodism, such as Watchnight and Lovefeast services, the separate seating of men and women in church, the role of women in the spiritual ministries, the importance of healing and the defence of open air preaching, are all defended in terms of Wesley's conception of Primitive Christianity. Despite this, however, Wesley repeatedly claimed that Methodism was not planned, and heavy emphasis was placed instead on the haphazard nature of the movement. Again, this is rhetorically significant. Wesley felt that Methodism should be interpreted as a divinely inspired movement that developed providentially – as opposed to the Romish Christianity fostered artificially by Constantine. The movement could claim to be 'truly' authentic and Wesley was keen to show that there was nothing programmatic about his use of Primitive Christianity. He therefore avoided writing an explicit treatise or essay on the subject and in this sense Wesley was not an ideologue.

Wesley approached the study of patristic evidence as he approached all bodies of knowledge, in the manner of an English liberal scholar. He attempted to extract, abstract and sum up complex sources in an intelligible way. This sprang from a deep theological conviction which was motivated by a personal relationship with God and the nourishment of one's own faith – a faith that was aided by acts of piety.[243] Here, the principle of practical piety coalesced with educative ideals to improve knowledge and literacy levels amongst his Methodist followers. Wesley's strenuous efforts to improve the lives of his flock are manifest in *Primitive Physic*, which was specifically designed to nourish the spiritual *and* physical wellbeing of ordinary people. Emphasis on an empirical methodology and espousal of plain style complemented and sprang from a theological commitment to holism and practical piety, but in the context of eighteenth-century England this methodology could potentially revive an ancient standard in physic. In turn, this standard provided an antidote to the esoteric systems of thought that Wesley believed dogged Georgian medical practice, a tendency he bitterly laments in Sections Eight and Nine of 'The Preface':

Men of learning began to set experience aside; to build physic upon hypothesis; to form theories of diseases and their cure, and substitute these in place of experiments. As theories increased, simple medicines were more and more disregarded and disused: till in a course of years, the greater part of them were forgotten… till at length physic became an abstruse science, quite out of the reach of ordinary men.[244]

An interesting parallel can be drawn here between the plain style of *Primitive Physic* and that of other vernacular medical texts in the eighteenth century such as *A Cheap, Sure, and Ready Guide to Health: Or, A Cure for a Disease Call'd the Doctor* (1742). This text, written by a 'Private Gentleman' and sold at the 'lowest rate' of 6d. states its intention of practical piety from the outset. The 'true' Christian healer writes in a style easily understood, not merely from a desire to popularise abstruse medical theory, but to make 'charity… his law and practice':

> There should be no mystery in physic, any more than religion: we have religion and law in a known tongue, and should have physic in the same.[245]

Buchan, author of the 'popular' text *Domestic Medicine*, makes a similar argument when he accuses physicians of concealing the art of physic and setting up a 'doctorcraft', akin to that Catholic tendency which sought to reduce religion to 'priestcraft'.[246]

In seeking to uncover an ancient standard set down in medicine by experiment, experience and plain facts, Wesley's medical manual drew strength from the traditions of Primitivism and practical piety. This chapter has identified how these traditions provided an impetus when writing *Primitive Physic*. The next chapter will shift its emphasis away from the theological motivation of *Primitive Physic* in order to investigate the ways in which this text suggested practical solutions to the problem of providing medical care to the sick in Georgian England – those sick who could not afford to 'swell the Apothecary's bill' or pay the doctor's 'spoil'.[247]

Notes

1. J. Wesley, *Primitive Physic: Or, An Easy and Natural Method of Curing Most Diseases,* 24th edn (London, 1792), iv; J. Wesley, *Sermon on Original Sin* (1759), in A.C. Outler (ed.), *The Bicentennial Edition of The Works of John Wesley* (Nashville: Abingdon Press, 1985), *Sermons,* Vol. II, 172–85: 184–5.

2. The arguments set down in this chapter have been treated in articles elsewhere. See, 'Experience and the Common Interest of Mankind: The Enlightened Empiricism of John Wesley's *Primitive Physic*', 41–53; 'Medicine and Moral Reform: The Place of Practical Piety in John Wesley's Art of Physic', *Church History* 73, 4 (December 2004): 741–58 and 'The

Limitation of Human Knowledge: Faith and the Empirical Method in John
Wesley's Medical Holism', *History of European Ideas,* 32 (2006), 162–72.

3. L.L. Keefer, 'John Wesley: Disciple of Early Christianity', *Wesleyan
   Theological Journal,* 19 (1984), 23–32.

4. T.A. Campbell, *John Wesley and Christian Antiquity. Religious Vision and
   Cultural Change* (Nashville: Kingswood Books, 1991), 21. For a discussion
   of the context of the revivial in patrology, see M.E. Fissell, 'Charity
   Universal? Institutions and Moral Reform in Eighteenth-Century Bristol', in
   L. Davison, *et al.* (eds), *Stilling the Grumbling Hive: The Response to Social
   and Economic Problems in England, 1689–1750* (New York: St Martin's Press,
   1992), 121–44.

5. George Bull had been a member of the same college as Wesley's father
   (Exeter). Before his election as Archbishop of Canterbury, William Wake had
   been a scholar and Canon of Christ Church. Wake's *Genuine Epistles of the
   Apostolic Fathers* (1693) and Bull's *Defensio Fidei Nicaenae* (1685) were prime
   examples of Anglican apologia, which drew on patristic writings. John
   Pearson's *Exposition of the Creed* (1659) also became a standard work of
   Anglican divinity. Pearson was Master of Trinity College, Cambridge, before
   becoming Bishop of Chester.

6. E. Duffy, 'Primitive Christianity Revived: Religious Renewal in Augustan
   England', in D. Baker (ed.), *Renaissance and Renewal in Christian History*
   (Studies in Church History, 14), (Oxford: Blackwell, 1977), 287–300.
   Anthony Horneck had been a member of The Queen's College, Oxford.
   Anthony Horneck and William Cave presented a rather idealised picture of
   the early Church, and although Wesley did not fully endorse this portrayal,
   both works were later abridged and included in *A Christian Library,* 1st edn
   (Bristol, 1749–55).

7. Campbell, *op. cit.* (note 4), 19–20.

8. J. Wesley, *An Address to the Clergy* (London, 1756) and *On Laying the
   Foundation of the New Chapel* (1777), in Outler, *op. cit.* (note 1), Vol. III,
   577–93. *An Address* was a reworking of Samuel Wesley's *Advice to a Young
   Clergyman* (London, 1735), written to Mr Hoole, a curate at Epworth. Like
   Samuel Wesley's earlier work, *An Address* was a prescriptive work of practical
   piety in its insistence of which texts the clergy should be familiar, but also in
   its concern for the welfare and education of those addressed. See Campbell,
   op. cit. (note 4), 46.

9. A.C. Outler, 'Introduction', in *op cit.* (note 1), Vol. I, 59.

10. Campbell, *op. cit.* (note 4), 27.

11. J.D. Walsh, 'John Wesley and the Community of Goods', in K. Robbins
    (ed.), *Protestant Evangelicalism: Britain, Ireland, Germany and America
    c.1750–c.1950. Essays in Honour of W.R. Ward* (Oxford: Oxford University
    Press, 1990), 25–50.

12. Wesley produced an abridged version of Abbé Claude Fleury's *The Manners of the Ancient Christians* (originally published in 1682, then translated into English in 1698), a text that described the early Church community and its disciplinary practices. For Wesley's version see J. Wesley (ed.), *The Manners of the Antient Christians, Extracted from a French Author,* 1st edn (Bristol, 1749).

13. Wesley, *Primitive Physic, op. cit.* (note 1), iii.

14. *Ibid.*

15. J. Wesley, *The One Thing Needful* (1734), Outler, *op. cit.* (note 1), Vol. IV, 351–9: 354.

16. J. Wesley, *The Trouble and Rest of Good Men* (1735), in Outler, *op. cit.* (note 1), Vol. III, 531–41: 533. P.W. Ott, 'Medicine as Metaphor: John Wesley on Therapy of the Soul', *Methodist History,* 33 (1995), 178–91: 184.

17. J. Wesley, *Sermon on Original Sin* (1759), in Outler, *op. cit.* (note 1), Vol. II, 185.

18. M. Schmidt, *John Wesley: A Theological Biography,* trans N.P. Goldhawk, 2 vols (London: Epworth Press, 1985), Vol II, 91.

19. R. Maddox, *Responsible Grace: John Wesley's Practical Theology* (Nashville: Kingswood Books, 1994).

20. The Incarnation represents the salvic centre, highlighting best the relationship between God and man, as outlined in Gal. 2: 19–20: 'With Christ I am nailed to the cross, yet I live now not I, but Christ in me'.

21. J. Wesley, *Heaviness through Manifold Temptations* (1760), in Outler, *op. cit.* (note 1), Vol. II, 222–35: 227.

22. R.L. Maddox, 'A Heritage Reclaimed: John Wesley on Holistic Health and Healing' in M.E.M. Moore (ed.), *A Living Tradition* (Nashville: Kingswood Books, forthcoming).

23. J.D.G. Dunn, *The Acts of the Apostles* (Peterborough: Epworth Press, 1996), 6.

24. Cited by R. Morgan, *Romans* (Sheffield: Sheffield Academic Press, 1995), 107. According to St Paul, we do not have bodies: we are bodies and must glorify God in our body.

25. I Cor. 6: 19, 6: 15; P. Brown, *The Body and Society: Men, Women and Sexual Renunciation in Early Christianity* (New York: Columbia University Press, 1988), 51.

26. J. Wesley, *The Good Steward* (1768), in Outler, *op. cit.* (note 1), Vol. II, 281–99: 285. Wesley was aware of the materialist implications of this notion, infamously promoted in the work of Julien Offray de la Mettrie, entitled *L'Homme Machine* (1748).

27. Ott, *op. cit.* (note 16), 182.

28. J. Wesley, *On the Fall of Man* (1782), in Outler, *op. cit.* (note 1), Vol. II, 400–12, 405.

29. G. Cheyne, *The English Malady,* 1st edn (London, 1733); R. Porter (ed.), *George Cheyne: The English Malady: Or, A Treatise of Nervous Diseases of all Kinds (1733)* (London: Routledge, 1991), 4.

30. S. Hales, *A Sermon Preached Before the Royal College of Physicians,* 1st edn (London, 1751), 6.

31. J. Wesley, *The Image of God* (1730), in Outler, *op. cit.* (note 1), Vol. IV, 290–303: 296.

32. *Ibid.,* n. 18. Outler observes that Wesley has updated an age-old discussion about Adam's mortality resulting from defiance. Had he obeyed, Adam would have carried out the physical demands made on his body, unhindered, until finally being transported to the spiritual and eternal life.

33. *Ibid.,* 297; Ott, *op. cit.* (note 16), 182.

34. Wesley, *ibid.,* 297.

35. 1 Cor. 15: 44, quoted in G. Cheyne, *An Essay on Regimen Together with Five Discourses, Medical, Moral and Philosophical: Serving to Illustrate the Principles and Theory of Philosophical Median, and Point Out Some of its Moral Consequences,* 1st edn (London, 1740), n.p.

36. Wesley in J. Telford (ed.), *The Letters of the Rev. John Wesley A.M.,* 8 vols (London: Epworth Press, 1931), Vol. VI, 327. Wesley used this phrase in a letter to Alexander Knox (October 1778).

37. Quoted in D.J. Melling, 'Suffering and Sanctification in Christianity', in J.R. Hinnells and R. Porter (eds), *Religion, Health and Suffering* (London: Kegan Paul, 1999), 46–64: 59.

38. J. Wesley (ed.), *Advice with Respect to Health,* 4th edn (London, 1789), 8.

39. Wesley thought that it was the fourth-century monk, Macarius the Egyptian, who had written the *Fifty Spiritual Homilies.* This was a common error in the eighteenth century and stemmed from Thomas Haywood's translation of the *Homilies* in 1721, entitled *Primitive Morality, or the Spiritual Homilies of St Macarius the Egyptian.* It is now thought that the *Homilies* were written in Syria, though debate still continues about their theological background and authorship. Wesley made a new translation of the *Homilies,* which was included in the *Christian Library.*

40. Hales, *op. cit.* (note 30), 10–11.

41. For a fuller explication of the radical bifurcation of body image that came to dominate histories of Western spirituality, see H. Ferguson, 'Me and My Shadows: On the Accumulation of Body-Images in Western Society. Part One – The Image and the Image of Body in Pre-Modern Society', *Body and Society,* 3 (September 1997), 1–31: 18, 20.

42. J. Wesley, *A Survey of the Wisdom of God in the Creation: Or, A Compendium of Natural Philosophy,* 5 vols, 3rd edn (London, 1763), Vol. I, 89–90.

43. Rom. 7: 23.

44. Rom. 8: 11 quoted in Brown, *op. cit.* (note 25), 48.

45. *Pneuma* was an eschatological gift that could liberate man from the bondage of Rabbinical Law. St Paul's mission to the Gentiles involved demonstrating that God loved them without the works of the law. Martin Luther's radical interpretation of this, and St Paul's phrase 'righteousness of God' (Rom. 1: 17), which he changed to 'righteousness from God', strongly asserted the gift of righteousness. It was this interpretation that Wesley responded to in 1738, as is now well known, during a reading of Luther's 'Preface' to Romans. Luther's recovery of 'Justification by Faith' moved Wesley's heart and subsequently led to his conversion experience. 'Justification by Faith' thus became a central doctrine to the Methodist movement. Morgan, *op. cit.* (note 24), 20, 142.

46. J. Wesley, *The Trouble and Rest of Good Men* (1735), in Outler, *op. cit.* (note 1), Vol. III, 531–41: 533.

47. A. Horneck, *The Happy Ascetick: Or the Best Exercise... To Which is Added, A Letter to a Person of Quality, Concerning the Holy Lives of the Primitive Christians,* 2nd edn (London, 1685), 482; V.H.H. Green, *The Young Mr Wesley: A Study of John Wesley and Oxford* (London: Epworth Press, 1961), 293.

48. *Ruach* is Hebrew for wind, breath or Spirit.

49. S. Beckwith, *Christ's Body: Identity, Culture and Society in Late Medieval Writings* (London: Routledge, 1993), 23.

50. Of interest here, though, is the fact that Scottish Calvinists resisted the introduction of smallpox inoculation in the eighteenth century on the basis that man should not intervene if it was God's will for people to die of this disease. Wesley was criticised by the Calvinists for the time he spent engaged in medical activity – time better spent, they argued, studying Scripture.

51. Melling, *op. cit.* (note 37), 59.

52. *Ibid.,* 62.

53. *Ibid.,* 56.

54. *Ibid.,* 62.

55. *Ibid.,* 63.

56. The spiritual writings of early Christians are filled with affirmations of suffering (voluntarily) for Christ's sake with fasting, hair-shirts and self-flagellation forming a significant part of Christian ascetic practice. Melling points out, however, that early Christian writers did not place a premium on self-inflicted suffering, but on the value of a voluntary acceptance of suffering. See Melling, *op. cit.* (note 37), 51.

57. *Ibid.,* 56.

58. Wesley, *Primitive Physic, op. cit.* (note 1), viii.

59. T. Sydenham, *The Works of Thomas Sydenham M.D,* trans. R.G. Latham, 2 vols (London: Sydenham Society, 1868), Vol. II, 90. See also P.W. Ott, 'John Wesley on Health as Wholeness', *Journal of Religion and Health,* 30

(1991), 43–57.

60. Wesley, *Primitive Physic, op. cit.* (note 1), iv.

61. *Ibid.*, iv.

62. Quoted in Melling, *op. cit.* (note 37), 56.

63. *Ibid.*, 57.

64. *Ibid.*, 58

65. *Ibid.*, 58.

66. Cyprian, *Epistles*, trans. C.H. Collyns (Oxford: Library of the Fathers of the Holy Catholic Church, 1844), 736, 783.

67. St Ignatius of Antioch, 'Epistle to the Trallians', in J.A. Kleist (ed.), *The Epistles of St Clement of Rome and St Ignatius of Antioch* (London: Newman Press, 1946), 36.

68. W. Cave, *Primitive Christianity: Or the Religion of Ancient Christians in the First Ages of the Gospel*, 6th edn (London, 1702), 'The Preface', iii.

69. This is recorded by Wesley in his journal. See *The Journal of the Rev. John Wesley, A.M.*, 4 vols. (London: J. Kershaw, 1827), Vol. I, 3; Vol. III, 205.

70. Schmidt, *op. cit.* (note 18), Vol. II, 80.

71. Horneck, *op. cit.* (note 47), 'The Preface' (preface unpaginated).

72. *Ibid.*, 484, 352.

73. Wesley, *Primitive Physic, op. cit.* (note 1), xii.

74. J. Wesley, *Upon our Lord's Sermon on the Mount: Discourse the Seventh* (1739–46), in Outler, *op. cit.* (note 1), Vol. I, 592–611.

75. J. Wesley, *Thoughts Upon Self Denial* (1760; repr. London, 1857), 56. This work had been extracted and amended from Bishop William Beveridge's *Private Thoughts Upon a Christian Life* (1709).

76. Wesley, *ibid.*, 57.

77. Quoted in *ibid.*, 43.

78. Wesley enjoyed a critical relationship with Thomas à Kempis. *Imitatio Christi* wielded much influence over him, but he was also suspicious of what he perceived to be its more severe forms of renunciation and mysticism. Wesley agreed with his father that the work needed to be contextualised, for it represented a severe withdrawal from the world at a particular moment in Christian history. He understood that the mystical element of *Imitatio Christi* was a dissolution of the historical, an escape from the ravages of temporality. This, however, did not prevent Wesley from extracting what was good about the work, which he amended and published as *The Christian Pattern: Or a Treatise of the Imitation of Christ* (London, 1735).

79. The Holy Club was attacked for its asceticism after the death of one of its members, William Morgan. This attack appeared in December 1732 in *Fog's Weekly Journal.* There is no proof that this individual had actually died as a result of extreme asceticism. An anonymous pamphlet, entitled *The Oxford Methodist, Being Some Account of a Society of Young Gentlemen in that City so*

Denominated (1733), defended the group by stating that Methodists were following rules which accorded with Scripture, the Primitive Church and the Anglican Church.

80. Wesley communicated this intention in a letter to Richard Morgan, dated 18 October 1732: 'we still endeavour to hold fast: I mean the doing what good we can…[to this we have added] the observing of the fasts of the Church, the general neglect of which we by no means apprehend to be a lawful excuse for neglecting them' (Wesley, *op. cit.* (note 36), Vol. I, 132).

81. St Clement, a first century Roman convert, used elements of Platonic and stoic philosophy to make this point – in contradistinction to those pagan philosophers who believed ascetic qualities to be exceptional. See E. Pagels, *Adam, Eve and the Serpent* (London: Penguin, 1988), 85.

82. Cited by K. Ware, 'The Preface', in Macarius (Pseudo-), G.A. Maloney (ed.) *The Fifty Spiritual Homilies* (New York: Paulist Press, 1992), xi.

83. *Ibid.*, xiv. Thus, Wesley could argue that New Birth could be an instantaneous or *gradual process*. The heart of the newly-born man is clean, but corruption remains in the soul as long as it is in the body. The new man, through God's grace, guards himself against his old nature and what ensues is a struggle for Christian (wholeness) perfection.

84. J. Wesley, *The Circumcision of the Heart* (1733), in Outler, *op. cit.* (note 1), Vol. I, 401–14: 404.

85. Macarius (Pseudo-), *op. cit.* (note 82), 108–14 (15: 20–33).

86. Ware, *op. cit.* (note 82), xv.

87. Macarius (Pseudo-), *op. cit.* (note 82), 108–14 (15: 20–33).

88. Wesley, *op. cit.* (note 42), Vol. I, 55.

89. Campbell has shown how Wesley developed a specialised vocabulary to describe the stages that Christians must go through in this struggle: 'the wilderness state', 'heaviness through manifold temptations', 'assurance of pardon' 'entire sanctification' and 'Christian perfection'. These terms litter the corpus of Wesley's written sermons. See Campbell, *op. cit.* (note 4), 55.

90. Wesley's later sermons, *The Mystery of Iniquity* (1783), *End of Christ's Coming* (1781), *General Spread of the Gospel* (1785) and *New Creation* (1785), are indicative of a more developed sense of Christian history, which changed over time. See Outler, *op. cit.* (note 1) Vol. I, 451–510.

91. Walsh, *op. cit.* (note 11), 36–7. Anthony Horneck's text did distinguish itself from that of William Cave by its willingness to concede to the possibility of corruption creeping into the golden age of Primitive Christianity: 'It is true, even among Christians in the purest ages, there were divers, who by their lives disgraced that noble religion' (Horneck, *op. cit.* (note 47), 537).

92. L.K. Keefer, 'John Wesley: Disciple of Early Christianity', 27–30. Like other primitivists, Wesley's view of Christian history followed that of the Biblical story. It was divided into three distinct epochs: a golden age, a fall and a

restoration. Where one placed the gridline for this division had been the subject of bitter religious dispute since the Reformation, with debates about 'authenticity' continuing well into the eighteenth century. See Campbell, *op. cit.* (note 4), 9.

93. Horneck, *op. cit.* (note 47), 482, 538–540.

94. *Ibid.*, 483.

95. Wesley used the early works of William Law to make the crucial point that perfection was not an end in itself. Rather it was the active pursuit of this goal and purity of intention that was vitally important.

96. J. Wesley, *The Character of a Methodist*, 3rd edn (Bristol, 1743).

97. Walsh, *op. cit.* (note 11).

98. Duffy, *op. cit.* (note 6).

99. Campbell has counted over one hundred and fifty citations in Wesley's work after 1738, but there are many more allusions left unacknowledged by Wesley. See Campbell, *op. cit.* (note 4), 43.

100. Keefer, *op. cit.* (note 3), 27–30.

101. J. Wesley, *On Laying the Foundation of the New Chapel*, (1777), in Outler, *op. cit.* (note 1), Vol. III, 585.

102. Keefer, *op. cit.* (note 3), 27–30.

103. Quoted in D. Valenze, 'Charity, Custom, and Humanity: Changing Attitudes towards the Poor in Eighteenth-Century England', in J. Garnett and C. Matthew (eds), *Revival and Religion since 1700: Essays for John Walsh* (London: The Hambledon Press, 1993), 59–78: 59; J. Wesley, *Causes of the Inefficiency of Christianity* (1789), in Outler, *op. cit.* (note 1), Vol. IV, 85–96. Wesley repeatedly lamented the commercialism, wealth and luxury of his age in sermons such as *The Danger of Riches* (1781) and *Danger of Increasing Riches* (1790) in Outler, *op. cit.* (note 1), Vol. III, 227–45 and Vol. IV, 177–86. Walsh has shown that Wesley's commitment to the 'community of goods' meant that he argued in favour of redistributing wealth accumulated from profit to the poor. This can be seen in his sermon *On the Use of Money* (1760) in Outler, *op. cit.* (note 1), Vol. II (1985), 266–80. See also Walsh, *op. cit.* (note 11).

104. Schmidt, *op. cit.* (note 18), Vol. I, 88.

105. Keefer, *op. cit.* (note 3), 27–30.

106. J. Cule, 'The Rev. John Wesley, M.A. (Oxon.), 1703–1791: "The Naked Empiricist" and Orthodox Medicine', *The Journal of the History of Medicine*, 45 (1990), 41–63.

107. R. Boyle, *Medicinal Experiments: Or, A Collection of Choice and Safe Remedies, For the Most Part Simple, and Easily Prepared*, 4th edn (London, 1703), n.p. In 1688, Boyle published a collection of recipes entitled *Receipts Sent to A Friend in America*. This collection was expanded and re-named *Medical Experiments* as a posthumous second edition in 1692. See B. Beigun

Kaplan, *'Divulging of Useful Truths in Physick': The Medical Agenda of Robert Boyle* (Baltimore and London: John Hopkins Press, 1993), 7. As Kaplan notes, this work exemplified a genre of medical recipe books popular in the mid-seventeenth century, which were written in the vernacular and designed as self-help manuals.

108. Boyle, *ibid.,* n.p.
109. R. Heller, 'Priest–Doctors as a Rural Health Service in the Age of Enlightenment', *Medical History,* 20 (1976), 361–83.
110. Rack, 'Doctors, Demons and Early Methodist Healing', in W.J. Sheils (ed.), *The Church and Healing* (Studies in Church History, 19), (Oxford: Oxford University Press, 1982), 137–52: 139. Felicity Heal modifies this view in her study of hospitality in early modern England. She argues that by the time one reaches the clerical diaries of the eighteenth century, George Herbert's advice about hospitality and charity as a means of curing souls was outdated: 'The good parson revelled in entertainment, and was on easy terms with most of his parish, but would have seen no purpose in providing them with general hospitality of any kind'. Heal does see that there were some clergymen who defended the apostolic ideal of open care but 'they were not normally the voices of mainstream Anglicanism: the greatest exponents of open hospitality were William Law… and John Wesley'. See F. Heal, *Hospitality in Early Modern England* (Oxford: Clarendon Press, 1990), 298.
111. 'Dedication to the Parochial Clergy of this Kingdom', in Anon., *The Family Guide to Health: Or, A Practice of Physic: In a Familiar Way,* 1st edn (London, 1767), iii–iv.
112. *Ibid.,* v.
113. Cule, *op. cit.* (note 106), 41–63.
114. G. Herbert, *The Country Parson,* 1st edn (London, 1671), 43.
115. Schmidt, *op. cit.* (note 18), Vol. I, 41. L. Tyerman argues that although Samuel Wesley held his ecclesiastical and political principles dearly, he was not a bigot – nor was he a Jacobite. See L. Tyerman, *The Life and Times of the Rev. Samuel Wesley, MA.* (London, 1866), 177–9.
116. Tyerman, *ibid.,* 51.
117. Rack, *op. cit.* (note 110), 139.
118. Bishop Gilbert Burnet noted that formerly there had been societies of this description amongst Puritan and dissenting religions, but Tyerman states that those springing up in this period belonged to the established Church. Tyerman, *op. cit.* (note 115), 215.
119. A. Wilson, 'The Politics of Medical Improvement in early Hanoverian London', in A. Cunningham and R. French (eds), *The Medical Enlightenment of the Eighteenth Century* (Cambridge: Cambridge University Press, 1990), 4–39: 15.
120. The idea for an infirmary in Westminster was conceived in 1716, but the

Charitable Society discontinued its activities for three years before resuming to found and open the Infirmary between the years 1719–20. Samuel Wesley was part of an enlarged personnel of 1719. See J.G. Humble and P. Hansell (eds), *The Westminster Hospital, 1716–1966* (London: Pitman Medical Publishing, 1966) where the Society Minutes are cited; C. Rose, 'Evangelical Philanthropy and Anglican Revival', *London Review*, 16 (1991), 35–65.

121. Cited from the Society Minutes in Humble and Hansell, *ibid.*, 6.

122. *Ibid.*

123. Wilson, *op. cit.* (note 119), 20.

124. Rose, *op. cit.* (note 120).

125. Wesley, *op. cit.* (note 36), Vol. I, 187.

126. L. Tyerman, *The Life and Times of the Rev. John Wesley, MA*, 3 vols (London, 1870–2), Vol. I, 114; Schmidt, *op. cit.* (note 18), Vol. I, 132–33; Campbell, *op. cit.* (note 4).

127. Tyerman, *op. cit.* (note 115), 215.

128. After the revolution of 1688, Horneck was appointed Chaplain to King William and Queen Mary. In 1693 he became Prebendary of Westminster.

129. Tyerman, *op. cit.* (note 115), 215.

130. *Ibid.* Samuel Wesley was helped by such initiatives when he was jailed for debt in 1705. See L. Tyerman and D. Rack, *Reasonable Enthusiast: John Wesley and the Rise of Methodism* (London: Epworth Press, 1992).

131. The Society for the Reformation of Manners became defunct in 1730 but was revived by John Wesley, amongst others. By 1766, the Society ceased to exist – as a result of legal action taken against it, which resulted in them paying £300 in damages. The Society could not recover this loss.

132. Tyerman, *op. cit.* (note 115), 226.

133. Cited by C. Rose, 'The Origins and Ideals of the SPCK 1699–1716' in J. Walsh, C. Haydon and S. Taylor (eds), *The Church of England c.1689–c.1833: From Toleration to Tractarianism* (Cambridge: Cambridge University Press, 1993), 172–90: 179.

134. Wilson, *op. cit.* (note 119), 20–5.

135. Rose, *op. cit.* (note 133). Philanthropic initiatives such as the charitable hospitals were an instance where Anglicans and Dissenters could and did work together.

136. Tyerman, *op. cit.* (note 115), 228.

137. *Ibid.*, 227.

138. Seen in the different views expressed in the work of Wilson and Rose. See Wilson, *op. cit.* (note 119) and Rose, *op. cit.* (note 133). Susan C. Lawrence sees how medical experts put their knowledge to charitable ends. See S.C. Lawrence, *Charitable Knowledge: Hospital Pupils and Practitioners in Eighteenth-Century London* (Cambridge: Cambridge University Press, 1996).

139. See Valenze, *op. cit.* (note 103), 63; M. Fissell, 'Charity Universal?

Institutions and Moral Reform in Eighteenth-Century Bristol', Davison, *et al.* (eds), *op. cit.* (note 4), 121–44.

140. Valenze, *op. cit.* (note 103), 63–4.

141. See B. Croxson, 'The Public and Private Faces of Eighteenth-Century London Dispensary Charity', *Medical History,* 41 (1997), 127–49: 129–8. See also Heal, *op. cit.* (note 110); Valenze, *op. cit.* (note 103), 63.

142. P. Bertucci, 'Revealing Sparks: John Wesley and the Religious Utility of Electrical Healing', *British Journal for the History of Science*, 39 (2006), 341–62; 350, 352.

143. *Ibid.*, 349.

144. *Ibid.*, 349.

145. An example of this 'social discipline' argument can be seen in K. Wilson, 'Urban Culture and Political Activism in Hanoverian England', in E. Hellmuth (ed.), *The Transformation of Political Culture: England and Germany in the Late Eighteenth Century* (Oxford: Oxford University Press, 1990), 165–84. Bronwyn Croxson argues that by restricting charitable acts to the 'industrious' or 'deserving' poor, charity could be used to impose order by rewarding acceptable behaviour. With regards to the Westminster Dispensary, she states that '…regulating the behaviour of patients may have been part of the medical regime', along with a regimen of care, which regulated diet, exercise and sleep. Croxson, *op. cit.* (note 141), 135. Many scholars have pointed to this element of social control in the Methodist movement – with particular reference to both John and Charles Wesley's desire to inculcate into the lower orders a disciplined 'work ethic'. This argument was famously put forward by E.P. Thompson in his essay 'Time, Work-Discipline and Industrial Capitalism', in *Customs in Common* (London: Penguin, 1993), 352–403 but also in his seminal text, *The Making of the English Working Class* (London: Penguin, 1963).

146. Cited by Tyerman, *op. cit.* (note 115), 221.

147. *Ibid.*, 213. See J. Wesley, *The Reformation of Manners* (1763), in Outler, *op. cit.* (note 1), Vol. II (1985), 300–23. Samuel Wesley's *Sermon* was published in the *Methodist Magazine* (1814), 648–65, 727–36.

148. Lawrence, *op. cit.* (note 138), 38.

149. R. Porter, 'The Gift Relation: Philanthropy and Provincial Hospitals in Eighteenth-Century England', in L. Granshaw and R. Porter (eds), *The Hospital in History* (London: Routledge, 1989), 149–78.

150. Porter argues that such acts of benevolence in Georgian England contrasted with those of the seventeenth century because they were stripped of their 'sectarian sting' and theological 'sniping'. Furthermore, 'an act of conspicuous, self-congratulatory, stage-managed *noblesse oblige* similarly underlay the infirmary'; *ibid.,* 152.

151. *Ibid.*, 162.

152. *Ibid.*, 163.

153. B. Mandeville, *An Essay on Charity and Charity Schools,* 4th edn (London, 1725), 24.

154. B. Mandeville, *The Fable of the Bees or Private Vices, Publick Benefits,* 2 vols (1723, 1728; repro. Indianapolis: Liberty Fund, 1988). For a full and illuminating discussion on this subject see E.J. Hundert, 'Sociability and Self-Love in the Theatre of Moral Sentiments: Mandeville to Adam Smith', in S. Collini, R. Whatmore, B. Young (eds), *Economy, Polity, and Society: British Intellectual History, 1750–1950* (Cambridge: Cambridge University Press, 2000), 31–47: 35. For Wesley's comment see, Wesley, *op. cit.* (note 69), Vol. II, 311.

155. Hundert, *ibid.*, 35.

156. T. Evans, *The History of Modern Enthusiasm from the Reformation to the Present Times,* 1st edn (London, 1752), 4.

157. *Ibid.*, 4.

158. Lawrence, *op. cit.* (note 138), 45.

159. *Ibid.*

160. Porter, *op. cit.* (note 149), 166. Porter observes that the Leicester Royal Infirmary had no fewer than two hundred copies of Dr James Stonhouse's *Friendly Advice to a Patient,* 12th edn (London, 1774) and *Spiritual Directions to the Uninstructed,* 14th edn (London, 1780).

161. T. Hitchcock, 'Paupers and Preachers: The SPCK and the Parochial Workhouse Movement', in Davison, *et al.* (eds), *op. cit.* (note 4), 145–66.

162. L. Haakonssen, *Medicine and Morals in the Enlightenment: John Gregory, Thomas Percival and Benjamin Rush* (Amsterdam: Clio Medica, 1997), 30. Margaret Pelling has made a similar point by tracing the etymological roots of the word 'profession' with regard to the medical profession. She has seen how this word derived its meaning from a religious context: a member of a religious order 'professed' when they took a public vow. After the Reformation, Pelling argues, this term began to acquire more 'secular' applications relating to themes of public commitment or open avowal. See Pelling, 'Medical Practice in Early Modern England: Trade or Profession?', in W. Prest (ed.), *The Professions in Early Modern England* (London: Croom Helm, 1987), 90–128.

163. W. Buchan, *Domestic Medicine: Or, A Treatise on the Prevention and Cure of Diseases by Regimen and Simple Medicines,* 2nd edn (London, 1772), xxx–xxxi.

164. Cited by Rousseau, 'John Wesley's "Primitive Physick" (1747)', *Harvard Library Bulletin,* 16 (1968), 242–56: 249.

165. Wesley, *Primitive Physic, op. cit.* (note 1), ix.

166. Boyle, *op. cit.* (note 107), 'The Authors Introduction to the First Volume', n.p. It must be stated here, however, that whilst the style, form and

motivation of *Primitive Physic* is very reminiscent of the earlier text written by Boyle, the actual remedies put forward by Wesley differ enormously. Wesley's 'receipts' were closely allied to the medical practice of his day.

167. Boyle, *ibid.*, 'Preface' n.p.

168. 'Dedication to the Parochial Clergy of this Kingdom', in Anon., *op. cit.* (note 111), iv.

169. Buchan, *op. cit.* (note 163), xxx–xxxi

170. *Ibid.*, xxxi.

171. Porter, *op. cit.* (note 149), 163.

172. D. Hartley, *Observations on Man*, 2 vols, 1st edn (London, 1749), Vol. II, 245–55, quoted in J. Priestley, *The History and Present State of Electricity, with Original Experiments,* 2nd edn (London, 1769), xxi.

173. Quoted from Boyle's *Usefulness of Natural Philosophy* by Kaplan, *op. cit.* (note 107), front cover, n.p. No bibliographical details are given by Kaplan.

174. Kaplan, *op. cit.* (note 107), 31, 130.

175. J.W. Haas, 'John Wesley's Views on Science and Christianity: An Examination of the Charge of Anti-Science', *American Society of Church History,* 63 (1994), 378–92: 384. Wesley was an avid reader of *The Philosophical Transactions,* the journal of the Royal Society, and they were abridged and listed on the advanced course at Kingswood School.

176. *Ibid.*, 384.

177. The very fact that Wesley was a theologian meant that many late-Victorian historians set him up in opposition to other Enlightenment scientists and philosophers. The tendency stemmed, primarily, from a nineteenth-century pre-occupation with a conflict between science and Christianity. In the *History of English Thought in the Eighteenth Century* (1881), Leslie Stephen claimed to see in Wesley 'that aversion to scientific reasoning that has become characteristic of orthodox theologians'. Here, Wesley is the very antithesis of John Locke, whom Stephen believed to be 'rationalist to the core' and whose *Reasonableness of Christianity* he represented as a type of 'constructive Deism'. See L. Stephen, *History of English Thought in the Eighteenth Century,* 2 vols, 3rd edn (London, 1902), Vol. II, 412, Vol. I, 100. Other nineteenth-century critics included Andrew Dickson White who stated in his *History of the Warfare of Science with Theology in Christendom,* 2 vols (New York, 1895) that Wesley subjected science to theology. These comments are only two of a large number of anti-science accusations made against Wesley and Methodism, accusations which filtered into twentieth-century historiography – most notably seen in Margaret Jacob, 'Christianity and the Newtonian Worldview', in D.C. Lindberg and R.L. Numbers (eds), *God and Nature: Historical Essays on the Encounter between Christianity and Science* (Los Angeles: University of California Press, 1986), 238–55. Haas, *op. cit.* (note 175), 379.

178   J. Redwood, *Reason, Ridicule and Religion: The Age of Enlightenment in England, 1660–1750* (London: Thames and Hudson, 1976), 116.

179. A. Cunningham, 'How the *Principia* Got its Name: Or, Taking Natural Philosophy Seriously', *History of Science*, 29 (1991), 377–92; J.H. Brooke, *Science and Religion: Some Historical Perspectives* (Cambridge: Cambridge University Press, 1991);
L. Stewart, 'Seeing Through the Scholium: Religion and Reading Newton in the Eighteenth Century', *History of Science*, 36 (1996), 123–65. For how this discussion relates to Wesley's *Survey of the Wisdom of God*, see B. Felleman, 'John Wesley's *Survey of the Wisdom of God in Creation*: A Methodological Inquiry', *Perspectives on Science and Christian Faith*, 58 (2006), 1–6.

180. Haas, *op. cit.* (note 175), 386. Again, Wesley inherited this tendency from his father, who had taken a keen interest in scientific matters. Samuel Wesley had been a member of the Spalding Gentlemen's Society, an organisation which included amongst its members Isaac Newton and Alexander Pope. This Society tackled literary, historical and scientific questions. Wesley's elder brother, Samuel (jnr) also belonged to this Society. See J.C. English, 'John Wesley and Isaac Newton's "System of the World"', *Proceedings of the Wesley Historical Society*, 48/3 (1991), 69–86.

181. See 'Introduction' to Robbins, *op. cit.* (note 11).

182. Wesley's high regard for Aristotle, whom he called a 'universal genius', must not be diminished in this context. Aristotle's natural philosophy formed a major part of the Oxford curriculum and Wesley, who made a distinction between this and scholastic Aristotelianism, expressed disappointment at Locke's faulty definition of Aristotle in Books 3 and 4 of his *Essay on Human Understanding*. For a full explication of this, see S. Mitsuo, 'Epistemology in the Thought of John Wesley' (PhD thesis: Drew University, 1980), 1–245, nn. 3, 81. On this, Rex D. Matthews has argued that it was Aristotle, rather than Locke, who was the major determining influence in the development of Wesley's epistemology, see R.D. Matthews, 'Religion and Reason Joined', (PhD thesis: Harvard University, 1986), 1–269; L. Bartels Felleman, 'John Wesley and Dr George Cheyne on the Spiritual Senses', *Wesleyan Theological Journal* (Spring 2004), 163–72.

183. K. Dewhurst, *John Locke (1632–1704), Physician and Philosopher: A Medical Biography with an Edition of the Medical Notes in his Journals* (London: Wellcome Historical Medical Library, 1963). Dewhurst notes that Locke's subsequent renown as a philosopher has eclipsed his medical activities to the extent that his medical practice has been obscured.

184. Quoted in Mitsuo, *op. cit.* (note 182), nn. 3, 85.

185. Kaplan, *op. cit.* (note 107), 31, 130, 226. On the same basis, Sydenham believed that only a general knowledge of anatomy was necessary, as it could yield no useful or practical application to medicine. The only useful task for

the physician was to compile a detailed series of disease histories, based on clinical observation.

186. Locke, (20 January 1692/3), quoted in *Some Familiar Letters between Mr Locke, and Several of his Friends*, 4th edn (London, 1742), 223–4. Thomas Molyneux was brother to William Molyneux, a Trinity College man who had founded the Dublin Philosophical Society in 1683. Locke met Thomas Molyneux in Leyden. See Dewhurst, *op. cit.* (note 183), 309.

187. Kaplan, *op. cit.* (note 107), 31.

188. Haas, *op. cit.* (note 175), 384; L.S. King, *The Medical World of the Eighteenth Century* (Chicago: University of Chicago Press, 1958).

189. Haas points out that it is Wesley's ambivalent attachment to the ideas of the anti-Newtonian John Hutchinson that has given rise to this interpretation. Hutchinson's work, *Moses Principia* (1724), claimed that the Bible was scientifically coherent and that the Hebrew language was God's way of enabling men to understand the physical world. Hutchinson believed that Newton had ignored or downplayed Scriptural principles, which could bring about true knowledge of the physical world. Haas sees how Wesley's views on Hutchinson were contradictory and subject to change, though only a few of the fifteen citations to Hutchinson in Wesley's works are neutral or favourable. On the whole, he found Hutchinson's work to be unsupported by Scripture and scientifically flawed. Haas concurs with Outler that Wesley used Hutchinson as a foil against Newtonianism; Wesley utilised aspects of Hutchinson's work to counter the threat of deism. Typically, Wesley extrapolated what was useful about the work and put it to practical effect. For a more detailed discussion of this see Haas, *op. cit.* (note 175), 390–1. See also, English, *op. cit.* (note 180).

190. R. Porter, *Enlightenment: Britain and the Creation of the Modern World* (London: Penguin, 2000), 136).

191. Brooke, *op. cit.* (note 179), 118.

192. Tyerman notes that Wesley studied Newton at Oxford. He also recommended that Newton's works be included on the curriculum at Kingswood school, which had been established to prepare young men for the Christian ministry in 1748. R.E. Schofield, 'John Wesley and Science in 18th Century England', *Isis,* 44 (1953), 331–40: 332. *The Compendium* affirmed Newton's account of the tides and praised the *Opticks*, whilst simultaneously dismissing the theory of gravitation. See Wesley, *op. cit.* (note 42), Vol. V, 93–117. For a very good discussion of Wesley's complex relationship to Newton's science, see J.C. English, 'John Wesley and Isaac Newton's "System of the World"', *Proceedings of the Wesley Historical Society,* 48 (1991), 71–3.

193. Wesley, *Primitive Physic, op. cit.* (note 1). See 'The Preface', sections 1, 11 and 13.

194. Wesley, *op. cit.* (note 42), 'The Preface', Section Six, n.p.

195. Kaplan, *op. cit.* (note 107), 56.

196. R. Harré, 'Knowledge', in G.S. Rousseau and R. Porter, (eds), *The Ferment of Knowledge: Studies in the Historiography of Eighteenth-Century Science* (Cambridge: Cambridge University Press, 1980), 11–54.

197. J. Wesley, *An Earnest Appeal to Men of Reason and Religion* (1743), in G.R. Cragg, *The Bicentennial Edition of The Works of John Wesley* (Nashville: Abingdon Press, 1989), Vol. XI, *The Appeals,* 37–94: 55–6.

198. *Ibid.,* Vol. XI, 46, 57. Initially, Wesley was confident in a syllogistic or demonstrative type of evidence for religious knowledge or faith and stated as much in a letter to his mother in July 1725. He believed that logical and demonstrative reason was the essential activity to perceive all truths: 'faith is a species of belief, and belief is defined "an assent to a proposition upon rational grounds". Without rational grounds there is therefore *no belief,* and consequently no faith'. Faith was an assent based upon rational grounds. However, in November 1725, Wesley modifies this stance and informs his mother that he had '…been under a mistake in adhering to that definition of faith which Dr Fiddes sets down as the only one'. Dr Fiddes's theory of assent takes science into account as well as faith but Wesley now believed that this was only part of the definition since faith is something distinct from science. Faith is an assent to what God has revealed and not what man has discovered – it necessarily relies upon God's grace. It is both a 'rational' and 'sensational' (spiritual sensationalist) form of knowledge. After November 1725, Wesley recognised that religious and scientific conviction rested upon *different types of evidence.* Moreover, that reason could provide a type of natural religion independent of revelation. See Wesley, *op. cit.* (note 36), Vol. I, 25. For a full but succinct summary of this shift in Wesley's epistemology of faith see Mitsuo, *op. cit.* (note 182), 16–19.

199. J. Wesley, *The Imperfection of Human Knowledge* (1784) in Outler, *op. cit.* (note 1), Vol. II, 567–86.

200. J. Wesley, *A Letter to the Right Reverend the Lord Bishop of Gloucester* (1763), in Cragg (ed.), *op. cit.* (note 197), Vol. XI, 459–538: 533. Wesley extracted this section from *A Letter to the Reverend Dr Conyers Middleton, Occasioned by his late Free Enquiry* (1749). This letter was in response to Bishop Warburton's tract, *Doctrine of Grace: Or, The Office and Operations of the Holy Spirit Vindicated from the Insults of Infidelity and the Abuse of Fanaticism* (1763). The first section of Warburton's work dealt with Dr Conyers Middleton, a semi-deist divine and Fellow of Trinity College, Cambridge. The latter part of the work deals specifically with the 'enthusiasm' of Methodism and Wesley. In Wesley's ministry of healing, Warburton claimed to see a fanaticism that threatened intelligent faith – the features of modern fanaticism, he argued, had come to replace seventeenth-century

'superstition'. See editors' 'Introduction' to Wesley's *Letter to the Right Reverend the Lord Bishop of Gloucester*, in Cragg, *op. cit.* (note 197), Vol. XI, 459–63: 462.

201. Locke (1695) in J.C. Higgins-Biddle (ed.), *The Reasonableness of Christianity: As Delivered in the Scriptures*, (Cambridge: Cambridge University Press, 1999), 154–5.

202. Kaplan, *op. cit.* (note 107), 30, 25.

203. *Ibid.,* 52–3.

204. J. Wesley, *The Desideratum: Or, Electricity Made Plain and Useful by a Lover of Mankind and of Common Sense* (London, 1759; repr. London, 1871), n.p. Hereafter referred to as *Desideratum.*

205. Wesley, *op. cit.* (note 42), Vol. I, 242, Vol. II, 8.

206. J. Ray, *The Wisdom of God Manifested in the Works of the Creation,* 10th edn (London, 1735), n.p.

207. J. Wesley, *A Letter to the Right Reverend the Lord Bishop of Gloucester*, in Cragg, *op. cit.* (note 197), Vol. XI, 534.

208. Wesley, *op. cit.* (note 42), 'The Preface', Vol. I, 91.

209. Wesley, *An Earnest Appeal*, in Cragg, *op. cit.* (note 197), Vol. XI, 57.

210. This is obviously some distance away from Locke's view in *An Essay Concerning Human Understanding* (1690). Man had an intuitive knowledge of his own existence; a demonstrative knowledge of God's existence and a sensory knowledge of everything else. Wesley believed that the divine element in man could discover the spirit of God: that spirit could influence spirit in a way analogous to matter influencing matter.

211. Outler, 'Introduction', in *idem., op. cit.* (note 1), Vol. I, 60.

212. *Ibid.,* i. 59–60. Wesley had been instructed in the philosophy of Malebranche by his father's friend, John Norris, who had been chief disciple of the French Cartesians. Outler observes that Wesley, more than any other eighteenth-century British theologian was heavily influenced by Malebranche's 'occasionalism'.

213. R.D. Matthews, '"With the Eyes of Faith": Spiritual Experience and the Knowledge of God in the Theology of John Wesley' in T. Runyon (ed.), *Wesleyan Theology Today. A Bicentennial Theological Consultation*, (Nashville: Kingswood Books, 1985), 409–26; F. Dreyer, 'Faith and Experience in the Thought of John Wesley', *The American Historical Review*, 88 (1983), 12–30.

214. Felleman, *op. cit.* (note 182). In this 'sense', Bartels Felleman argues, Wesley was tracing an 'anti-Lockean' source to develop this notion.

215. Maddox, *op. cit.* (note 22).

216. Felleman, *op. cit.* (note 182).

217. J. Wesley, *An Earnest Appeal*, in Cragg, *op. cit.* (note 197), Vol. XI.

218. *Arminian Magazine*, 2 (February 1779), 89–91, Quoted in Haas, *op. cit.*

(note 175), 382–3.

219. Wesley, *op. cit.* (note 42), Vol. I,. 10.

220. *Ibid.*, 10–11.

221. Cheyne, *op. cit.* (note 35), ii.

222. Hartley's physiology of 'vibrations' in the nerves, which caused association, owed much to Cheyne's mechanical explanation of the body.

223. Wesley, *op. cit.* (note 42), Vol. I, 21, 51–2. There was considerable debate over whether nerves were solid or tubular. Cheyne believed that nerves were solid and drew on Newton in this belief. Newton had described the nerves as being composed of 'solid, pellucid and uniform Capillamenta' along which the 'vibrating motion of the Aetherial Medium' was propagated. Cited by Guerrini from 'Query 24', which was added to the 1717–18 edition of Newton's *Opticks*. A. Guerrini, *Obesity and Depression in the Enlightenment: The Life and Times of George Cheyne* (Oklahoma: University of Oklahoma Press, 2000), 133. Boerhaave, on the other hand, believed that the nerve was tubular and contained the 'animal spirits'.

224. Kaplan, *op. cit.* (note 107), 71.

225. Wesley, *op. cit.* (note 42), i. 54.

226. Wesley's great grandfather, Bartholomew Westley, used a peculiar plainness of speech according to Tyerman. See L. Tyerman, *The Life and Times of the Revd Samuel Wesley*, 3 vols (London, 1866), 28. Wesley was indebted to his father's 'plain' style sermons, but Outler sees how the adoption of this can be attributed to his discovery in Oxford of the sermons of seventeenth-century divines, especially those of Benjamin Calamy, William Tilly and John Tillotson. Outler notes that Wesley knew of the rivalry between 'plain' and 'ornate' styles of preaching and took a partisan stand on the issue. The ornate style of English sermonising, of which Lancelot Andrews and Jeremy Taylor were the best exponents, was too baroque for Wesley's taste. The Puritans elevated the sermon to its place as mediator of grace, thus regarding preaching as an act of prophecy: 'The essence of preaching in this tradition was *biblical exposition.* The prophet–preacher's prime task was to find and expound a word from God to his hearers' (22). This meant that clarity and simplicity became prized virtues in the rhetoric of 'plain' style. See Outler, 'Introduction', *op. cit.* (note 1), Vol. I, 22–7. However – and many thanks to Dr Jeremy Gregory for pointing this out to me – by the time Wesley was preaching Anglicanism, he incorporated and subsumed the plain style, with many Anglican divines choosing it as their preferred method. When Wesley decided to provide his preachers with a manual on the subject, he chose to abridge an anonymous text entitled *The Art of Speaking in Publick: Or An Essay on the Action of an Orator as to his Pronunciation and Gesture* (1727). He renamed this *Directions Concerning Pronunciation and Gesture* (Bristol, 1749).

227. Outler, 'Introduction', *op. cit.* (note 1), Vol. I, 28.

228. Whilst Wesley was a student at Christ Church awaiting ordination as a priest, Samuel Wesley wrote to him urging his son to read Chrysostom's *De Sacerdotio*. 'Master it' and 'digest it' was the advice. Cited by Campbell, *op. cit.* (note 4), 25.

229. Quoted in Outler, 'Introduction', *op. cit.* (note 1), Vol. I, 26.

230. *Ibid.*

231. M. Schmidt, 'John Wesley's Place in Church History', in K.E. Rowe (ed.), *The Place of Wesley in the Christian Tradition* (Metuchen: The Scarecrow Press, 1976), 67–93.

232. Quoted in Tyerman, *op. cit.* (note 126), Vol. II, 183.

233. G. Lawton, *John Wesley's English: A Study of his Literary Style* (London: George Allen & Unwin, 1962), 197.

234. *Ibid.*, 14.

235. Eusebius of Caesarea, *The History of the Church,* trans. G.A. Williamson (London: Penguin, 1989), 3.

236. Ott, *op. cit.* (note 16), 179.

237. T. à Kempis, *Imitatio Christi* (London: Penguin, 1952), 33.

238. Morgan, *op. cit.* (note 24), 88.

239. Schmidt, *op cit.* (note 18), Vol. I, 132.

240. Wesley, *op. cit.* (note 69), Vol. I, 170–1 (28 February 1736).

241. G.V. Bennett, 'Patristic Tradition in Anglican Thought, 1600–1900', *Oecumenica* (1972), 63–85.

242. J. Wesley, *A Plain Account of the People Called Methodists* (London, 1748), 4.

243. Schmidt, *op. cit.* (note 18), Vol. III, 107.

244. Wesley, *Primitive Physic, op. cit.* (note 1), vi–vii.

245. Anon., *A Cheap, Sure and Ready Guide to Health: Or, A Cure for a Disease Call'd the Doctor,* 2nd edn (London, 1742), n. p.

246. Buchan, *op cit.* (note 163), xvii.

247. Wesley, *Primitive Physic, op. cit.* (note 1), x.

3

Experience and the Common Interest of Mankind: Physic, an Art or Science in Eighteenth-Century England?

If it be enquired, but are there not books enough already, on every part of the art of medicine? Yes, too many ten times over, considering how little to the purpose the far greater part of them speak. But besides this, they are too dear for poor men to buy, and too hard for plain men to understand. Do you say, 'But there are enough of these collection of Receipts'. Where? I have not seen one yet, either in our own or any other tongue, which contains only safe, and cheap, and easy medicines. In all that have fallen into my hand, I find many dear and many far-fetched medicines: besides many of so dangerous a kind as a prudent man would never meddle with. And against the greater part of those medicines there is a further objection: they consist of too many ingredients. The common method of compounding and re-compounding medicines, can never be reconciled to Common Sense… How often, by thus compounding medicines of opposite qualities, is the virtue of both utterly destroyed? Nay, how often do those joined together destroy life, which singly might have preserved it? This occasioned that caution of the great *Boerhaave*, against mixing things without evident necessity, and without full proof of the effect they will produce when asunder: seeing (as he observes) several things, which separately taken, are safe and powerful medicines, when compounded, not only lose their former powers, but commence a strong and deadly poison.

John Wesley, 'The Preface', *Primitive Physic.*

The *Balsam of Honey* a tickling Cough stops,
To *Maredant* the *Scurvy* submits;
There's what's his Name's wonderful *Viperine Drops*,
And *Henry* for Hysteric Fits;
But *Physic*, like Music, bears Fashion's decree,
Of Modish Distempers they tell us;
Licentiates, or not so, yet ev'ry *M.D.*
Pronounces us *Narvous* or *Bilous*.

George Alexander Stevens, *The Specifick* (1788).[1]

John Wesley's dialogue with the Ancients and Moderns in *Primitive Physic*

Wesley had taken a keen interest in science, anatomy and medicine as a student and Fellow at Oxford. This, as V.H.H. Green has shown, was reflected in his reading at the time, but also by the fact that he busied himself translating 'specifick Remedies' for his tutor, Mr Henry Sherman.[2] His attention had been drawn to Cheyne's *An Essay of Health and Long Life*, and he subsequently arranged his habits according to the advice given in this essay. Wesley's intellectual curiosity in the area of science and medicine was nourished at Oxford but fitted into a bigger context of increased interest and education within those disciplines. This was particularly notable in Oxford, where the Philosophical Club left an enduring legacy.

Wesley's medical curiosity soon found a suitable outlet when his concern for the spiritual undernourishment of the poor extended into an interest in their physical welfare. Close contact with them increased his awareness of the need for medical attention, and in a letter to his friend the Revd Vincent Perronet, Wesley explained how he had decided to 'prepare and give physic' out of sheer necessity:

> At length… I thought of a kind of desperate expedient: 'I will prepare and give them physic myself'. For six or seven and twenty years, I had made anatomy and physic the diversion of my leisure hours; though I never properly studied them, unless for a few months when I was going to America, where I imagined I might be of some service to those who had no regular physician among them. I applied to it again. I took into my assistance an apothecary, and an experienced surgeon; resolving, at the same time, not to go out of my depth, but to leave all difficult and complicated cases to such physicians as the patients should choose. I gave notice of this to the Society; telling them that all who were ill of chronical distempers (for I did not care to venture upon acute) might, if they pleased come to me at such a time, and I would give them the best advice I could and the best medicines I had… In five months, medicines were occasionally given to above five hundred persons. Several of these I never saw before; for I did not regard whether they were of the Society or not. In that time, seventy-one of these, regularly taking their medicines, and following the regimen prescribed (which three in four would not do), were entirely cured of distempers long thought to be incurable. The whole expense of medicines, during this time, was nearly forty pounds.[3]

This was in 1746 and that same year he opened Dispensaries in London (Moorfields) and Bristol.[4] In Stroud, a subscription dispensary was functioning by 1755. The dispensaries, served by a physician and two surgeons, accepted approximately five hundred patients per year.[5] Commenting on the success of the Dispensary in Bristol to his friend Ebenezer Blackwell, Wesley says:

> Our number of patients increases in Bristol daily. We have now upwards of two hundred. Many have already desired to return thanks, having found considerable change for the better already. But we are at a great loss for medicines; several of those we should choose being not to be had at any price in Bristol.[6]

One year later, as a result of this overwhelming response, *Primitive Physic* was produced from a list of receipts, drawn up by Wesley from his medical reading and experiences. These 'receipts' were used to guide lay preachers and other Methodist helpers when visiting the sick.[7] W.F. Bynum has pointed out that Wesley's *Primitive Physic* (along with Buchan's *Domestic Medicine* and Tissot's *L'Avis au People sur sa Santé*) was aimed at individuals in a higher economic stratum than the average hospital patient. Evidence of this can be seen by the fact that Wesley assumed his readers would be able to recognise specific conditions, such as scurvy and consumption, as well as being able to distinguish between ordinary and dry asthma and, even more subtly, between slow and intermittent fevers. Guerrini suggests Buchan's audience, who paid six shillings, compared to one shilling paid for *Primitive Physic*, 'occupied the social stratum between Wesley's literate workers and Cheyne's fashionable elite, comprising those upwardly mobile members of the "middling ranks" who aspired to Bath if they did not attain it'.[8]

Having made a commitment to the lower orders, literate or otherwise, Wesley was not going to be deterred from practising physic by disgruntled physicians jealously guarding their 'professional' status. In a letter written to Archbishop Thomas Secker, he declared that:

> For more than twenty years, I have had numberless proofs, that regular physicians do exceeding little good. From a deep conviction of this, I have believed it my duty… to prescribe such medicines to six or seven hundred of the poor as I knew were proper of their several disorders. Within six weeks, nine in ten of them, who had taken these medicines, were remarkably altered for the better; and many of them were cured of disorders under which they had laboured for ten, twenty, forty years. Now, ought I to have let one of these poor wretches perish, because I was not a regular physician? [T]o have said, 'I know what will cure you; but I am not of the college; you must send for Dr. Mead?' Before Dr. Mead had come in his chariot, the man might have been in his coffin. And when the doctor was come, where was his fee? What! he cannot live upon nothing! So, instead of an orderly cure, the patient dies; and God requires his blood at my hands.[9]

A number of important issues are highlighted in this letter, which was written in 1747. The first is Wesley's deep-seated doubt about the medical practice of his day: an examination of this scepticism will be undertaken shortly. The second important point is the confidence and conviction with which Wesley carried out his medical practice – though it must be stated that he was adamant in his resolve to leave complex cases to fully trained physicians, a point made in the above-cited passage taken from his letter to the Revd Perronet. Wesley was keen to reiterate this in 'The Preface' to *Primitive Physic*, where he advises the patient to consult 'a Physician that fears God' for complicated disorders.[10]

It is impossible for historians now to verify in any objective way Wesley's claim to have cured so many of those burdened with long-term ill health. This declaration may very well raise a sceptical smile, but it would be anachronistic for modern scholars to judge the medical efficacy of Wesley's remedies. As historians, we cannot seek recourse to clinical evidence for any of his 'cures', yet the positive way in which medical advice was received by his beneficiaries points to some measurable effect in itself.[11] To his patient Wesley provided comfort and hope as well as advice on regimen and specific therapies. This was as much as any Georgian medical practitioner could expect to achieve. The effect of Wesley's 'cures' may also be attributed to the fact that Methodism as a movement helped to restore a sense of dignity and wellbeing amongst the poor in a context where they were ignored or actively despised. At any rate, there is evidence to show that Wesley's medical advice did provide some sort of alleviation and relief to those suffering from a range of symptoms and diseases.

The third, and final, issue raised in Wesley's letter is his preoccupation with duty and authority. With regard to dispensing physic as an 'irregular', Wesley risked being heavily criticised by the Royal College of Physicians. An attempt to counter potential criticism on this score is made by invoking his duty to God; a duty, he argues, which is to be esteemed over and above all other 'worldly' authority – even that of the Royal College. Wesley does this, in spite of the fact that he was licensed by the Church to dispense physic as a clergyman and need not have worried about breaching College authority.[12] In his *Sermon Preached before the Royal College of Physicians* in 1751, Stephen Hales makes a similar point: 'God, who *maketh all our bed in our sickness… has not only created medicines out of the earth…* but has also ordained the physician to prescribe the kind and proportion of the medicine....'[13]

The physician has been *ordained* and Hales, an unqualified medical practitioner, is referring to himself here. He is citing Scripture, but his point is overtly political. Wesley's letter to Archbishop Secker is significant too for its pre-emptive and rhetorical manoeuvre. Divine authority is sought via the Archbishop to counter criticism and justify his foray into a discipline for which he had no formal qualification.[14] The very fact that Wesley felt the need to elicit sanction in this way suggests that he was worried about transgressing authority and coming into conflict with the Royal College of Physicians. As G.S. Rousseau points out, Wesley was 'deferential' to physicians both in life and in *Primitive Physic.*[15]

This deference did not prevent Wesley from making caustic observations about the way in which medical practice was conducted in eighteenth-century England. In the same way that he sought to revive the primitive purity and simplicity of the early Church, Wesley wanted to rediscover an ancient standard in the art of physic. That is, clinical observation, something which he believed had been lost in an age of speculative philosophy and abstruse medical theory. After presenting the reader with his Miltonian cosmography in the first three sections of 'The Preface', Wesley then begins the task of explicating the history of medicine using, by way of example, Ancient Greece, Rome and other 'barbarous nations', including the Native Americans of his own day. Amongst those who had travelled to the New World it was well documented and generally agreed that Native Americans enjoyed greater longevity because of their healing practices. In 1725, Wesley read Daniel Le Clerc's *Histoire de la Médecine* (1696) while an undergraduate at Oxford.[16] This text had given him a vivid, if partisan, sense of medical historiography. The medical historiography in 'The Preface' to *Primitive Physic* shared much in common with other physicians who had written texts or taken an interest in the history of medicine, such as Le Clerc, John Freind, Richard Mead and Francis Clifton.[17] Ludmilla Jordanova argues that these histories of medicine had three distinguishing features: firstly, they were based on something akin to research; secondly, that they developed a narrative thread, but did not necessarily list individuals or works; thirdly, that they attempted to account for the shape of the medical past. They were polemical and 'profoundly permeated by local concerns' whilst also reaching wider audiences.[18] The historiography Wesley sets out in 'The Preface' to *Primitive Physic* only consists of six pages, but it nevertheless fits into Jordanova's conception of eighteenth-century medical historiography. Furthermore, it is sharply rhetorical and permeated by local, contemporary concerns.

Wesley had gone to Georgia in 1735 intending to instruct the indigenous population in Christianity, but they had taught him by example how to care for the sick, and in 'The Preface' he notes that the Native Americans were complete strangers to disease. The traditional method, he argues:

[I]s the method wherein the art of healing is preserved among the *Americans* to this day. Their diseases are exceedingly few; nor do they often occur by reason of their continual exercise and (till of late) universal temperance. But if any are sick, or bit by a serpent, or torn by a wild beast, the fathers immediately tell their children what remedy to apply. And it is rare, that the patient suffers long; those medicines being quick, as well as generally, infallible.[19]

Drawing on this, Wesley goes on to describe how such simple healing methods led to 'Experience and Physic' growing up together in Europe; remedies were subject to 'trial', through which 'the cure was wrought'.[20] The 'Author of Nature' taught man the use of many medicines 'by what is vulgarly termed Accident':

> [P]hysic was wholly founded on experiment. The *European*, as well as the American, said to his neighbour, Are you sick? Drink the juice of this herb and your sickness will be at an end... has the snake bitten you? Chew and apply that root, and the poison will not hurt you. Thus, ancient men, having a little experience joined with common sense, and common humanity, cured themselves and their neighbours of most distempers, to which every nation was subject'.[21]

By contrast, the philosophical age of eighteenth-century Europe had inverted this process by replacing experience and experiment with hypotheses. Simple remedies had been discarded and medicine had become far removed from common observation:

> [I]n the process of time, men of philosophical turn were not satisfied with this. They began to enquire how they might *account* for these things? How such medicines wrought such effects? They examined the human body, and all its parts; the nature of the flesh, veins, arteries, nerves; the structure of the brain, heart, lungs, stomach, bowels; with the springs of the several kinds of animal functions. They explored several kinds of animal mineral, as well as vegetable substances. And hence the whole order of physic, which had obtained to that time, came gradually to be inverted. Men of learning began to set experience aside; to build physic upon hypothesis; to form theories of disease and their cure, and to substitute these in place of experiments.[22]

Wesley's critique here is similar to that made by Francis Clifton in *The State of Physick, Ancient and Modern Briefly Consider'd: With a Plan for the Improvement of It* (1732). Clifton's text utilised Le Clerc and Freind's historiographies by emphasising the value of ancient medicine over and above modern medical theories.[23] In so doing, Clifton deployed that common rhetorical device used in eighteenth-century discussion and commentary: the battle between the ancients and moderns. Clifton was also eager to show that his 'plan for the improvement' of physic contained a pious element and was written for the general good of mankind.[24]

Wesley is not objecting to theory *per se* in the above quotation. Nor is he opposed to medical advance, and his position in the quarrel between the ancients and moderns is somewhat complex. His critique is levelled against those who 'invert' the 'order of physic' by setting 'experience aside' and who build 'physic upon hypothesis' – as opposed to basing it on an empirical, experimental approach. Physic, he argues, has become an 'abstruse science, quite out of the reach of ordinary men'. With profit the main concern, Wesley was convinced that physicians attempted to increase the difficulty of their art with technical terms to keep the 'bulk of mankind at a distance'.[25]

The sentiments expressed in 'The Preface' by Wesley are strangely reminiscent of the letter, (cited in Chapter 2), written by Locke to Dr Thomas Molyneux:

> I wonder, that after the pattern Dr Sydenham has set them of a better way, men should return again to that Romance way of Physic. But I see it is easier and more natural for men to build castles in the air of their own, than to survey well those that are to be found standing. Nicely to observe the history of diseases, in all their changes and circumstances, is a work of Time, Accurateness, Attention and Judgment.[26]

Primitive Physic is, indeed, a work of time, accuracy, attention and judgement. Wesley was concerned, not to build 'castles in the air' of his own, but to 'survey well those' remedies that have been empirically validated as useful cures for disease. Like Locke, Wesley detested the commercial element that had crept into medical practice. He condemned those physicians interested only in 'profit' and 'honour', particularly those who were eager to cash-in on compound medicines. This practice, he insisted, was designed to 'prolong the distemper' only to 'swell the Apothecary's bill' so that he and the doctor could 'divide the spoil':

> Physicians now began to be had in admiration, as persons who were something more than human. And profit attended their employ, as well as honour; so that they had now two weighty reasons for keeping the bulk of mankind at a distance, that they might pry into the mysteries of the profession. To this end, they increased those difficulties by design, which began in a manner by accident. They filled their writings with abundance of technical terms, utterly unintelligible to plain men. They affected to deliver their rules, and to reason upon them, in an abstruse and philosophical manner. They represented the critical knowledge of Astronomy, Natural Philosophy... some of them insisting on that of Astronomy, and Astrology too, as necessarily previous to... understanding the art of healing. Those who

understood only, how to restore the sick to health, they branded with the name of Empirics. They introduced into practice abundance of compound medicines, consisting of so many ingredients, that it was scarce possible for common people to know which it was that wrought the cure: abundance of exotics, neither the nature nor name of which their own countrymen understood: of chymicals, such as neither had skill, nor fortune, nor time to prepare: yea, and of dangerous ones, such as they could not use without hazarding life… and thus both their honour and gain were secured.…[27]

The above passage bears some resemblance to Boyle's critique of that esoteric knowledge associated with alchemy. Boyle believed that knowledge, once obtained, should be disseminated widely to benefit society as a whole.[28] Prompted by the same principle of practical piety, Wesley was also reacting negatively to those 'Gentlemen of the Faculty' who wished to shroud their art in mystery and secrecy. The Royal College of Physicians 'deliver their rules' and 'reason upon them' in an 'abstruse and philosophical manner' to protect their professional status, prestige and income. Wesley's critique here also echoed that of Dr Thomas Dover, one of the few physicians he praises in 'The Preface'. Dover had bitterly condemned the Faculty of physicians in his 'popular' medical work, *The Ancient Physician's Legacy to his Country* (1742). The Royal College of Physicians, he suggests, were like moles working underground 'lest their practices should be discovered to the populace'.[29]

The majority of mankind, Wesley argues, has been prevented from helping themselves 'by design', and indeed, were discouraged from even attempting to self-medicate. *Primitive Physic* was his way of offering to the poor a 'cheap' and 'safe' form of medicine, which was easy to dispense. This did not spring merely from a popularising impulse, but was inspired by the example of Primitive Christianity and, specifically, Eastern Christianity, where the cult of 'unmercenary healer' was strong. Here, physicians refused payment for medical practice and usually worked as doctors to the poor.[30] In reminding the reader of this Christian precept, *Primitive Physic* bore some likeness to another vernacular text entitled, *A Cheap, Sure and Ready Guide to Health: or, a Cure for a Disease Call'd the Doctor*, a manual written in 1742 by 'a Private Gentleman' and sold at the 'lowest rate'. The subtitle of this text is particularly informative as it sets out to instruct the patient on 'How to Prevent Being Cheated and Destroyed by the Exactions and Unmerciful Usage of Ignorant and Oppressive Physicians and Apothecaries'.[31] In the 'Introduction', the anonymous writer reminds his reader that the 'Christian healer' should be a dispenser of life, not death. The physician, he argues, should refrain from demanding 'tall fees'. Using the Christian ideal of unmercenary healer, this author sought to expose the abuse of contemporary physic whilst securing health at a reduced cost: 'The medicines, which this nation affords in great plenty, are withheld from the poor by the exorbitant prices....'[32]

Contemporary medicine, this 'gentleman' complains, has an abundance of expensive, useless and dangerous drugs, such as 'juleps', 'compound waters', 'syrups', 'barks', 'purging salts' and 'volatile spirits' – all of which bring vast profit to the apothecary. *Primitive Physic* certainly shares many of its assumptions with this text, but Wesley's medical manual also differs in that it offers much more than a collection of 'simples'. Unlike *A Cheap, Sure and Ready Guide to Health*, which sets itself up in opposition to contemporary medical practice, *Primitive Physic* draws on authoritative sources to make use of those very medicines denounced by the anonymous author.

There is no doubt that a caricatured version of eighteenth-century medical practice is presented by Wesley in 'The Preface' to *Primitive Physic*. Not all physicians 'designed' to keep mankind in medical ignorance and a significant number of 'orthodox' practitioners wrote medical manuals intended to be less theoretical and more practical in orientation. Some physicians quickly realised that a great deal of money could be made out of texts explicitly aimed at a wider audience and Buchan's *Domestic Medicine* is only one example of the many successful volumes that flooded the market. Joan Lane argues that the commercial success of 'quacks' even provoked envy amongst qualified practitioners. Vast amounts of money could be made from manuals dealing with the treatment of sexually transmitted diseases, for example.[33] Remedies and cures for sexually related diseases are notably sparse in *Primitive Physic*, though this did not diminish its sales. Judging from his journal and private correspondence, Wesley, in fact, preferred to treat sexually transmitted diseases individually or in a more *ad hoc* manner.

Wesley's observation about the prevalence of medical theory holds true by virtue of the fact that humoral explanations had been recast in mechanical terms. This process can be seen in the very title of Dr Jeremiah Wainewright's *A Mechanical Account of the Non-Naturals* (1708). Yet Wesley himself adapted the language and concepts of mechanical philosophy when it suited his purpose, as is indicated in a passage taken from his *Compendium*:

> The diseases of the *fluids* lie chiefly in the blood, when it is either too thick and sizy, whereby its motion becomes too languid and slow, whence spring diseases owing to obstruction: or too thin. From the former cause arises leprosies, schirrhis, lethargies, melancholy, hysteric affections. And it at the same time... abound in acid salts, the sharp points of these tear the tender fibres and occasion the scurvy, Kings-Evil, consumption; with a whole train

of painful distempers. Fevers in general arise from the too great thinness of the blood.[34]

In using this language he fitted into a much bigger trend, noted by Anita Guerrini, who argues that physicians and patients both continued to discuss illness in traditional humoral terms of 'balance', 'imbalance', 'surfeit' and 'deficiency': 'these terms were translated into fashionably mechanical language by 1700, but their meaning remained largely unchanged from Galenic times'.[35] The shift from humoral to mechanical theory was identified by many contemporaries and can be seen in the following extract from a text, written by the eminent and leading physician Sir Richard Blackmore, entitled *A Treatise of the Spleen and Vapours* (1725):

> The primitive Doctors... imagined that all hypochondriacal symptoms were derived from a collection of black Dregs... separated from the Blood and lodged in the Spleen, whence, as they supposed, noxious Reeks and cloudy Evaporations were always ascending to the superior regions.[36]

New discoveries in medicine and anatomy, Blackmore argued, could now explain the symptoms of hypochondria in terms of defects or obstructions in the nerves. Galenic medicine was given a new direction by Thomas Willis who, like Boyle, believed in a chemical version of mechanical philosophy. Willis contended that mental and bodily disturbances lay in defective nerves – lack of tone or elasticity, due to clogging or obstructions, which checked the flow of 'animal spiritis'. Willis's theory of disease was partly mechanistic and partly chemical in that he believed both physiological and pathological processes were forms of fermentation brought about by the vibratory motion of loosely combined particles, which were able to recreate new combinations. The influence of Thomas Willis can be seen in the work of Archibald Pitcairne, Cheyne and Hartley, although many other eighteenth-century physicians built on this theory.[37]

Humoral theory transformed itself into the language of mechanics and was espoused by physicians like Pitcairne, Cheyne and Boerhaave, all of whom believed that good health was less dependent on the four humoral fluids and more akin to bodily hydraulics. Attendant to this theory of hydraulics was a concern with the flow and quality of bodily fluids, which could be hindered by the presence of accidental obstructions. Porter has highlighted this significant change in the work of Cheyne:

> Cheyne thus devoted prime attention to the valves, veins, and pipes, conveying air, aliment, chyle and other 'juices'. All such vessels required the widest possible bore and had to remain unclogged. Tubes, however, readily

scaled up, or grew swollen, or partially blocked by accretions, nodules, swellings, inflammations, and other obstructions....[38]

The biggest cause of obstructions was an improper lifestyle and diet. Poor diet could see the fluids becoming 'viscous', thick, 'glewy' or 'sizy'. Coagulating blood or 'glewy' juices, combined with 'lax fibres', could clog up the channels and prevent the body from functioning properly.[39] Boerhaave believed that an obstruction was 'the shutting up of a canal, and denying the passage to a liquid which should go and flow through the same, whether it be vital, sound, or depraved, proceeding from the size of the matter that should pass, exceeding the cavity of the canal through which it should be let pass'. The reasons for obstructions were manifest but could be caused by external compressions 'outwardly pressed' making the fibres and vessels constricted.[40]

The theory of obstructions, of which Boerhaave, Pitcairne and Cheyne were the most famous exponents, meant that from the very outset physicians claimed to know the cause of disease.[41] This, argues Guerrini, was the mark of a 'rational' physician.[42] Cheyne observed that Pitcairne had demonstrated 'the necessity of obstructions rather happening in the arteries than in the nerves, and in the nerves rather than veins; and how these obstructions are produced'. But Cheyne also argued that physicians had not yet 'traced the continuation of the arteries, veins, and nerves, so far as they go....' Furthermore, he believed that the medical professions had not yet reached a perfect understanding of the human body. If Cheyne posited the body in terms of a machine, he did not seek to reduce the phenomena of nature or life to a mechanical interplay of material components, a point made by Porter:

> Cheyne was no anatomist... or micro-scopist, and did not advance a detailed micro-physiology of the nervous fibres. He did not particularly envisage them as hollow pipes through which fluids coursed to conduct messages through the body; nor did he postulate them mainly as electrical conductors. Rather he frequently drew upon the model of the well-tuned musical string, which, when struck or plucked, would vibrate with a proper pitch and so convey the right signal.[43]

It was this model of the body as well-tuned instrument or machine that appealed specifically to Wesley. Cheyne, in fact, had ambivalent feelings about metaphysical theories and this was stated in the 'Preface' to *An Essay of Health and Long Life*:

> I have been often contented with plain and obvious facts to account for appearances, and the cautions thence deduced; when, according to the

humour of the present age, I might have run into refined speculations of metaphysicks or mathematicks; being contented with the *crasso modo philosophari*; because we shall never be able to search out the works of the Almighty to perfection, so as to penetrate the internal nature of things. I have consulted nothing but my own experience and observation on my own crazy carcase and the infirmities of others I have treated, in the following rules, their reasons and philosophy....[44]

In his *Essay*, Cheyne insisted that he had deployed as little subtlety and 'refinement in my explications... as the present state of natural philosophy could admit'.[45] In addition to this, Cheyne's *The English Malady* contained lengthy patient case histories, as well as a medical autobiography. On this basis, as Porter has shown, Cheyne worried that his book would be dismissed as a 'Quacks Bill' because it contained too many patient cases.[46]

Cheyne realised that a purely metaphysical, hypothetical or materialist approach had limited appeal, a discovery he made after the muted response to his *A New Theory of Continual Fevers* (1701).[47] This work had set out to give free rein to the physiological ideas developed by his mentor and tutor at Edinburgh, Pitcairne, which redefined medical theory and practice for the treatment of fevers in the language of Newtonian mathematical formulations.[48] Although he still regarded it as a 'solid' and 'just' foundation for an explanation of the fevers, when writing his *Essay* in 1724, Cheyne described *A New Theory* as 'a raw and inexperienced performance'.[49]

Frequently it was the case, as W.F. Bynum has noted, that medical writing in Britain was avowedly theory-free.[50] This can be partly attributed to the fact that discoveries in the new sciences wielded little impact on medical practice – a point bemoaned by many eighteenth-century physicians, including Dr Richard Mead who vigorously attempted to transform physic from 'art' to 'science'. Mead, who completed his medical training at Leyden and became acquainted with Boerhaave, fully endorsed the Newtonian stamp of authority in Cheyne's *New Theory* and applauded the work for its mathematical learning. This, he argued, had helped to distinguish Cheyne's method from empiricists and quacks. But despite Mead's unadulterated praise for *New Theory*, his own Newtonian tract, which sought to provide *A Mechanical Account of Poisons* (1702), contained very little mathematics.[51]

Contemporary mistrust of speculative systems, combined with the fact that science wielded little influence over medicine, meant that for a large part of the eighteenth century, physicians were obliged to think about disease in the same way as 'non-professionals' – or at least until later discoveries had been made in chemistry, physiology and pharmacology. It was not until the nineteenth century that 'popular' medicine came to define itself as 'alternative' medicine, distinct from professional orthodoxy.[52] Doctors not only continued to seek recourse to the five senses in diagnoses, but there was also a dynamic interplay of medical and lay-knowledge, both of which were coloured by religion and, on occasion, folkloric 'superstition'.[53] Furthermore, the politics of Georgian medicine, combined with the imperatives of a consumer-led market, meant that many patients listed their symptoms and confidently enunciated their own diagnoses.[54] The physician's model of illness thus largely coincided with that of the patient and was not always determined by objective theories of disease. Rather, it was determined by a patient's personal experience of illness.[55] Steven Shapin sees how patients knew very well what was meant by the terms 'clysters' and 'electuaries'. They understood what diseases rhubarb and Jesuit Bark should be used for and why a physician might advocate bleeding. This 'common culture', smoothed the way between patients and doctors, making interaction here more meaningful.[56] Moreover, it was the joint ownership of 'dietetic culture' that gave physicians great authority, providing that their advice on this score was deemed to be common sense. Shapin sees, however, that this cultural sharing sometimes presented doctors with problems when attempting to assert clinical expertise. Here, their advice might seem like nothing more than common sense or, conversely, everything else but.[57] By contrast, Guenter B. Risse makes a crucially significant point when he sees how patients were less able to exercise their purchasing power in hospitals where physicians still had considerable authority. This, he says, allowed for more 'continuity of observation and care as well as compliance with the prescribed therapeutic regimen'. In hospital, patients were virtually imprisoned, which empowered physicians to observe illness at all times 'without even the need to intervene prematurely with dramatic therapeutic strategies'.[58]

The interplay between patient and practitioner, combined with a more commercialised form of medical pluralism, meant that religion and medicine continued to be inextricably linked throughout the period. Even those most wedded to mechanical theories, such as Pitcairne, regarded theology as an indispensable anchor of natural philosophy and religion as the essential glue of society.[59] M. Benjamin has shown that religion and medicine had a symbiotic relationship in the eighteenth century. She suggests that although it may have been the case that 'Gentlemen of the Faculty' fell out with clergymen over theoretical detail, 'they generally saw eye to eye in practice; the purveying of medicines and attendance on the sick and dying being instances of appropriate duties for both'.[60] This proximity is personified in Cheyne, an unlicensed, but 'rational', medic who, despite mixing with Society's fashionable élite, was an open pietist and friend to the Methodists.

According to Porter, Cheyne should have been dismissed as an interloper, 'no better than a quack'.[61]

In terms of career choice, the clergyman and physician carried equal status. The Methodist movement, in fact, contained more medical men than one might have expected given its inability to attract other 'professional' groups.[62] Between clergyman and physician there existed many intellectual, social and practical links – their close alliance can be seen in much of the literature of the period. Jonathan Andrews and Andrew Scull have seen how clerical–medicine continued well into the period with a significant number of Georgian clergymen offering both spiritual consolation and material medicine to their flock. Meanwhile:

> Methodists and other evangelicals, some of whom enthusiastically espoused new medical techniques such as electricity and shock therapies, were also actively seeking out those troubled individuals, seeing it as very much their responsibility to intercede in the lives of the imprisoned, the sick, and the afflicted.[63]

Andrews and Scull suggest that Methodist power resided in its ability to step into areas where 'neither doctors nor the Anglican clergy were well represented'.[64]

Many scholars in the area of history of medicine have amply demonstrated the fluidity of eighteenth-century medical practice and its association with religion. In so doing, they have done a great deal to modify Geoffrey Holmes's characterisation of the period between 1660 and 1740 as being an age of 'professionalism' or 'coming of the doctor'.[65] Margaret Pelling argues that medical 'professionalism' was more imagined than real – the reality being that a small élite of highly educated physicians practised in London.[66] Whilst acknowledging the tripartite division of physician, surgeon and apothecary, these scholars have also shown how doctors, non-qualified medical practitioners and patients operated in the same cognitive world of humoralism and the system of non-naturals, in other words, the body of medical knowledge left by antiquity.[67] Medical practitioners were required to think about disease in similar ways drawing from a common tradition, though Guerrini has seen how the many pamphlet wars in this period also highlight deep divisions among physicians over practice and sources of authority. Although there was something of an identifiable medical profession by the early nineteenth century, Lane argues that medicine struggled to become more orthodox during the eighteenth century. An important step to 'professionalisation', she says, was the publication of medical registers in 1779. This register was published by a London physician, Samuel Foart Simmons, and referred to as the *Medical Register* or

Simmons's Register. It was arranged on a county basis and even covered
Britain's colonies. Included in the register were physicians, hospitals, asylums
and dispensaries. Lane observes that the register highlighted an uneven
national coverage of doctors with physicians being concentrated mainly in
county towns – usually attached to hospitals or spas. The register enabled
patients to choose their practitioners and for doctors to contact each other.[68]

'Professionalism' was piecemeal and uneven but what had changed since
the late-sixteenth- and early-seventeenth-centuries was an appeal, at least, to
natural law with emphasis on a 'rational' or mechanical medical vocabulary,
though, again, this process was by no means uniform. If medicine was a
prime example where practitioners attempted to use a different language to
display 'expertise', Susan C. Lawrence has indicated that a great deal of
technical knowledge crossed occupational and social boundaries.[69] There was
an abundance of dictionaries and guides, such as Dr Robert James's *A
Medicinal Dictionary... with a History of Drugs* (1743), available to patients
so that they could familiarise themselves with medical terms. Particular
medical words, such as 'belly', 'guts' and 'jaw', might sound like 'lay' terms
to modern ears, but Lawrence cautions historians against regarding them as
being used purely to accommodate the patient. This type of language, she
argues, was 'chameleon-like' in character: 'practitioners chose to use "lay"
terms not because they were the patient's words, but because they were
perfectly acceptable anatomical referents', technical enough to serve the
required clinical purpose.[70]

The Royal College of Physicians sought to distinguish itself by using a
philosophical and medical learning that was expressed in technical jargon
and Latin prose. This was the mark of a learned physician, whose work could
automatically be differentiated from that of the irregular or quack.
Physicians needed to show that they understood the underlying causes of
health and disease. Indicative of this knowledge was the display of
iatromechanical expertise, which, as Shapin suggests, was a powerful vehicle
for 'cultural product-differentiation'.[71] An anti-theoretical or overtly
empiricist stance carried with it a lack of respect for intellectual, political and
medical authority – although College approval of Sydenham and Dr John
Radcliffe somewhat complicates this picture.[72] College élitism was
undergirded by the practice of only granting fellowships to those medical
men who had obtained their degrees from Oxford and Cambridge.[73] In
reality, the expiration in 1695 of the Licensing Act ended College censorship
of medical books, while the House of Lords' 'Rose decision' in 1704 lost the
College its monopoly on prescribing medicines and legitimised the medical
practice of apothecaries in London.[74] This legislation dramatically
undermined the Royal College of Physicians' regulatory function, which

already had difficulty suppressing unlicensed medical activity, particularly that of the clergy.[75]

Pelling observes that the Royal College of Physicians dealt with unlicensed practitioners by positing a unified body of medical knowledge. This was an entirely deliberate move. It was, she argues, a barrier that the College sought to erect for a variety of epistemological, social and economic motives: 'this effort by the College was in opposition both to the diffuseness of the knowledge relevant to medicine, and to the structure of medicine as an occupation'.[76] The College felt under threat by vernacular medical sources and so a 'unified' but select body of knowledge was put forward.[77] This knowledge was narrowly defined, compared to the flourishing medical pluralism of the early-modern period and herein lies part of the reason for negative responses to *Primitive Physic*. Orthodox practitioners regarded its plain style, empirical method and syncretic medical approach as a blatant flouting of authority. It was thus viewed with suspicion, despite the fact that Wesley was careful to underpin all of his remedies with authoritative medical sources.

Although the new sciences wielded little impact on eighteenth-century medical practice, it was the case that medics such as Pitcairne and Cheyne followed the example set down by Thomas Willis and Robert Boyle. But if humoral theory became less Galenic and more iatrochemical, corpuscularian or mechanical in its basis, the toolkit of medical practice continued to include bloodletting, stimulants, emetics, purgatives and modifications in lifestyle with an awareness of environmental factors.[78] Patient treatment therefore changed less than the theory surrounding it – as can be seen in the work of Cheyne, whose mechanical theory did little to undermine his traditional 'holistic' method, which relied on empiricism and included regimen.[79] In terms of theorising about disease, language changed to become more philosophically, scientifically and medically specified, particularly amongst those physicians anxious to guard their 'professional' status. Yet even this development was patchy; patients and practitioners were required to interpret the meaning of illness in a culture where, as Phyllis Mack points out, different 'paradigms of bodily pain, both in its physical nature and spiritual meaning, were in coexistence and competition'.[80] This in turn saw a convergence in the language of disease, religion and other folkloric traditions. As Porter suggests, 'physic and faith still criss-crossed at innumerable points'.[81] By the late-eighteenth century, however, mechanical explanations, which left a space for religion, were judged incapable of accounting for the full complexity of nature. Physicians like John Hunter and scientists such as Priestley substituted mechanical explanations with a philosophy of 'vitalism' that was shorn of its theological, though not spiritual, power. Exponents and practitioners of this philosophy believed that nature had its own inherent vital force, which was distinguished from inorganic matter.

Until these developments began to alter the landscape of scientific and medical practice, interpretations of illness and disease continued to be crammed with religious meaning, as C.J. Lawrence makes clear:

> In the eighteenth century the orthodox held that, in God's creation, the natural and the moral law were one... the body was healthy when things were in their proper place. Transgression of the natural laws which produced health, by overeating, drunkenness or promiscuity, for example, led to a similar moral chaos, signalled by vomiting, sweating or diarrhoea; by matter out of place... sickness could thus be a sign of sin.[82]

Natural phenomena, such as storms and earthquakes, were regarded providentially, while epidemics or threats of the plague were seen as judgements sent by God. Death was an ever-present danger and contemporaries like Hogarth, Swift and Fielding satirised their suspicion that the medical profession and mortality were close allies.[83] In this atmosphere it was easy for unscrupulous practitioners of 'fringe' medicine to cash-in on the association between 'orthodox' doctor and death.[84] Disease and human frailty dominated the minds of our ancestors and against this backdrop the afterlife offered some hope of compensation for the brevity of earthly existence.[85] This, in part, helps to explain the widespread appeal of *Primitive Physic*: Wesley's text offered hope both in this life and the hereafter.

Religion and medicine converged on a conceptual level for Wesley, but the remedies contained within *Primitive Physic* are empirically based from beginning to end. This division between theological conception and empirical method is reflected in the way he organised his text. We have seen already that the opening paragraphs of 'The Preface' are concerned to explicate Wesley's holistic concept of healing. The rest of 'The Preface' and the main body of *Primitive Physic* are characterised by an empirical and naturalistic mode. The theoretical structure of *Primitive Physic* is informed by the commonly used regimen of non-naturals, while the remedies are underpinned by contemporary medical practice. In this respect, *Primitive Physic* conforms to a predictable pattern and differs very little from the *modus operandi* of most eighteenth-century medical texts, which also usually included acknowledging the Divine Author in the preface.

Rousseau has suggested that critics of *Primitive Physic* may have found the 'religious tone of the baroque cadences of its preface' distasteful though he gives no evidence for this statement. Yet an acknowledgement of God and attendant concession to the post-lapsarian condition of man was a common device deployed in prefaces to eighteenth-century medical texts. This can be seen in the following extracts taken from the work of three well-known and eminent physicians of the time. The extracts are in chronological order and are taken from Dr Mead's *A Treatise Concerning the Influence of the Sun and Moon upon Human Bodies and the Diseases Thereby Produced* (1704), Sir Richard Blackmore's *Dissertations on a Dropsy* (1727) and Dr James's *A Medicinal Dictionary* (1743):

> [T]he wisdom, goodness, and wonderful continuance of the Omnipotent Creator of the World... who while he made ample provision for all living things, established this difference between brutes and rational creatures; that whereas those enjoy the common gifts of Nature, he has permitted us, besides, to investigate their properties and uses, and to contemplate the labyrinth of his divine works....

> It is highly probable, if not certain, that had our first parents persevered in a state of innocence... they would never have seen natural corruption; for death being the off-spring and wages of sin, the sanction annexed to the divine positive Law to secure *Adam's* obedience, it is reasonable to believe that Enoch and Elijah, had not sin prevented it, would have been translated from earth to heaven, without dissolution of the body. And when after their defection our parents became mortal, or obnoxious to death, the punishment threatened to disobedience, yet the execution of the sentence was mercifully suspended through a long, succession of years before *Noah's* flood; and it is not repugnant to reason that men at that time did not at their death suffer a violent separation of soul and body, but seemed not so much to dye, as by a gentle and gradual decay to cease to live... [now man has] degenerated from the simplicity and primitive manners of their predecessors to become soft and voluptuous....

> Providence having, in the beginning, furnished Mankind with a large store of remedies in the animal, vegetable, and mineral kingdoms, their uses and application seem to have been originally discovered by inspiration or accident.[86]

Even the most 'rational' of physicians, such as Mead, felt the need to include a nodding glance to his creator, though it is clear that his purpose is very different from that of Wesley – indicated in his statement that God has granted man permission to investigate the *properties* of nature. The second extract is interesting because Blackmore has presented a full-blooded account of the Genesis story. This prose is positively purple and Wesley's account in *Primitive Physic* looks less 'baroque' and more 'rational' by comparison. 'The Preface' in *Primitive Physic* comes closest to that of the physician James, particularly in its assumption that: 'the Author of Nature

112

taught us the use of many other medicines, by what is vulgarly termed Accident'.[87]

Significantly, for all Wesley's approbation regarding the virtue of ancient or simple practices, his medical manual rarely utilises 'popular' medicine. Nor does *Primitive Physic* draw on Native American medicine, which is, perhaps strange, given his glowing praise of its method. Wesley's endorsement of both ancient and contemporary 'popular' medicine was more rhetorical than actual. In reality, *Primitive Physic* adopted, elaborated and simplified those authoritative medical sources that were validated by leading contemporary physicians. Like those 'Gentlemen of the Faculty', Wesley had nothing but contempt for the egregious quack. In common with Locke, Wesley was an unorthodox practitioner who, with some hypocrisy, disapproved of irregular medical practice. In this sense, perhaps it could be said that Wesley was a frustrated medic, at least in terms of what he understood a true doctor should be.

Wesley justified his medical activity by pointing to his concern for those people who wanted to self-medicate and risked doing so badly because they were subject to the unscrupulous practice of nostrum-mongers.[88] The 'mass' production of nostrums and patent medicines in Georgian England has been vividly depicted by Porter, who shows how new drugs, such as Dr James's Powders, Turlington's Pills, Daffy's Elixir, Godfrey's Cordial and Anderson's Scots Pills, were widely advertised in the press and sold in numerous outlets.[89] This was noted by George Alexander Stevens, whose satirical song, *The Specifick* (1788), observed how the 'News-papers puff ev'ry Nostrum to town'.[90] In 1783, the government devised a tax on the drugs peddled by non-qualified practitioners, but eminent physicians were keen to cash-in on the huge amounts of money that could be exploited from this market. Here the line between 'orthodox' and non-orthodox was not so clear-cut and, as Lane points out, qualified practitioners, such as John Pechey or John Taylor, made lucrative livings as 'quacks'. Even distinguished qualified men, such as Robert James, Hans Sloane, Richard Mead and Edward Jenner, promoted remedies bearing their names, though these products were more exclusive and aimed at the upper end of the market.[91] These physicians may have despised quacks but did not shrink from using the same methods to exploit the profit-making potential of marketing such cures. Hence, Dr Hans Sloane advertised the medicinal value of his drinking chocolate, while Dr Mead peddled rabies powder.

Sales of these products reached epidemic proportions despite the fact that they could be lethal. Oliver Goldsmith, himself a physician, self-dosed to such an extent on Dr James's Powders it was widely believed that this contributed to his death. Dr William Hawes, a noted apothecary-physician to the London Dispensary and founder of the Royal Humane Society, wrote a tract on his death, entitled *An Account of the Late Dr Goldsmith's Illness, so Far as it Relates to the Exhibition of Dr James's Powders...* (1774). Hawes attributed Goldsmith's death to the consumption of 2ozs of Dr James's Powders and condemned the 'universally fashionable' nature of this lethal drug.[92] Porter notes that during the seventeenth century, patients could medicate themselves quite safely on harmless simples and herbal remedies. By contrast, the eighteenth-century self-medicator had access to cheap but potent and lethal medical brews. Utterly unrestricted by law, many of them were laced with opium and alcohol.[93]

Later editions of *Primitive Physic* sought to address this problem by providing cheap alternatives or Wesley's own version of the commonly-used nostrums. His recipes for Daffy's Elixir, Turlington's Balsam and Anderson's Scots Pills were intended to offer cheaper and safer options – though he was keen to point out to his reader that the alternatives put forward in *Primitive Physic* were just as effective. For Dr James's Powders he says:

> Instead of giving half a crown a packet, for these powders, you may at any Druggist's, get Dr. *Hardwick's* fever powder, for a shilling an ounce, which, if it be not the same, will answer just the same end.

Commenting on the Emetic Tartar Vomit, for which Wesley provides his own recipe, he makes the following observation about the Georgian medical market:

> 'Some of the quack doctors mix powdered ginger with emetic tartar, and call it the *ginger vomit.* I do not know that this is any injury to the medicine. But some of the low country Druggists adulterate it with chalk, or magnesia; these articles are only hurtful by preventing the purchasers knowing exactly the quantity they ought to take. It is therefore necessary to apply to the Apothecaries or Druggists on whose veracity you can depend. Mr. *Durban* an eminent Chymist in *Bristol*, prepares the best emetic tartar I have ever met with, either in town or country, and many Druggist shops are supplied with it by him.[94]

Wesley's distrust of nostrums was based on his suspicion of compound medicines generally. He disliked the fact that patients were unable to verify both the quantity and quality of the ingredients involved. Adulteration was also another problem that concerned him, and the 'veracity' of druggist or apothecary was essential to ensure quality and safety. The virtue of those medicines contained in *Primitive Physic*, he argued in the 'Postscript' to the 9th edition of 1761 (written in 1760), lay in the fact that the reader could be:

[S]ure of having them good in their kind, pure, genuine, unsophisticate. But who can be sure of this, when the medicines he uses are compounded by an Apothecary? Perhaps he has not the drug prescribed by the Physician, and so puts in its place 'what will do as well'. Perhaps he has it; but it is stale and perished: yet 'you would not have him throw it away. Indeed he cannot afford it'. Perhaps he cannot afford to make up the medicine as the Dispensary directs, and sell it at the common price. So he puts in cheaper ingredients: and you take neither you nor the Physician knows what! How many inconveniences must this occasion! How many constitutions are ruined hereby! How many valuable lives are lost! Whereas all these inconveniences may be prevented, by a little care and common sense, in the use of those plain, simple Remedies, which are here collected.[95]

Wesley took a dim view of the whole gamut of Georgian medical practitioners and made his feelings perfectly plain. The physicians he admired, however, are described in 'The Preface' to *Primitive Physic* as 'lovers of Mankind who have endeavoured, even contrary to their own interest, to reduce physic to its ancient standard....'[96] Those he held in esteem were the 'great and good Dr Sydenham' and his pupil Dr Dover who, Wesley remarks, 'has pointed out simple medicines for many diseases'. Wesley endorses here Dover's manual on self-medication, *The Ancient Physician's Legacy*, but there is no doubt that he would have approved of the fact that Dover offered his medical services to the poor.[97] Guerrini notes with some sarcasm the error of Wesley's endorsement of Dover, whose commercially driven medicine, she says, should not be equated with ancient medical practice. Yet Wesley extrapolated what he thought was useful about Dover's work to aid his own purpose. He thus chose to ignore the commercial aspect of Dover's medical practice by emphasising the simplicity of his approach and its legacy to Sydenham. He noted and approved of Dover's aim to help patients self-medicate, and the element of practical piety deployed to provide a service to the sick–poor.

Wesley displayed his admiration for the 'learned and ingenious' Cheyne by reworking much of the advice and 'Rules' set out in *An Essay of Health and Long Life*, but use was made too of Cheyne's *The English Malady, An Essay on Regimen* and *The Natural Method of Curing Most Diseases* (1742).[98] Regarding the work of Cheyne, Wesley makes the following observation:

Dr Cheyne... doubtless would have communicated [much] more to the world, but for the melancholy reason he gave one of his friends, that prest him with some passages in his works, which too much countenanced the modern practice, 'O Sir, we must do something to *oblige the Faculty*, or they will tear us in pieces'.[99]

Wesley is, of course, referring to that 'modern practice' of speculative system-building and probably has Cheyne's *New Theory* in mind, which he had read at Oxford in 1725.[100] But Wesley inadvertently put his finger on an essential truth; in fact, it was the Newtonian tenor of this text and its connection to Pitcairne that gained Cheyne his appointment as Fellow of the Royal Society.[101]

Many scholars who have noted the influence of Cheyne over *Primitive Physic* have criticised Wesley for 'lifting' sections of the *Essay* when writing his own medical text, though even a cursory glance over Wesley's work alerts the reader to its many influences. *Primitive Physic* draws heavily on Sydenham's 'cool regimen', both in its general sense but also in its application for treating smallpox. He adapts Sydenham's histories of clinical observations and these are often inserted into the text or footnotes. The multiple influences of Locke can be seen, not least in Wesley's use of the empirical method. Locke had also collected a great number of recipes and made copious notes about his medical reading and experiments in 'commonplace' books.[102] The additions and deletions that Wesley makes to subsequent editions of *Primitive Physic* reflect the fact that he picked up medical knowledge and tips like a collector, making cautious changes to his text along the way.

Primitive Physic draws from an array of eighteenth-century European medical sources and celebrated physicians, including Dr Richard Mead, Dr John Huxham, Dr John Fothergill, Dr Alexander Monroe, and the Dutch physician and botanist, Herman Boerhaave. Citing such authorities was Wesley's way of reassuring the reader but it also gave his medical manual an aura of legitimacy. His medical writing was greatly affected by the Swiss professor of medicine, Samuel Tissot, particularly Tissot's *L'Avis au People sur sa Santé*. Tissot lived in Lausanne, but his text went to at least nine editions throughout Europe. *L'Avis* sprang from a concern about depopulation in Switzerland and Tissot did not really intend for his text to become popularised. He wrote it in order for clergymen to mediate important medical advice and information to a wider audience.[103] Though Wesley did not obtain any of the remedies for the first publication of *Primitive Physic* from *L'Avis*, he incorporated Tissot's work into subsequent editions. He also (anonymously) produced an abridged version of *L'Avis* in 1769 and entitled it *Advice with Respect to Health*. This text proved to be in just as much demand as *Primitive Physic*, reaching ten editions in less than six years.

In the 'Introduction' to *Advice*, Wesley praised Tissot for his plain language, use of regimen, and empirical approach to medicine. He commended Tissot too for his humanity – those qualities singled out by Wesley were already amply demonstrated in *Primitive Physic*. He was not completely uncritical of *L'Avis* and castigated Tissot for an excessive use of clysters (enemas), and his 'violent fondness for bleeding', which Wesley thought was recommended 'on the most trifling occasions'.[104] Wesley's critique of venesection, as well as other points of criticism, involves an interesting intertextual relationship between *Primitive Physic* and *Advice with Respect to Health*. Frequently, Wesley appended Tissot's advice with a number of his own prescriptions and opinions in the form of footnotes. By contrast, many of the remedies presented in the editions of *Primitive Physic* following the publication of *L'Avis* were backed up by citing Tissot as an authority.

In the *Advice*, Wesley wishes to undercut and mitigate Tissot's constant recommendation of bleeding for diseases like pleurisy and quinsy by adding asterisked footnotes directing the reader to remedies given for those conditions in *Primitive Physic*. For pleurisy, Wesley recommends 'a poultice of boiled nettles' which, he says, will cure without bleeding.[105] *Advice* is peppered throughout with recommendations that the reader refer to Wesley's *Primitive Physic*. Despite this, *Primitive Physic* – in the editions following 1762 – is keen to use Tissot's name and authority to give credence to the remedies put forward. Even when Wesley has been critical of Tissot's recourse to bleeding for pleurisy and quinsy, he continues to utilise other remedies suggested by the Swiss doctor for those very diseases. Thus, he recommends the following remedy in *Primitive Physic* for the 'Pleurisy':

> 547. Or, a plaister of *flour of brimstone* and *white of an egg*: tried. This seldom fails – See Dr. *Tissot*, page 38.[106]

Again, Wesley draws on Tissot's *L'Avis* to give credibility to the following remedy for the 'Quinsy':

> 568. Or, draw in, as hot as you can bear, (for ten or twelve minutes together) the fumes of red rose-leaves, or camomile-flowers, boiled in water and vinegar: or a decoction of bruised hemp-seed.'
>
> This speedily cures the sore-throat, peripneumony and inflamation of the uvula – See Extract from Dr. *Tissot*, page 41.[107]

His reservation about some of Tissot's methods did not prevent him from extrapolating what was good or useful about *L'Avis*, and this manoeuvre is typically Wesley.

In general, Wesley took a conservative stance on the practice of venesection, but he was adamant that its use in the case of pleurisy was futile. His position here was informed by advice given to him by Dr Cockburn, a friend of his brother, Charles. Wesley recalled what Cockburn had told him some years previously:

> Sir, I never bleed a pleurisy. I know no cause, I know no one intention it
> answers which I cannot answer as well or better without wasting the strength
> of my patients.[108]

Wesley never forgot this advice, which was further reinforced by his own
experience:

> I have not seen a man in a pleurisy these twenty years (and I have seen not a
> few) whom I could not cure, not only without bleeding, but without any
> internal medicines whatever.[109]

Wesley's doubts about the efficacy of bleeding can be seen again when he
directs the reader of *Advice* to his own medical manual in order to obtain a
remedy for 'inflammation of the breast'. Tissot had advised his reader to
bleed the inflammation but Wesley states that 'the application set down in
the *Primitive Physic*, cures without bleeding at all'.[110] The following remedy
is given in *Primitive Physic* for this disease:

> 90. Boil a handful of *camomile* and as much *mallows* in milk and water.
> Foment with it between two flannels as hot as can be borne every twelve
> hours. It also dissolves any knot or swelling in any part.[111]

Wesley took a critical stance on Tissot's excessive use of venesection, but
he also severely reprimands Tissot for recommending internal medicine for
scabies in *L'Avis*:

> Can it be thought that so great a man as Dr Tissot never saw the transactions
> of our Royal Society? But if he had seen them, how could he utterly forget
> the paper communicated by Dr Mead, which puts beyond all possible
> dispute, being a matter of ocular demonstration, that the itch is nothing but
> animalcules of a peculiar kind, burrowing under the scarf-skin....[112]

Wesley is keen to use orthodox medical sources to counter what he regards
as a glaring medical error. He draws attention to this error in the footnote
attached to the 'Itch' in *Primitive Physic*:

> This distemper is nothing but a kind of small lice which burrow under the
> skin. Therefore inward medicines are absolutely needless – is it possible any
> physician should be ignorant of this?[113]

Another contentious point in *L'Avis* for Wesley is Tissot's
recommendation of Peruvian bark as an 'infallible' remedy for
'mortifications' and 'intermittent fevers'. The 'Bark', also known as 'Peruvian
bark', 'Jesuits bark' or 'Cinchona' had been brought to Europe by Jesuit
missionaries in the seventeenth century. It was used for numerous illnesses,
including palpitations of the heart and the 'ague' (malaria). Its active

ingredient, now known to be quinine, was used primarily to suppress the malarial parasite.[114] On the condition of 'intermittent fevers' or the 'ague', Wesley drew from his own experience to call Tissot's usage into question.

He argued that Peruvian bark did little to help him when he had taken it for 'Tertian ague' as a young man. He had been cured 'unawares' by drinking a large quantity of lemonade:

> I myself took some pounds of it when I was young for a common tertian ague and that, after vomiting: yet it did not, would not, effect a cure. And I should probably have died of it had I not been cured unawares by drinking largely of lemonade.[115]

Referring to a more recent bout of illness for which the bark had been used, Wesley says:

> In the last ague which I had, the first ounce of bark, was, as I expected, thrown off by purging. The second being mixed with salt of wormwood, stayed in my stomach. And just at the hour the ague should have come, began a pain at my shoulder-blade. Quickly it shifted its place, began a little under my left breast and there fixt. In less than an hour I had a short cough; soon after, a small fever. From that time the cough, the pain and the fever continued without intermission. And every night, very soon after I lay down, came first a dry cough for forty or fifty minutes: then an impetuous one till something seemed to burst, and for half an hour more, I threw up thick fetid pus. Here was expedition! What but a ball could have made quicker than this infallible medicine? In less than six hours it obstructed, inflamed, and ulcerated my lungs, and by this summary process, brought me into the third stage of a true pulmonary consumption… look at me and beware of the bark![116]

Ironically, although Wesley is keen to point out the specific remedy he had used to self-medicate whilst suffering under this condition, there is no mention of lemonade as a course of treatment in *Primitive Physic* for the 'Tertian ague'.[117]

Wesley's invective against Tissot's use of the bark for intermittent fevers is on shaky ground. A. Wesley Hill attempts to provide some defence here by suggesting that Wesley was concerned about the varying quality and impure nature of the anti-malarial factor contained within crude bark. This anti-malarial ingredient varied in quantity making it insufficient for any one administration to have any discernible effect.[118] Moreover, the bark was frequently prescribed in the form of an indigestible powder and Wesley justifies his antipathy to the drug by stating:

I mean the Bark in substance. If you love your lives, beware of swallowing ounce after ounce of indigestible powder. To infusions or decoctions I have no objection.[119]

He insisted that the remedy in its powdered form was unsafe and therefore useless. Wesley would not be swayed from this belief, probably because he had suffered such a bad experience when taking the remedy. A. Wesley Hill says that a possible explanation for his incalcitrance here could be due to the fact that:

Wesley was allergic to quinine or some other alkaloid contained in the bark. It is not sufficient to say that he took it in the form of an indigestible powder and therefore it did him no good, for he speaks of some more profound effect it had upon him when he says: 'I should probably have died of it'. Then, when he ceases using it and drinks plenty of lemonade, he has immediate relief and comes to the unfortunate conclusion that his lemon-juice has wrought the cure and that the bark is of no value in ague.[120]

In many ways Wesley's instincts about the dubious nature of powdered bark were correct. All too often there existed unsafe and bogus preparations of this remedy. Hans Sloane discovered that a cheaper and unsafe version, 'bark of the cherry' was dipped into tincture of aloes and passed off as the bark.[121]

Wesley had reservations about some of Tissot's recommendations but this did not prevent him from extracting what was useful about *L'Avis* when producing the *Advice*. He retrenched and appended the practice of clysters, venesection and use of bark, but stated that 'one might retrench, without any loss….'[122] Wesley's careful retrenchment of Tissot's *L'Avis* amply illustrates the fact that patient safety was a consideration uppermost in his mind. In fact, none of Wesley's remedies were harmful or dangerous, despite the criticisms levelled at *Primitive Physic* and many of his preparations consisted of natural ingredients. In the 'Postscript' to the 5th edition of 1755, Wesley stresses that *Primitive Physic* recommends to 'men of plain, unbiased reason':

[S]uch remedies as air, water, milk, whey, honey, treacle, salt, vinegar, and common *English* herbs, with a few foreign medicines, almost equally cheap, safe and common.[123]

This statement is substantially accurate, but it must be pointed out that *Primitive Physic* is not just a list of 'herbals' or 'simples'.

Wesley, in fact, makes great use of a range of ingredients commonly used by eighteenth-century physicians, such as vitriol, tartar, tar-water, balsam of peru, balsam of tolu, gum storax and gum guaiacum. For someone who was so vehemently opposed to excessive drugging, Wesley's *Primitive Physic* recommends and makes use of many of the medicines listed below by the author of *Domestic Medicine*. Buchan suggested that every well-equipped home should have supplies of:

Adhesive plaster	Gum ammoniac	Oil of almonds	Spirits of wine
Agaric of oak	Gum arabic.	Olive oil	Spirits of nitrate
Ash coloured	Gum asafoetida	Pennyroyal water	Spirits of vitriol
Ground liverwort	Gum camphor	Peppermint water	Syrup of lemons
Burgundy pitch	Ipecacuanha	Rhubarb	Syrup of oranges
Cinnamon water	Jalap	Sal ammoniac	Syrup of poppies
Crabs claw	Jesuit's bark	Sal prunell	Tamarind
Cream of tartar	Liquid laudanum	Seneka root	Vinegar of squills
Elixir of vitriol	Liquorice root	Senna	Wax plaster
Flowers of sulphur	Magnesia alba	Snake root	Valerian root
Gentian root	Manna	Spirits of harts.	Yellow basilicum
Glauber's salts	Nitre or salt petre	Horn ointment [124]	

This list contains many herbals and simples, but has a distinctively eighteenth-century feel and is a world away from Boyle's *Medicinal Experiments*. Animal, including human, *materia medica* was beginning to be replaced by newer minerals and chemicals: aconite, castor oil, magnesia, tartrate of iron, oxide of zinc.[125] The medical practice indicated by this list is also very different from that type of 'kitchen physic' espoused by the apothecary John Hill in his *The Family Herbal; Or, An Account of all those English Plants, which are Remarkable for their Virtues* (1755).[126]

Unlike many of his contemporaries, who still clung to the notion of vicious humours or acrid blood, Wesley did not recommend purging or bleeding patients to extremitus.[127] In *Primitive Physic* he condemned the overuse of the three active treatments: bleeding, blistering and cathartics. More importantly, the edition of 1755 dramatically reduces its use of the 'Herculean remedies', such as opium and steel, Peruvian bark and the commonly used quicksilver. Quicksilver, or mercury, was used to treat a number of diseases, including syphilis.

Dover, dubbed the 'Quicksilver doctor', was an avid prescriber of mercury. Drawing on Dr Freind's *Emmenologia* (1703), Dover believed that it was a 'balsam' for the blood, which could also open 'obstructions'. He recommended it for hysteria, scrofula, intestinal inflammations, ulcers, asthma and iliac passion (appendicitis) – Cheyne recommended it for scorbutic ulcers and gout.[128] Dover even dispensed mercury for infertility problems and thought that it was a general 'cure-all' medicine.[129] As a treatment, College physicians believed that mercury was only applicable for treating asthma and iliac passion. Dover thus found himself at the centre of much criticism and controversy on this matter.[130]

Wesley's cautious use of this treatment was more in keeping with orthodox medicine than one might have expected. He reduces its recommendation from 1755 but suggests using quicksilver for 'The Asthma': '45. Or, take an ounce of *Quicksilver* every morning....'[131] Quicksilver is also suggested for the iliac passion: '437. ... take, ounce by ounce, a pound or a pound and a half of *quicksilver* – (see Dr. *Tissot* page 120).' Here, Wesley seeks recourse to the authority of Tissot, but this remedy was already presented in the first edition of *Primitive Physic*, long before Tissot's *L'Avis* was published. It is likely that Wesley drew his authority here from Dr Mead, who had stated that 'pounds' of mercury could be given for the iliac passion to good effect.[132]

In the 1755 edition of *Primitive Physic* where Wesley reduces the use of 'Herculean' medicines, 'except in very few cases', he issues the following caution:

> It is because they are not safe, but extremely dangerous, that I have omitted (together with Antimony) the four *Herculean* medicines, Opium, the Bark, Steel and most preparations of Quicksilver. *Herculean* indeed! Far too strong for common men to grapple with. How many fatal effects have these produced even in the hands of no ordinary Physicians! With regard to the four of these, the instances are glaring and undeniable. And whereas Quicksilver the fifth, is in its native form as innocent as bread or water: has not the art been discovered, so to *prepare* it, as to make it the most deadly of all poisons? *These*, Physicians have justly termed edged Tools. But they have not yet taught them to wound at a distance: and honest men are under no necessity of touching them, or coming within their reach.[133]

Wesley Hill argues that the statement here referring to the 'innocent' nature of quicksilver in its native form is both irresponsible and unfortunate.[134] Yet this observation was based on Boerhaave's investigative work into the effects of mercury. Boerhaave's *Some Experiments Concerning Mercury* (1734) sought to show the physical and chemical properties of this element. Apart from discovering that mercury was an element which could not be broken down or split into other metals, the result of Boerhaave's experiments showed that metallic mercury given orally was not absorbed by the ailmentary tract but harmlessly excreted. Mercury compounds, however, were toxic and thus poisonous.[135] Mead had demonstrated this in *A Mechanical Account of Poisons* (1702), where he argued that 'pure mercury is not poisonous or corrosive' but that mercury sublimate was noxious. Its poisonous nature depended on how it was compounded with other substances.[136]

Wesley continued to recommend small amounts of the bark, quicksilver and steel for exceptional illnesses. He curtailed his recommendation of opium after the 1755 edition of *Primitive Physic*, though Laudanum continued to be prescribed for a number of serious conditions such as the ague.[137] Opiates were widely recommended by eminent physicians and avid supporters throughout the Georgian period; many did not believe that opium was habit-forming.[138] In 1679 Dr Sydenham claimed that medicine would be crippled without it, though he also cautioned against prescribing it for certain conditions, suggesting its limited or intermittent use in cases of 'bloody urine' and rheumatic fever. Any use of opium, moreover, needed to be preceded by a cathartic.[139] Sydenham's positive endorsement of this drug was echoed throughout the Georgian period, for example in Dr John Jones's *Mysteries of Opium Reveal'd* in 1700 – the title almost has a religious feel to it – and Dr George Young's *Treatise on Opium* in 1753.[140] Young's work supported the theory that opium heated, rarified and expanded the blood. Therefore it should not be administered for inflammatory diseases because an accelerated flow of heated, rarified blood would expand the blood vessels and make inflammations worse. Young advised extreme caution when using this drug because, in the wrong hands, it was a 'slow poison'.

Opium was prescribed as a remedy for innumerable diseases, such as diarrhoea, vomiting, coughs or gout, and was used as a diaphoretic, and obviously, an analgesic.[141] While some eighteenth-century physicians did report cases of opium addiction resulting from excessive therapeutic use, this was not regarded as a serious medical or social problem.[142] On the contrary, John Jones actually eulogised the psychological effects of opium which:

> [C]auses a brisk gay and good Humour… Promptitude, Serenity, Alacrity, and Expediteness in Dispatching and Managing Business… Assurance, Ovation of the Spirits, Courage, Contempt of Danger, and Magnanimity… prevents and takes away Grief, Fear, Anxieties, Peevishness, Fretfulness… [it] causes Euphory, or easie undergoing of all Labour, Journeys & c… lulls, sooths, and (as it were) charms the Mind with Satisfaction, Acquiescence, Contentation, Equanimity & c.[143]

Wesley, in fact, was amongst a small number when he surmised its addictive and debilitating nature. Andreas-Holger Maehle observes, with regard to the psychic effects of opium, that there was no specific tool or theory available in the eighteenth century to carry out a thorough investigation into the psychological effect of this drug. Indeed, J.C. Kramer points out that opium addiction was a phenomenon not fully recognised until the nineteenth century – although John Jones, despite his unstinting advocacy, was the first to describe this side-effect.[144]

The medical and scientific debates in which Wesley engaged with physicians illustrates the depth and breadth of his knowledge. His anxiety about the use of dangerous drugs is a good example of this, but another can be seen in Wesley's published extract and introductory commentary on Dr Cadogan's *A Dissertation on the Gout and all Chronic Diseases* in 1774 which, he insisted, was the most masterly work on the subject.[145] Cadogan was physician to the London Foundling Hospital and Fellow of the Royal College of Physicians. His dissertation had evoked a great deal of controversy from a number of physicians, primarily for its denial of the importance of heredity in this disease. Wesley took Cadogan to task for denying the place of heredity, but his stance on this issue was a great deal more complex and sophisticated than one might have expected from a non-professional. Wesley believed that heredity played an important role in the condition. Like Cadogan, however, he disagreed with most other contemporary physicians by insisting that a combination of regimen and medicine could mitigate, if not cure, this disease. Wesley argued that very few of the 'chronic' distempers associated with gout could properly be called hereditary, springing instead from an intemperate and indolent lifestyle.

Wesley did not simply cull from leading authoritative medical texts to source his remedies in *Primitive Physic*, but had a critical dialogue with physicians, using his experience to make cautious changes to subsequent editions. Alterations made to later editions were given due care and consideration, as is made plain in the 'Postscript' to the 5th edition of 1755:

> Those alterations are still in pursuance of my first design, to set down cheap, safe, and easy medicines; easy to be known, easy to be procured, and easy to be applied by plain, unlettered men. Accordingly, I have omitted a considerable number, which though cheap and safe, were not so common or well known; and have added at least an equal number, to which that objection cannot be made: which are not only of small price, and extremely safe, but likewise easily to be found, if not in every house or yard, yet in every town, and almost every village throughout the kingdom.[146]

Wesley's medical activity should not be equated with that of the most eminent or leading doctors of his day, but if we compare his method to other eighteenth-century physicians we can see how exacting and rigorous it really was. Physicians sought to defend their profession by denouncing all trespassers as empirics or quacks and a show of philosophical learning distinguished their practice from quackery. Wesley was forced to fend off sharp attacks from physicians and other critics, the most celebrated attack came in 1776 from Dr Hawes whose criticisms of *Primitive Physic* were unfair.

Wesley's response to those who dismissed him as an empiric was to state that those who knew how to restore health to the sick were always branded with this name. His 'unorthodoxy' was a lack of formal qualifications and it is for this reason that he would not have considered himself an exponent of alternative medicine but a cautious prescriber within the boundaries of 'orthodox' medicine.[147] His empiricism alerted the public to the dangers of misapplied theory. Like Sydenham, he delighted in the comfort of empiricism; the 'tried remedy' would have lasting appeal because it reassured patients.[148] In the editions after 1755, he introduced footnotes commenting on particular remedies and in the 'Postscript' attached to the 9th edition of 1761 (written in 1760) he makes the following statement:

> During the observation and experience of more than five years, which have passed since the last impression of this Tract, I have had many opportunities of trying the virtues of the ensuing Remedies. And I have now added the word *Tried* to those which I have found to be the greatest efficacy.[149]

Those editions after 1772 contained an asterisk against his preferred articles:

> Most of those medicines which I prefer to the rest, are now marked with an Asterisk.[150]

He criticised doctors who replaced experience with hypothesis and speculation, but his own emphasis on the empirical tradition did not mean that he was backward-looking. Nor was empiricism without its own theoretical baggage. Like Boyle and Sydenham, Wesley was convinced to the point of arrogance that his method was free from theory, though this approach was thoroughly Baconian and Lockean, characterised by a belief that true knowledge could only come from experience. Empiricism could lead to a steady progress in clinical medicine rather than research being based on *a priori* hypotheses. Bacon urged physicians to study natural philosophy by making a series of specific inquiries, so that the accumulated mass of facts could produce a general explanation. Locke makes this position clear as he urges fellow medic Thomas Molyneux to extend Sydenham's method:

> That which I always thought of Dr Sydenham living, I find the world allows him now he is dead... I hope the age has many who will follow his example, and, by the way of accurate practical observation, as he has so happily begun, enlarge the History of Diseases, and improve the Art of Physic; and not, by speculative Hypotheses, fill the world with useless, though pleasing visions....[151]

Following on from Bacon, Boyle, Sydenham and Locke, Wesley makes a virtue of the empirical method in *Primitive Physic*. Careful clinical observation was a simple and safe means of arriving at probable knowledge, based on experience.

Here too, the meaning of the word 'primitive' in *Primitive Physic* has given rise to much confusion. Wesley believed in simplicity. He also wanted to restore that ancient standard in physic, which privileged experiment and experience over and above theory. However, Wesley was not merely peddling traditional herbal remedies to hark back to a golden age. His aim was to show that progress in medicine could only be made through experimentation and observation, trial and error. If he pointed to the role of accident in discovering cures, he did not wish to reduce medicine to a vulgarised notion of this idea.[152] Rather, he saw the importance of designed and controlled experiment; this was the basis of real medical progress and here his ideas represented a type of Burkean enlightened empiricism.

His praise of those 'modern' philosophers and medics who 'improved' natural philosophy attests to this, as does Wesley's approval of new discoveries, such as the circulation of blood and blood transfusions. In addition to this, Wesley's *Compendium* makes clear from the outset its enlightenment objective: 'As man ought to know himself best, we begin our treatise here' by contemplating the human body.[153] In his sermon, *What is Man?* (1788), Wesley again sought recourse to medical imagery and language to argue that contemplation of the human body, with God's assistance, was perfectly permissible. To the question 'what am I?' Wesley makes the following statement:

> Here is a curious machine, fearfully and wonderfully made. It is a little portion of *earth*, the particles of which, cohering I know not how, lengthen into innumerable fibres a thousand times finer than hairs. These, crossing each other in all directions, are strangely wrought into membranes; and these membranes are as strangely wrought into arteries, veins, nerves, and glands; all of which contain various fluids, constantly circulating the whole machine... but besides this strange compound of the four elements, earth, water, air and fire, I find something in me of a quite different nature, nothing akin to any of these. I find something in me that *thinks*, which neither earth, water, air, fire, nor any mixture of them can possibly do. Something which sees, and hears, and smells, and tastes, and feels, all which are so many modes of thinking. It goes further: having perceived objects by any of these senses it forms inward ideas of them. It *judges* concerning them, it sees whether they agree or disagree with each other. It *reflects* upon its own operations. It is endued with imagination and memory. And any of its operations, judgment in particular, may be subdivided into many others.[154]

The influence of Locke's *Essay* can be clearly discerned in this passage. But the concept of ethereal fire energising the blood given in this sermon echoes the 'Introduction' to Wesley's *Compendium*, where Harvey's *Exercitatio Anatomica de Mortu Cordis et Sanguinis in Animalibus* (1628) is cited as a work which far outstrips that of the ancients.

His approval of contemporary discoveries in both science and medicine makes Wesley's position in the debate between the ancients and moderns rather complicated, as the following extract from the *Compendium* demonstrates:

> And how many things in all bodies, as well as in the human, which eluded all the art and industry of the Antients, have the moderns discovered by the help of *microscopes*? Altho' these are not properly a modern invention: it being certain that something of this kind was in use, many hundred years ago. There are several works of great antiquity still extant, the beauties of which cannot even be discerned, much less could they have been wrought, by the finest naked eye... such is that seal, now in the cabinet of the King of France, allowed to be at least fifteen hundred years old, six-tenths of an inch long, and so far broad, which to the naked eye presents only a confused group, but surveyed with a microscope, distinctly exhibits trees, a river, a boat and sixteen or seventeen persons.[155]

Unlike Sydenham, Wesley did not disapprove of using microscopes. Such modern discoveries in tandem with developments in anatomy could assist man in the search for scientific and medical knowledge. Furthermore, like Boerhaave, Wesley did not see any contradiction in adopting a Hippocratic empirical approach and combining this with a mechanistic language that could describe the body and diseases. Wesley understood that there were sufficient points of contact between the two concepts, and in this sense his technique was not simply eclectic but consciously aped Boerhaave's 'syncretic' method.[156]

Emphasis on simplicity saw Wesley denounce status-seeking professionals who wished to make profits from compound medicines. He held firm to his method of taking one remedy at any given time and refused to use compound medicines because he believed they contained too many dangerous ingredients. As we have seen from the passage given at the beginning of this chapter, Wesley drew his authority here from Boerhaave, but it was the case that other physicians such as Dr John Fothergill preferred 'elegant simplicity' over and above the 'multifarious compounds prescribed by other physicians'.[157] The physician, Dr George Young also opposed compound medicines on the basis that it proved impossible to ascertain exactly which medicinal property was taking its effect on the patient. Boyle had made this very same point in 1692, arguing that compounds could hinder health rather than aid it:

> I think it… not unreasonable to suspect that, where a great many ingredients are blended into one medicine, one or other of them may have other operations, besides that designed by the physician: it may awaken some sleeping ferments, and if not produce a new distemper, may excite and actuate some other hostile matter, that lay quiet in the body before… I have had so many unwelcome proofs of this in myself, that it engages me to be the more careful to caution others against the like inconvenience.[158]

When dispensing medicines, Young insisted that the following factors needed to be taken into account: the patient's constitution – various constitutions provoked very different reactions – the disease and to precisely what stage the disease had developed, plus a careful consideration of the exact dosage of any drug administered:

> These difficulties are not a little increased by that absurd, tho' fashionable practice of blending, in one compound, a farrago of all the simples which authors have classed together for that disease. How impossible it is for the prescriber to know which ingredient was useful, which unnecessary or hurtful?[159]

Young sees how this was made worse by the fact that physicians constantly changed their prescriptions every time they visited the sick. Modern medicine takes for granted the positive synergistic effect produced by a combination of drugs, but it was generally true that eighteenth-century compounds could be protracted and dangerous.[160] Porter argues that Georgian pharmacy left a great deal to be desired:

> Quack nostrums were often quite unsafe. Polypharmacy – complex drug cocktails, in which certain ingredients were supposed to counter the deleterious effects of others – was open to glaring abuses. Violent purgatives and lead – or mercury – based medicines caused spasm and colic, often relieved by belladonna or other concoctions that induced further poisoning.[161]

Wesley was right to point out the danger of polypharmacy: many died as a result of it.[162]

Georgians were forced to confront the possibility of death on every side, but it was also the case that there existed widespread confidence in the efficacy of medicine to ameliorate physical suffering and positively determine good health. Unlike Puritan concepts of enduring physical suffering and illness, when writing *Primitive Physic,* Wesley consciously espoused the principles of enlightened thinking. This included a defiance of death and a belief that infant mortality or death in childbirth could be avoided through human knowledge and skill. Hence Jordanova remarks, 'the claim that individuals could and should manage their own health through the regulation of lifestyle were central tenets of Enlightenment thinking'.[163] *Primitive Physic* not only represents an enlightened approach to medicine, but Wesley's practical application of the cool regimen came to be sublimated into a moderate liberal hypothesis of hygienic treatment, potently symbolised in 1842 with Edwin Chadwick's *Report on the Sanitary Conditions of the Labouring Population*. It did much to direct public attention to the importance of health, hygiene and temperance and some of Wesley's remedies could still be found in the US Pharmacopoeia in 1903.

Wesley's adoption of a 'cool vegetable regimen' pointed to the natural environment as a rich source of possible treatment and cure. This 'cool' regimen incorporated the primal elements and *Primitive Physic* used natural remedies to unite man with those elements. This optimism reached its climax with the espousal of electrical therapy, representative of that most powerful primal element, fire, and Wesley was as much a pioneer here as he was in the area of preventative medicine. The interconnected themes of regimen and its incorporation of the primal elements, including electricity, are subjects that will be looked at later. For now it is important to pay some attention to the criticism evoked by Wesley's medical manual, *Primitive Physic*, and in particular that of Dr William Hawes.

Contemporary reaction to *Primitive Physic*: or the case of Dr William Hawes examined[164]

In his biography *The Life and Times of the Revd John Wesley* (1872), Tyerman makes the following observation about the lack of response to *Primitive Physic*:

> It is a remarkable incident that the medical profession, so generally impatient of medical empirics, allowed Wesley's work to circulate for nearly thirty years before any of their honourable fraternity deigned to take notice or to denounce it.[165]

The modern scholar of the history of medicine, G.S. Rousseau, not only seems to take this observation on board when he suggests that Tyerman's comment is 'well taken', but further endorses it in the following statement:

> Though thousands of sick and healthy laymen bought Wesley's book, few scientists took notice of it. It was not debated by the learned physicians as was, for example, Berkeley's treatise on tar water.[166]

Considering the wars that had taken place over Berkeley's Tar Remedy, Ward's Pill and Drop, and James's Fever Powders, Rousseau argues:

> [T]he reasons are sufficiently clear. No other similar work of the century was so popular or had sold so many copies, and once poor folk brought it into their homes (as they did from the start) there was no getting it out. Moreover, Wesley offered his readers many alternative cures (an average of six or seven) for each disease. If one failed, another might succeed. No physician could therefore justifiably charge him with suggesting too few remedies.[167]

Rousseau has raised three important points which will be investigated here. The first point concerns the issue of orthodox reaction to *Primitive Physic*. It is therefore necessary to examine exactly why those physicians or their 'honourable fraternity' had not bothered to respond to the text for 'nearly thirty years'. The second point raised by Rousseau involves looking at whether Wesley's work was really accepted and conceded to on the basis of its popularity with the 'poor folk'. The third and final point that needs to be addressed is the issue of whether Wesley's eclectic method staved off or attracted criticism.

Concerning the first point, it may have been the case that College or orthodox physicians failed to respond to the author of *Primitive Physic* because Wesley could not be addressed personally. John Wesley's name did not appear on the title page of the text until the 9th edition of 1761 ('Postscript' dated as 1760). It must have been common knowledge that the author of this manual was Wesley, but the best that could be achieved in this circumstance was an implicit criticism of the text in general, addressed to 'the author of *Primitive Physic*'. This, however, would have been a fairly pointless exercise. Taken as a whole, most of the remedies contained within the text were ubiquitous, if not 'orthodox'. Without being able to conflate the recommendation, usage or efficacy of any given remedy with that unique set of doubts and fears gathered around the figure of John Wesley, an attack on this work would have been difficult. Indeed, criticism which called into question the medical practice of *Primitive Physic* could only ever become a petty, hair-splitting exercise – as will be demonstrated in the explication of Dr Hawes's critique.

Before the 9th edition of *Primitive Physic*, established physicians and Faculty members might have considered themselves above that type of invective and innuendo associated with hudibrastics. But here the association between Wesley's 'quack' medicine and equally 'unorthodox' religion had entertained the Georgian public for some time. The mock epic written in 1767 by Nathaniel Lancaster, *Methodist Triumphant*, a satire based on Henry More's *Enthusiasmus Triumphatus*, provided a vivid depiction of

Wesley exhorting a crowd to denounce reason. Of particular significance is the fact that this scenario takes place in the field around Bedlam.[168] Here, Wesley personifies religious mountebank and medical interloper, and it is wholly appropriate that he is placed in his natural habitat: the irrational environment of Bedlam. Bishop Warburton's *The Doctrine of Grace: Or, The Office and Operations of the Holy Spirit Vindicated from the Insults of Infidelity and the Abuses of Fanaticism* (1763) also parodied Wesley's medical proclivities by wryly alluding to his healing gift for turning fools into madmen.[169]

Wesley's foray into medicine had been noted and disapproved of by a range of critics. This disapproval was not based on medical disagreement: attacks were sectarian and increasingly so after 1761, when it became clear that Wesley had written *Primitive Physic*. Small wonder Wesley wished to remain anonymous when publishing *Primitive Physic, Advice* and *Desideratum*. Evidently he anticipated this reaction and believed it would damage the reception of those medical and scientific works before they had a chance to establish validity on their own terms. Proof of this can be seen in the bitter and scathing assault published by Dr Hawes in his *An Examination of the Rev Mr John Wesley's Primitive Physic* (1776).

Rousseau is absolutely right when he suggests that Hawes's animosity stemmed from the fact that Wesley, as Methodist preacher, had the audacity to practise medicine when he was not a *bona fide* member of the medical profession. He argues that it was 'Wesley's cloth and not his medicine' that was 'the target of Hawes's invective', the majority of which was 'unfair and stated in hyperbolic language'.[170] This was noted by the Revd Samuel Romilly Hall, who believed that *Primitive Physic* had been unwisely ridiculed and much maligned:

> A medical gentleman of Leeds, reputed as eminently intelligent and skilful in his profession, has declared to me that the unfriendly criticisms, so freely given on Wesley's 'Primitive Physic', are altogether unwarrantable. He affirms, that, judged in comparison with other non-professional works of the same class, and of the same date, the 'Primitive Physic' is incomparably superior to anything that he knows.[171]

We have seen already how *Primitive Physic* not only compares favourably with 'non-professional' works, but with the 'professional' practices of leading medical authorities.

Hawes's celebrated attack was published in the form of a pamphlet, which set out to show that a:

> [G]reat number of the prescriptions therein contained are founded on ignorance of the medical art, and of the power and operations of medicine;

and that it is a publication calculated to do essential injury to the health of those persons who may place confidence in it.[172]

By the time Hawes wrote this tract, *Primitive Physic* had reached its 16th edition. Tyerman observes that *An Examination* was 'in the highest degree ironical' and indeed, it must have been, judging by Hawes's assertion that he bore Wesley no personal animosity.[173] Hawes's pamphlet, in fact, was a sectarian, political and even *ad hominem* denunciation of Wesley's work.

This leads on to the second point raised by Rousseau: that orthodox opinion accepted Wesley's text based simply on its popularity with the 'poor folk'. Rousseau's assertion here is countered by the declaration made by Hawes in *An Examination* to criticise the manual on this very basis. In the 'Advertisement' given at the beginning of the volume, Hawes's prose sounds a rather shrill note when discussing this point:

> I have made Quacks of all denominations my sworn enemies: but what medical man of honour and reputation, would wish to be upon tolerable terms with the murderers of the human race?[174]

In similarly dramatic tones he states that it is the popularity of *Primitive Physic* that impels him to protect readers from the:

> [I]njudicious collection of pretended remedies for almost every disorder that can affect the human frame… those who rely on Mr Wesley's pamphlet, will often be led to trifle with the most dangerous diseases, and while they are forming vain expectations of obtaining relief from his insufficient prescriptions, may be led to neglect timely application for real and effectual assistance… a book that has passed through so many editions as the *Primitive Physic*, must have been attended to by great numbers; and as the recipes in it are often so injudicious, absurd, and so strongly characterised by ignorance of the human body, and of the power and operation of medicines, they may have been productive of great mischief.[175]

Hawes wants to alert the public to the danger of Wesley's book. It is strange, given Hawes's scrupulous attention to every aspect of *Primitive Physic* in its numerous editions, that he should have neglected to overlook Wesley's repeated admonishment to call 'without delay' in 'complicated cases… a Physician that fears God'.[176]

It was precisely the popularity of *Primitive Physic* that gave Hawes a much-needed justification to write *An Examination* in the first place. Hawes was by no means unique on this score and established physicians sought to protect their status by denouncing anything that smacked of irregularity or medical pluralism. This belies the third, and final, point highlighted by Rousseau: that the lack of orthodox response to *Primitive Physic* was due to

Wesley offering 'his readers many alternative cures'. As far as Hawes was concerned, a 'great number of the prescriptions' contained within *Primitive Physic* were 'founded on ignorance of the medical art, and of the power and operations of medicine'. He criticised Wesley for having the temerity to offer his own 'tried' and tested remedies, but is equally dismissive when *Primitive Physic* utilises a range of medical sources to provide alternative cures.

This can be seen in the following observation that Hawes makes about a suggested remedy in *Primitive Physic* for the 'Tertian ague'. Wesley recommends applying to each wrist 'a plaister of *treacle* and *foot* – Tried'. Hawes begins his critique by misquoting the disease for which this remedy had been suggested and brought it under a general heading for the 'Ague'. He then goes on to trivialise Wesley's 'tried' and tested method: 'As the word tried is affixed to this footy application, it may be presumed that Mr. Wesley or his chimney-sweeper, have experienced its efficacy.'[177]

By contrast, where Wesley has put forward a range of remedies, drawing on medical authorities, Hawes makes the following acerbic comment:

> Mr. Wesley, in many parts of his *Primitive Physic*, proves himself an adept in plagiarism; and many authors, there is no doubt, from whom he has borrowed, would do him no credit, had he mentioned their names....[178]

Hawes, it would seem, wants to cut the criticism both ways: he despises *Primitive Physic* for its eclectic list of receipts, which, he alleges, has no basis in the discipline of medicine. On the other hand, he castigates Wesley's conscientious use of eighteenth-century medical sources.

Popularity was no protection against 'professional' criticism and, in fact, could elicit ridicule or censure. Even 'regular' physicians, who were licensed from the College to practice medicine, could be berated for what appeared to be 'unorthodox' medical practices that appealed to popular audiences – hence Dr Dover was denigrated as the 'Quicksilver doctor' for peddling a medicine best left to quacks. Dover also suffered abuse for his recommendation of the 'Toad Powder' when treating asthma. Dr Henry Bradley, a surgeon who also wrote a *Treatise on Mercury* (1733) in which he sought to show 'the danger of taking it crude', bitterly repudiated Dover's use of this remedy in a tract entitled *Physical and Philosophical Remarks on Dr Dover's Late Pamphlet* (1733):

> I can only say of our Nostrum-Monger as the facetious Dr. Baynard said of his Dr. Stew-Toad, as he calls him, that he was one who set up for miracle and mystery; and always makes honey of a dog's tird. This martyrs more toads than Popery has done hereticks.[179]

Hawes ridicules Wesley for including precisely this remedy in *Primitive Physic*:

> Of all Mr. Wesley's remedies for the convulsive asthma, *powder of toad* is the most curious; but it is suited to the credulity of the frequenters of the Foundry.[180]

Yet we know that this remedy was not Wesley's, but Dr Dover's, and it is clear that Wesley drew on this source because he acknowledges Dover in 'The Preface'.

The worst example of Hawes's prejudice can be seen in his attempt to discredit *Primitive Physic* with his assertion that Wesley had a 'total incapacity to produce any medical treatise calculated to be of the least service to Mankind'.[181] This statement is particularly vicious and intended to inflict the deepest of wounds. Any author reading such a comment could not fail to be affected by the callous, cold and calculating nature of it. This was Wesley's Achilles' heel: to produce a medical treatise for the 'interest of Mankind' was the primary reason for his writing *Primitive Physic*.

Hawes had been alerted to the existence of *Primitive Physic* when 'a sensible writer, who signed himself ANTIDOTE, in the *Gazetteer* of December 25 1775' had 'justly animadverted upon' a 'destructive prescription' contained within *Primitive Physic*. It was, argues Hawes, 'this gentleman's observations which first led me to peruse Mr. Wesley's *Primitive Physic*....' [182] The 'destructive prescription' alluded to here revolved around a typographical error in *Primitive Physic*. 'To one Poisoned' Wesley had prescribed '... one or two drachms of *distilled verdigrease*: it vomits in an instance'.[183] The error exposed here is Wesley's prescription of 'one or two drachms' instead of 'one or two *grains*' of the verdigris. One drachm was equivalent to sixty grains or one-eighth of an ounce and so this was a considerable difference in weight. 'ANTIDOTE' severely reprimanded Wesley for this gross error and this was printed in the *Gazetteer* and quoted in *An Examination* by Hawes:

> [A]t reading such a prescription... I could scarce believe my eye-sight for some time, nor can at present by any means account for the ignorance and presumption of a man who deals out as an antidote, one of the most active poisons in nature, in such an enormous dose... it is very probable that your dose of two drachms would effectively poison 20 or 30 people, or operate very sensibly on every man, woman, and child in one of your largest congregations.[184]

Hawes reproduces Wesley's response to 'ANTIDOTE', which was addressed 'To the Printer of the Gazetteer' on 28 December 1775. The speed with which Wesley responded to this serious allegation indicates that he regarded the matter with some concern:

> Between twenty and thirty editions of the *Primitive Physic*, or 'A Rational and Easy Method of Curing Most Diseases', have been published either in England or Ireland. In one or more of these editions stand these words: 'give one or two drachms of verdigris'. I thank the gentleman who takes notice of this, though he might have done it in a more obliging manner. Could he possibly have been ignorant (had he not been willingly so) that this is a mere blunder of the printer? That I wrote *grains* not drachms? However, it is highly proper to advertise the public of this; and I beg every one that has the book would take the trouble of altering that word with his pen....[185]

Unsurprisingly, Hawes is not impressed with this response. He accuses Wesley of evading the issue:

> Mr. Wesley above says, that this dangerous error stands in *one or more of the twenty or thirty editions of the Primitive Physic*... but this appears to be a most artful evasion; for this error is in the fifth, the eighth, and the sixth editions....[186]

Hawes's criticism is justified here and this, combined with Wesley's rather hard-faced and 'evasive' response, brings several issues to light. The first issue concerns Wesley's evasiveness. It could be argued, by way of explanation rather than defence, that Wesley was not so much evasive as vague. Wesley could often be vague on points of detail. He sometimes misquoted texts, including his own, largely because he committed so much information to memory. Moving on horseback from place to place, combined with his heavy workload of writing, editing and practical commitments, meant that Wesley was forced to rely on a working memory, rather than a considered recourse to written records – though, obviously, he demonstrated his ability to do this as and when appropriate. As a result, the occasional inaccuracy crept into his work – particularly when it involved making quick-fire editorial decisions about amendments and abridgements. At such times Wesley could be slap-dash.

Wesley's critic in the *Gazetteer* was keen to reproach him on this very point, making the following objection:

> Some people *run as they read*. Mr. Wesley's whole progressive life stands as a proof that he is one of that species of readers. In that mode he hath read the Scriptures, and in that mode doth he read every book.[187]

Wesley's response to 'ANTIDOTE', which was again addressed 'To the Printer of the Gazetteer' and dated 25 January 1776, is worth citing at length because it demonstrates exactly where he thought the emphasis should be placed:

> For several years, while my brother and I travelled on foot, our manner was for him that walked behind to read aloud some book of history, poetry, or philosophy. Afterwards for many years (as my time at home was spent mostly in writing) it was my custom to read things of a lighter nature, chiefly when I was on horseback. Of late years, since a friend gave me a chaise, I have read them in my carriage. But it is not in this manner I treat the Scriptures: these I read and meditate upon day and night. It was not *in running* that I wrote twice over the *Notes* on the New Testament… containing above 800 quarto pages… I add a word concerning the former objection. I do still in a sense run as I read. I make haste, though I do not hurry. It behoves me to do, as my work is great and my time is short. For how much can a man expect to remain who has seen between seventy and eighty years? And may I not plead for some indulgence even on this account, if I am mistaken in more points than one?[188]

Evidence of Wesley's mistakes can even be seen in the statement he gave to 'ANTIDOTE' in the first instance. It is quite apparent that Wesley is unable to trace exactly when and in which edition this typographical error makes its first appearance. Hawes quickly detects Wesley's prevarication here and seizes upon it immediately. He correctly points out that the error arises in 'the fifth, the eighth, and the sixth editions'. Wesley's claim that the error had been made in only 'one or more' out of 'twenty or thirty' editions is patently untrue. Firstly, because *Primitive Physic* had only gone to sixteen editions by the time Hawes made his *Examination*. Secondly, the remedies presented for 'one Poisoned' were added at a later date to be included in the fifth edition of 1755. It is something of a surprise that Hawes did not pick up on these discrepancies. It is equally surprising that Wesley was so vague on this matter, and Hawes may have been right about the evasive nature of his opponent's response.

When replying to 'ANTIDOTE' about the 'destructive prescription', Wesley did not relay the remedy verbatim but gave an *ad hoc* version for the sake of speed and efficiency of time. The most interesting aspect of Wesley's vagueness during this debate can be seen in the way he misquotes the subtitle of *Primitive Physic*. Instead of giving it as 'An Easy and Natural Method of Curing Most Diseases', he presents it as 'A *Rational* and Easy Method of Curing Most Diseases'. It would be nice, though far-fetched, to think that Wesley's replacement of the word 'Natural' for 'Rational' in this context was entirely calculated. Yet even if it was not a deliberate move, this slippage provides a wonderful and unexpected glimpse into Wesley's mind.

Substituting this particular word is significant because we can see how it became a tool that Wesley sought to use against his 'rational' critics. The word 'rational' is a marker of credibility and Wesley's misquote of the subtitle to *Primitive Physic* duplicates, in microscopic form, the language he consciously adopted in his *Appeals to Men of Reason and Religion*.

Leaving aside the typographical error made in *Primitive Physic* concerning the dosage of verdigris, the actual practice of administering this poison (a type of corroded copper substance) was commonplace. It had been prescribed as a vomit, amongst a range of other uses, medical and otherwise, for several centuries. In terms of remedy and intended dosage, Wesley's recommendation was not out of place. This is further underlined when looking at the prescription in the context of those other remedies put forward for 'one Poisoned' in *Primitive Physic*. It is only by looking at its relationship to the other recommendations listed that we can get a sense of what Wesley was trying to achieve:

> 550. Let one poisoned by *arsenic* dissolve a quarter of an ounce of *salt of tartar* in a pint of water, and drink every quarter of an hour as much as he can, till he is well.

> 551. Let one poisoned by *opium* take thirty drops of *Elixir of Vitriol* in cold water, every quarter of an hour, till the drowsiness or wildness ceases:

> 552. Or, a spoonful of *lemon-juice.*

> 553. Let one poisoned with *mercury sublimate* dissolve an ounce of *salt of tartar* in a gallon of water, and drink largely of it… this will entirely destroy the force of the poison, if it be used soon.[189]

Wesley's use of 'verdigris' as a poison to counter poisoning was potentially very dangerous. The dosage had to be just right and this is exactly why he incurred the wrath of 'ANTIDOTE' and Hawes after the error was exposed in *Primitive Physic*. The patient needed to vomit and expel the original poisonous substance via secondary poisoning. However, Wesley was acutely aware of the danger involved when using poisonous substances, especially those 'Herculean' remedies.[190] Despite the fact that many physicians advocated using hemlock, for example, Wesley disapproved of using this poison. What is interesting about the other receipts listed above is the fact that he seeks to provide remedies for the ubiquitous so-called 'cure-all' medicines commonly used in the eighteenth century: opium, mercury and, to a much lesser extent, arsenic.

Wesley was very keen to point out to his patients that they lived in an age when many cures could be lethal poisons in the wrong hands. He thus advised extreme caution when handling any of the active ingredients used in medical practice. By contrast, he also understood that poisonous chemicals, if used correctly, could provide efficacious remedies. Boyle had argued that 'turning poisons into medicines' could advance medicine considerably, but here Wesley applied the same logic to this matter as other eighteenth-century practitioners.[191] In *A Mechanical Account of Poisons,* Mead argued that the patient who had been poisoned by mercury sublimate, could mitigate its effect by swallowing:

> [T]he same compound resublimed with *live mercury* in the proportion of four parts to three… [after which] it loses its corrosiveness to that degree as to become not only a safe, but in many cases a noble medicine… thus a violent poison is mitigated into a vomit or purge.[192]

There was a close relationship between poison and cure in the eighteenth century and this obviously reached full fruition with the inoculation of patients against smallpox. Given Wesley's strong feelings regarding the issue of exercising caution when using poisonous ingredients, it must have been acutely embarrassing for him when the recommended dose for verdigris was exposed as a potentially fatal blunder.

There can be no justification for the way in which Wesley blamed his printer for the typographical error. Wesley enjoyed complete control and authority as an editor over his own work. He had ultimate responsibility for ensuring that such errors were rectified before going to print. The writer who published under the pseudo-name 'FLY-FLAP' made this same point and joined in on the debate. His remarks were duly printed in the *Gazetteer*: 'the weak attempt to throw blame upon the printer, is as uncandid as it appears improbable'.[193] Such a dangerous error should have been spotted immediately. The defensive way in which Wesley responded to his critics over this issue indicates that he understood perfectly well the hazard to which he had exposed his readers. Yet his advice that those who possessed corrupted copies of *Primitive Physic* simply take 'the trouble of altering that word with his pen' was altogether inadequate – not least because he had to rely on the fact that these individuals were also readers of the *Gazetteer*.

Hawes condemned Wesley for not expressing sufficient grief or anxiety over the blunder. More importantly, he reproached Wesley for the triumphant tone he adopted regarding the increased sales of *Primitive Physic* that had resulted from the controversy. In a letter to the *Gazetteer*, dated 31 January 1776, Wesley issued the following statement. Clearly, this had enraged Hawes:

> In one respect, I am much obliged to the Gentlemen, (or Gentleman) who spends so much time upon the *Primitive Physic;* and would humbly intreat them to say something about it, (no matter what) in half a dozen more of

your papers. If nothing was said about it, most people might be ignorant that there was any such tract in the world. But their mentioning it, makes more enquire… and so disperses it *more and more.*[194]

Wesley was certainly very astute at working out exactly how the machinery of publicity could be turned to his advantage. Doubtless, this came from his long-standing experience as a controversial figure. But this reaction was more defensive than triumphant: it is highly likely that Wesley thoroughly objected to his work being subjected to such scrutiny and recoiled at having it brought under the spotlight in this way. This style of defensive rebuttal was one that was repeated again, shortly after the publication of *An Examination*. Here, Wesley reacted with characteristic brazenness and deference in equal measure.

In the immediate aftermath of *An Examination* Wesley addressed a letter to 'Mr. Hawes, Apothecary and Critic' in the *Lloyd's Evening Post*. This letter was dated 22 July 1776:

My bookseller informs me that since you published your remarks on the *Primitive Physic…* there has been greater demand for it than ever. If, therefore, you would please publish a few further remarks, you would confer a farther favour upon your humble servant.[195]

Wesley must have known that his terse riposte to a work that was as detailed and self-righteous as *An Examination* would have infuriated Hawes no end. Yet in spite of this public show of obstinacy, Hawes's criticism impacted upon and influenced those editions of *Primitive Physic* following the 16th in a number of very important ways. No mention is made of Hawes in the 'Postscript' written in 1780 for the 20th edition of 1781, but Wesley must have had this man in mind when he made the following statement:

Since the last Correction of the Tract, near twenty years ago, abundance of objections have been made to several parts of it. These I have considered with all the attention which I was master of: and in consequence hereof, have now omitted many Articles, and altered many others. I have likewise added a considerable number of Medicines, several of which have been but lately discovered: and several (although they had long been in use) I had never tried before. But I still advise, 'in complicated cases, or where life is in immediate danger, let everyone apply without delay, to a Physician that fears God'. From one who does not, be his fame ever so great, I should expect a curse rather than a blessing.[196]

Wesley is still quite defensive here, but the tone of his 'Postscript' is less defiant and more conciliatory. The defiant public demeanour adopted in the *Gazetteer* and *Lloyd's Evening Post* thus gave way to an act of private deference in *Primitive Physic.* Moreover, Wesley took a great deal of Hawes's criticism on board. Certainly, he was eager to ensure that the blunder exposed by 'ANTIDOTE' was rectified as a matter of urgency. It is also very probable that Hawes's scathing commentary regarding the use of 'Toad Powder', despite the fact that its origin resided with Dover, led to its omission.

Another remedy that had been listed in *Primitive Physic* before Hawes chose to subject the text to close scrutiny was a recommendation for 'Bleeding at the Nose'. This seems a trivial omission, but is worth relaying as it provides us with some deeper sense of Wesley's response to Hawes's critique. For 'Bleeding at the Nose' Wesley had prescribed the extraordinary 'remedy' of placing a 'red hot poker under the nose'. Even compared to the most obscure medical practices of the period, this suggestion strikes a slightly ludicrous, Shandean note. There certainly appears to be no medical source that can account for this remedy. With caustic wit, Hawes makes the following observation:

> The *red-hot poker* (prescription no. 83) is undoubtedly new; and I am confident no one will dispute the honour of its invention with Mr. Wesley. I shall, however, beg leave to recommend this caution in the use of it, that no one should attempt the application, who has not a very steady hand, lest the patient should bear the marks of his effectual cure....[197]

An accident of this kind could not be so easily remedied by any of the recommendations put forward in *Primitive Physic.* One hopes that this remark at least raised a smile from Wesley before he discreetly dropped the remedy from subsequent editions.

Hawes influenced later editions of *Primitive Physic* in less obvious ways. This included a more concerted and comprehensive effort to cite medical sources. Wesley took Hawes's accusation of plagiarism on board to such an extent that he backed up remedies that had been listed in the 1st edition of *Primitive Physic* with medical sources which had been written at a much later date. He therefore used the authority of Buchan and Tissot to add credibility to those receipts that had been presented in the 1st edition – some of which had been informed by his own medical experience or suggestions given to him by close friends and other lay preachers. Wesley was keen to show the appropriate deference to medical authorities in the aftermath of Hawes's criticism. In addition, he was concerned to be more specific both in terms of his descriptions of diseases and in his directions regarding treatment.

That Wesley deferred to Hawes's medical authority by taking on board many of his criticisms was compounded by the fact that he did not seek to address some of the doctor's own shortcomings. With his extensive medical knowledge gained through reading and experience, Wesley could have challenged Hawes very easily on a number of issues. Hawes's medical practice carried its own necessary limitations, while his claim to 'professionalism' was tenuous to say the least. But Wesley was not interested in debating trivial points of esoteric medical doctrine, any more than he was interested in sectarian theological disputes. Indeed, as an elder in Abraham Rees's Presbyterian Church, and as someone who loathed Wesley's doctrine of Christian Perfection, Bertucci reminds us that Hawes's attack was both theologically and politically inspired – Hawes also took sides with the Dissenter, Caleb Evans, in the political controversy that followed Wesley's *A Calm Address to Our American Colonies* (1775).[198] Wesley detested religious sects and sought instead to achieve a general Christian alliance that recognised different opinions but which was based on a union of affection and practical piety. Similarly, when it came to medicine, he wished to emphasise a pragmatic method; an approach that drew on common experience and which could be easily assimilated – an approach that echoed his *eirenic* theological stance. Like Boyle, Wesley was theologically and medically eirenic: he liked to downplay doctrinal differences by emphasising what men had in common.

Wesley's pragmatic and optimistic vision of health was grounded in an unshakable belief that the common and 'plain' man could be proactive and responsible for his own welfare. This emphasis on individual empowerment mirrored a theological conviction that man could potentially work towards his own salvation. The correlation between physical and spiritual health, albeit in the context of man's fallen state, was revealed to those who adopted a life of simplicity and discipline – a life that could mitigate original sin. In Chapter 2 the theological implications of regimen were explored in terms of its relationship to Primitive Christianity. The purpose of the next chapter is to examine the 'rational' and practical concerns of regimen and the non-naturals: what this meant to Wesley and how it was linked to the bigger picture of environmental medicine and hygiene in eighteenth-century England.

Notes

1. J. Wesley, *Primitive Physic*, 24th edn (London, 1792), ix–x; G.A. Stevens, *The Specifick* (London, 1788), in *English Poetry Full-Text Database*, [Windows CD-ROM], (Cambridge: Chadwyck-Healey, 1993).

2. V.H.H. Green, *The Young Mr Wesley: A Study of John Wesley and Oxford* (London: Epworth Press, 1963), 75 n. 9. This was in July 1725 and Green has noted that amongst other scientific works read during his period at Oxford was D. Le Clerc's *Histoire de la Médecine* (1696), G. Cheyne's *A New Theory of Acute and Slow Continual Fevers; Wherein, Besides their Appearances and Manner of Cure, Occasionally, the True Structure of the Glands, and the*

Manner and Laws of Secretion, the Operation of Vomative, Purgative and Mercurial Medicines are Mechanically Explain'd (London, 1724), F. Fuller's, *Medicina Gymnastica, or a Treatise Concerning the Power of Exercise with Respect to the Animal Economy* (1728). He also read works by Francis Bacon, Robert Boyle, John Keill, John Locke and Edmund Halley.

3. J. Wesley, *The Letters of the Rev. John Wesley A.M.,* J. Telford (ed.), 8 vols (London: Epworth Press, 1931), Vol. II, 307; L. Tyerman, *The Life and Times of the Rev. Samuel Wesley, MA,* 3 vols (London, 1866), Vol. I, 526.

4. Wesley, *ibid.*, 307. This is recorded by Wesley in his *Journal* for December 1746 (N. Curnock [ed.], *The Journal of the Revd John Wesley, A.M,* 8 vols (London: n.p., 1909–16), Vol. III, 273). Many scholars have shown that there is no direct relationship between charity and the needs of the poor – see B. Croxson, 'The Public and Private Faces of Eighteenth-Century London Dispensary Charity', *Medical History,* 41 (1997), 127–49: 149. However, it is abundantly clear that Wesley did make this connection and felt compelled to provide charity in the form of medical care to those who needed it. It is also evident from the enormous demand for *Primitive Physic* that there was a need for medical advice and information amongst the literate poor.

5. This is linked into a point made by Guenter B. Risse when he says that the growth of hospitals and dispensaries meant that medical practitioners could observe large numbers of patients, thus increasing their understanding of diseases. G.B. Risse, 'Medicine in the Age of Enlightenment', in A. Wear (ed.), *Medicine in Society: Historical Essays* (Cambridge: Cambridge University Press, 1992), 149–95. Though not a qualified physician, contact with the dispensaries undoubtedly increased Wesley's medical understanding.

6. Cited by L. Tyerman, *The Life and Times of the Rev. John Wesley, MA.,* 3 vols (London, 1870–2), Vol. I, 527.

7. E.B. Bardell, 'Primitive Physick: John Wesley's Receipts', *Pharmacy in History,* 21 (1979), 111–21: 116. The 1745 pamphlet, *Collection of Receipts for the Use of the Poor,* was enlarged and corrected to a 119-page book, *Primitive Physic,* including a 24-page preface. The diseases increased from 93 to 243, whilst the remedies increased from 227 to 725 – by the 23rd edition this had increased to 288 diseases listed and 824 remedies. Wesley's name did not appear on the volume until the 9th edition.

8. See W.F. Bynum, 'Health, Disease and Medical Care', in G.S. Rousseau and R. Porter (eds), *The Ferment of Knowledge: Studies in the Historiography of Eighteenth-Century Science* (Cambridge: Cambridge University Press, 1980), 211–54; A. Guerrini, *Obesity and Depression in the Enlightenment: The Life and Times of George Cheyne* (Oklahoma: University of Oklahoma Press, 2000), 185.

9. Wesley, *op. cit.* (note 3), Vol. II, 95. Originally the letter was addressed to

'John Smith' and formed a series of replies to six letters – 'John Smith' was Secker's *nom de plume* – though in recent years there has been some discussion as to whether 'John Smith' really was the Archbishop.

10. Wesley, *op. cit.* (note 1), x.

11. Irvine Loudon points out that very little can be known about the clinical aspect of 'rank-and-file' medical practitioners. See I. Loudon, *Medical Care and the General Practitioner, 1750–1850* (Oxford: Clarendon Press, 1986). Though given by Wesley himself, there is ample evidence in his letters and journals to show how 'patients' responded to the medical advice he dispensed.

12. Porter points out that whilst the College did little to promote medical pluralism, it was unable to restrict it. Its jurisdiction extended only to a seven-mile radius from London and it barely exercised its authority to debar interlopers: 'And when it acted, the College suffered reverses. Following the House of Lords' judgment in the Rose Case (1704), the College lost its monopoly of prescribing medicines; henceforth apothecaries might also prescribe and act as doctors'. The apothecary could practise physic but only charge a fee for medicines. Apothecaries relied on the sale of their medicines and this, in part, explains why they tended to make their prescriptions fairly lengthy. See R. Porter, 'The Eighteenth Century', in L. Conrad, *et al.* (eds), *The Western Medical Tradition* (Cambridge: Cambridge University Press, 1995), 371–475: 449. In theory, the College regulated medical practice within their jurisdiction, but provincial practice was regulated by episcopal licences. See H.D. Rack, 'Doctors, Demons and Early Methodist Healing', in W.J. Sheils (ed.), *The Church and Healing* (Oxford: Oxford University Press, 1982), 137–52: 138–9. Elsewhere, Porter argues that it was only those 'irregulars' who brazenly trespassed upon the privileges of the London College who found themselves in court. For the most part, lay and irregular medical practice was legal. R. Porter, 'The Patient in England, *c*.1660–*c*.1800', in A. Wear (ed.), *Medicine in Society: Historical Essays* (Cambridge: Cambridge University Press, 1992), 91–118.

13. S. Hales, *A Sermon Preached before the Royal College of Physicians,* 1st edn (London, 1751), 9–10.

14. Of interest here is the fact that Archbishop Thomas Secker was also a medic who had studied medicine under Boerhaave at Leyden, graduating in 1721. Secker put his medical knowledge to use by tending to his parishioners when he was a rector of Houghton-le-Spring (1724–7). This medical interest continued throughout his ecclesiastical life. See J. Cule, 'The Rev. John Wesley, M.A. (Oxon.), 1703–1791: "The Naked Empiricist" and Orthodox Medicine', *The Journal of the History of Medicine*, 45 (1990), 41–63: 43.

15. G. Rousseau, 'John Wesley's "Primitive Physick" (1747)', *Harvard Library Bulletin,* 16 (1968), 242–56: 250.

16. Green, *op. cit.* (note 2), 75.

17. John Freind, medic and scientist, gave chemistry lectures at Oxford when Wesley was an undergraduate, though there is no evidence to prove that Wesley actually attended. I am thankful to Professor Paul Kent of Christ Church, Oxford, for this information.

18. L. Jordanova, *The Sense of a Past in Eighteenth-Century Medicine* (Reading: University of Reading, 1999), 6–7. Freind's *The History of Physick, From the Time of Galen, to the Beginning of the Sixteenth Century, Chiefly with Regard to Practice* (1725–6) was written in prison – Freind was suspected of being involved in the 'Atterbury plot'. Jordanova points out that this work was dedicated to Richard Mead, who had looked after Freind's patients whilst he was imprisoned and who aided Freind's subsequent release.

19. Wesley, *op. cit.* (note 1), v.

20. *Ibid.*

21. *Ibid.*, vi.

22. *Ibid.*, vi.

23. Jordanova, *op. cit.* (note 18), 10.

24. *Ibid.*

25. Wesley, *op. cit.* (note 1), vii.

26. Locke, (20 January 1692/3), quoted in *Some Familiar Letters between Mr Locke, and Several of his Friends,* 4th edn (London, 1742). James C. Riley makes the following important point about the legacy of Sydenham and his ideas: 'After his death a myth developed about the power and clarity of his ideas. John Locke advanced that myth by consistently praising Sydenham, even though the two men had disagreed on a number of issues, such as the utility of purges, or the gathering of meteorological observations'. Sydenham's reputation was further increased when Locke sent a questionnaire to physicians throughout Europe which, amongst other questions, sought to find out about the esteem physicians had for Sydenham. Riley thus argues that 'when eighteenth-century physicians cited a mythical view of Sydenham's achievements to justify their own... ideas' they affirmed the power of a carefully cultivated effort to build up Sydenham's reputation. J.C. Riley, *The Eighteenth-Century Campaign to Avoid Disease* (London: Macmillan, 1987), 12. This is an interesting perspective given Wesley's rhetorical and practical use of Sydenham in *Primitive Physic.*

27. Wesley, *op. cit.* (note 1), vii, x.

28. B. Kaplan, *"Divulging of Useful Truths in Physic": The Medical Agenda of Robert Boyle* (Baltimore and London: John Hopkins Press, 1993), 30.

29. T. Dover, *The Ancient Physician's Legacy to his Country,* 6th edn (London, 1742), 106.

30. D.J. Melling, 'Suffering and Sanctification in Christianity', in J.R. Hinnells and R. Porter (eds), *Religion, Health and Suffering* (London: Kegan Paul,

1999), 46–64: 59–60. These physicians were known as the 'Anargyroi' and Melling shows that many were venerated as saints in the Orthodox calendar: 'Their icons with their traditional insignia, the spatula, medicine chest and loose doctor's mantle [were] seen in churches and houses'. They provided an important model of Christian sanctity and social service, 60.

31. Anon., *A Cheap, Sure and Ready Guide to Health: Or, A Cure for a Disease Call'd the Doctor,* 2nd edn (London, 1742).

32. *Ibid.,* 1.

33. J. Lane, *A social History of Medicine: Health, Healing and Disease in England, 1750–1950* (London: Routledge, 2001), 8–9.

34. J. Wesley, *A Survey of the Wisdom of God in the Creation: or, a Compendium of Natural Philosophy,* 5 vols, 3rd edn (London, 1763), Vol. I, 84.

35. Guerrini, *op. cit.* (note 8), 98.

36. Quoted in R. Porter, 'Barely Touching: A Social Perspective on Mind and Body', in G.S. Rousseau (ed.), *The Languages of Psyche: Mind and Body in Enlightenment Thought* (Berkeley: University of California Press, 1990), 45–80: 56.

37. For a fuller discussion of this see A. Wear, 'Early Modern Europe – 1500–1700', in Conrad, Neve, Nutton (eds), *op. cit.* (note 12), 251–361. See also K. Dewhurst, *John Locke (1632–1704), Physician and Philosopher: A Medical Biography with an Edition of the Medical Notes in his Journals* (London: Wellcome Historical Medical Library, 1963), 6–11, who points out that although Locke's medical practice was thoroughly Baconian he espoused an iatrochemical vision of medicine. Locke had attended the lectures of Thomas Willis at Christ Church, Oxford in 1664.

38. R. Porter, 'Introduction', in *George Cheyne: The English Malady: Or, A Treatise of Nervous Diseases of all Kinds (1733),* (Tavistock Classics in the History of Psychiatry), (London: Routledge, 1991), ix–xlix: xix–xx.

39. *Ibid.,* xxi.

40. H. Boerhaave, *Boerhaave's Aphorisms: Concerning the Knowledge and Cure of Diseases* (London, 1742); originally published as *Aphorismi de Cognoscendis et Curandis Morbis in Usum Doctrinae Domesticae Digesti* (Leyden, 1728).

41. See Cheyne, *op. cit.* (note 2), 19–22.

42. Guerrini observes that Cheyne sought no recourse to experimental proof or anatomical confirmation to support his claims: 'His work was devoid of even Pitcairne's minimal anatomical demonstration'. Guerrini, *op. cit.* (note 8), 57.

43. Porter, *op. cit.* (note 38), xix, xxi.

44. G. Cheyne, *An Essay of Health and Long Life,* 6th edn (London, 1725), vi–vii.

45. *Ibid.,* vi.

46. Porter, *op. cit.* (note 38), xxxix n. 132, I.

47. This work was explicitly Newtonian and underpinned Pitcairne's assertion of certain, rather than probable, knowledge.

48. Pitcairne arranged for its publication to heighten medical debates on the issue and advance Cheyne's career. See A. Guerrini, 'A Club of Little Villains: Rhetoric, Professional Identity and Medical Pamphlet Wars', in M. Mulvey-Roberts and R. Porter (eds), *Literature and Medicine During the Eighteenth Century* (New York: Routledge, 1993), 226–44.

49. Cheyne, *op. cit.* (note 44), ii.

50. Bynum, *op. cit.* (note 8).

51. Guerrini, *op. cit.* (note 8), 67.

52. A. Wear, 'Puritan Perceptions of Illness in Seventeenth-Century England', in R. Porter (ed.), *Patients and Practitioners* (Cambridge: Cambridge University Press, 1985), 55–99; J. Barry, 'Piety and Patient: Medicine and Religion in Eighteenth-Century Bristol', *idem*, 145–75; G. Smith, 'Prescribing the Rules of Health: Self-Help and Advice in the Late Eighteenth Century', *idem*, 249–82.

53. Porter, 'The Eighteenth Century', *op. cit.* (note 12), 371–475; R. Porter, *Health For Sale: Quackery in England 1660–1850* (Manchester: Manchester University Press, 1989); Porter, *op. cit.* (note 52); R. Porter (ed.), *The Popularization of Medicine 1650–1850* (London: Routledge, 1992).

54. R. Porter, 'The Rise of Physical Examination', in W.F. Bynum and R. Porter (eds), *Medicine and the Five Senses* (Cambridge: Cambridge University Press, 1993), 179–97.

55. Guerrini, *op .cit.* (note 8), 98.

56. S.Shapin, 'Trusting George Cheyne: Scientific Expertise, Common Sense, and Moral Authority in Early Eighteenth-Century Dietetic Medicine', *Bulletin of the History of Medicine*, 77 (2003), 263–97: 264.

57. *Ibid.*, 268.

58. Risse, *op. cit.* (note 5), 185.

59. Guerrini, *op. cit.* (note 8), 45.

60. M. Benjamin, 'Medicine, Morality and the Politics of Berkeley's Tar-Water', in A. Cunningham and R. French (eds), *The Medical Enlightenment of the Eighteenth Century* (Cambridge: Cambridge University Press, 1990), 165–93: 171.

61. Porter, in *op. cit.* (note 38), xv.

62. Barry, *op. cit.* (note 52); Smith, *op. cit.* (note 52).

63. J. Andrews and A. Scull, *Undertaker of the Mind: John Monro and Mad-Doctoring in Eighteenth-Century England* (California: University of California Press, 2001), 79.

64. *Ibid.*, 396, n.25.

65. Loudon, *op. cit.* (note 11); M. Pelling, 'Medical Practice in Early Modern England: Trade or Profession?', in W. Prest (ed.), *The Professions in Early*

Modern England (London: Croom Helm, 1987), 90–128. G. Holmes, *Augustan England: Professions, State and Society, 1680–1730* (London: George Allen & Unwin, 1982). It should be remembered, perhaps, that Holmes's work was responding to those nineteenth-century critics who exaggerated the eccentricity of Georgian medical practice by way of contrasting it unfavourably to their own age.

66. Pelling, *op. cit.* (note 65), 90.
67. Wear, *op. cit.* (note 52); Guerrini, 'A Club of little Villains' (note 48).
68. Lane, *op. cit.* (note 33), 9–15.
69. S.C. Lawrence, 'Anatomy and Address: Creating Medical Gentlemen in Eighteenth-Century London', in V. Nutton and R. Porter (eds), *The History of Medical Education in Britain* (Amsterdam: Rodopi, 1995), 199–228: 214.
70. *Ibid.*, 215.
71. Shapin, *op. cit.* (note 56), 271.
72. Guerrini, *op. cit.* (note 8), 37. Sydenham was eligible for a College Fellowship in 1676 but did not apply for it. Radcliffe was appointed Fellow of the College in 1687.
73. Non–Anglicans or Dissenters, whose religious beliefs barred them from the English Universities, usually trained in Edinburgh or on the Continent (Leyden, Rheims and Padua).
74. See note 12 of this Chapter for details regarding the 'Rose decision'. See also, Porter, 'The Eighteenth Century', *op. cit.* (note 12), 449; Guerrini, *op. cit.* (note 8), 49.
75. M. Pelling, 'Knowledge Common and Acquired: The Education of Unlicensed Medical Practitioners in Early Modern London', in Nutton and Porter (eds), *op. cit.* (note 69), 250–79.
76. *Ibid.*, 270.
77. *Ibid.*
78. R. Porter, *The Enlightenment in National Context* (Cambridge: Cambridge University Press, 1981), 139–40.
79. Porter, 'The Eighteenth Century', *op. cit.* (note 12), 415.
80. P. Mack, 'Religious Dissenters in Enlightenment England', *History Workshop Journal,* 49 (2000), 1–23: 8.
81. Porter, 'The Eighteenth Century', *op. cit.* (note 12), 413; Porter, *op. cit.* (note 78), 139–40.
82. C.J. Lawrence, *Medicine in the Making of Modern Britain, 1700–1920* (London: Routledge, 1994), 12.
83. R. Porter, 'Death and the Doctors in Georgian England', in R. Houlbrooke (ed.), *Death, Ritual and Bereavement* (London: Routledge, 1989), 77–94: 77.
84. M.M. Roberts, '"A Physic Against Death": Eternal Life and the Enlightenment – Gender and Gerontology', in Roberts and Porter (eds), *op. cit.* (note 48), 151–67: 152.

85. Houlbrooke, 'Introduction', in *op. cit.* (note 83).

86. R. Mead, *A Treatise Concerning the Influence of the Sun and Moon upon Humane Bodies and the Diseases thereby Produced,* 1st edn (London, 1704), 1; R. Blackmore, *Dissertations on a Dropsy, a Tympany, the Jaundice, the Stone and Diabetes,* 1st edn (London, 1727), iii; R. James, *A Medicinal Dictionary; Including Physic, Surgery, Anatomy, Chymistry and Botany… Together with a History of Drugs,* 1st edn (London, 1743) n.p.

87. Wesley, *op. cit.* (note 1), v.

88. Porter, 'The Patient in England', *op. cit.* (note 12), 107.

89. Porter, *Health For Sale, op. cit.* (note 53); Porter, 'The Patient in England', *op. cit.* (note 12), 110. Dr James's Powder was sold to cure the fever whilst Dr Benjamin Godfrey claimed that his cordial could cure fevers, fluxes, smallpox, measles, rheumatism, coughs and colds.

90. Stevens, *op. cit.* (note 1).

91. Lane, *op. cit.* (note 33), 9.

92. W. Hawes, *An Account of the Late Dr Goldsmith's Illness, So Far as it Relates to Dr James's Powders,* 4th edn (London, 1780), 7.

93. Porter, 'The Patient in England', *op. cit.* (note 12), 111.

94. Wesley, *op. cit.* (note 1), 116.

95. *Ibid.,* xviii.

96. *Ibid.,* viii.

97. K. Dewhurst, *The Quicksilver Doctor: The Life and Times of Thomas Dover, Physician and Adventurer* (Bristol: John Wright & Sons, 1957).

98. Wesley, *op. cit.* (note 1), viii; G. Cheyne, *An Essay of Health and Long Life,* 1st edn (London, 1724); *The Natural Method of Curing Most Diseases of the Body, and the Disorders of the Mind Depending on the Body,* 1st edn (London, 1742). Wesley described Cheyne's *Natural Method* as 'one of the most ingenious books which I ever saw. But what epicure will ever regard it? For "the man talks against good eating and drinking"!', *op. cit.* (note 3), Vol. I, 11, n.1.

99. Wesley, *op. cit.* (note 1), viii.

100. Green, *op. cit.* (note 2).

101. Guerrini, *op. cit.* (note 48), 235.

102. Dewhurst, *op. cit.* (note 37), 27.

103. S.A. Tissot, *L'Avis au Peuple sur sa Santé,* 2nd edn (London, 1765). This was the version that Wesley used and subsequently abridged as *Advice with Respect to Health* (London, 1769). The title of Wesley's abridgement was altered for the 6th edition of 1797 to *The Family Physician: Or, Advice with Respect to Health, including Directions for the Prevention and Cure of Acute Diseases, extracted from Dr Tissot.* Wesley was also very familiar with Tissot's other works, including *Onanism* (1760), *Treatise on Epilepsy* (1770), *Diseases of the Men of the World* (1770) and *Nervous Diseases* (1782).

104. Wesley, *Advice with Respect to Health, ibid.*, iii–v.

105. *Ibid.*, 43 n. *.

106. Wesley, *op. cit.* (note 1), 83.

107. *Ibid.*, 86.

108. Wesley, *Advice, op. cit.* (note 103), 29; A.W. Hill, *John Wesley Among the Physicians: A Study of Eighteenth-Century Medicine* (London: Epworth Press, 1958), 61.

109. Wesley, *Advice, op. cit.* (note 103), 29; *The Journal of the Rev. John Wesley, A.M,* 4 vols (London: J. Kershaw, 1827), Vol. II, 310; Hill, *op. cit.* (note 108), 61.

110. Wesley, *Advice, op. cit.* (note 103), 29.

111. Wesley, *op. cit.* (note 1), 31.

112. Wesley, *Advice, op. cit.* (note 103), iii–v.

113. Wesley, *op. cit.* (note 1), 71 n. *.

114. Hill, *op. cit.* (note 108), 64.

115. Wesley, *Advice, op. cit.* (note 103), vii. See also, Tyerman, *op. cit.* (note 6), Vol. II, 345. Agues were divided into the following categories and Wesley explains the division in asterisked footnotes in *Primitive Physic*: 'An *Ague* is an Intermitting Fever, each fit of which is proceeded by a cold shivering, and goes of in a sweat'. A Tertian ague 'returns every other day' and a Quartan Ague 'misses two days; coming on *Monday* (suppose) and again on *Thursday*'. See Wesley, *op. cit.* (note 1), 19–22nn.

116. Wesley, *Advice, op. cit.* (note 103), vii.

117. He does recommend it for the 'Quartan Ague', ordinary ague and intermittent fever.

118. Hill, *op. cit.* (note 108), 64.

119. Wesley, *Advice, op. cit.* (note 103), vi–viii; Hill, *op. cit.* (note 108), 65.

120. Hill, *op. cit.* (note 108), 65.

121. K. Dewhurst, *Dr. Thomas Sydenham (1624–1689): His Life and Original Writings* (London: The Wellcome Historical Medical Library, 1966), 41. Dewhurst points out that this, combined with its association with the Jesuits, explains why Sydenham was initially suspicious about this drug. It was in his *Observationes Medicae* (1676) that Sydenham identified the specific quality of bark.

122. Wesley, *Advice, op. cit.* (note 103), vii.

123. Wesley*, op. cit.* (note 1), xvi.

124. Cited by Porter, 'The Patient in England', *op. cit.* (note 12), 107.

125. Porter, 'The Eighteenth Century', *op. cit.* (note 12), 424. Chapter 5 will show where it did continue to exist.

126. John Hill was a somewhat eccentric character who, in many ways, personifies the colourful complexity of eighteenth-century medicine. Calling himself 'Sir John, member of the Swedish order of Vasa', he was apprenticed to an

apothecary before setting up a small shop in St Martin's Lane, Westminster. He studied botany and travelled the country in search of rare plants. After trying his hand at an unsuccessful career on the stage, Hill attempted to get himself nominated to the Royal Society. Failing to get the requisite nominations, he attacked the Society in a series of satirical pamphlets. Because his farce, 'The Rout', was hissed off the stage in London, Hill waged a pamphlet war against Garrick. Through his patron, Lord Bute, he became superintendent of the Royal Gardens at Kew. See, G.F.R. Barker, 'Hill, John....', in *Dictionary of National Biography* [Windows CD-ROM], (1890; Oxford: Oxford University Press, 1995).

127. Cule, *op. cit.* (note 14), 46.

128. Some scholars have described the 'iliac passion' as being a non-specific obstruction of the bowel, rather than appendicitis.

129. Dewhurst, *op. cit.* (note 97), 155.

130. Dover's extensive use of mercury led to him being blamed for the death of a well-known actor, Barton Booth, who had died of mercury poisoning under Dover's supervision. See Dewhurst, *op. cit.* (note 97), 155–8.

131. Wesley, *op. cit.* (note 1), 26.

132. R. Mead, *A Mechanical Account of Poisons in Several Essays,* 1st edn (London, 1702), 104.

133. Wesley, *op. cit.* (note 1), xvi.

134. Hill, *op. cit.* (note 108), 10.

135. Dewhurst, *op. cit.* (note 97), 164.

136. Mead, *op. cit.* (note 132), 106.

137. Laudanum could be a water-opium solution or Sydenham's Laudanum liquidum, which consisted of opium and Spanish wine.

138. Thomas Willis had warned of the dangers of opium poisoning in 1692 and suggested that it be used for serious diseases only. Cheyne also advised the patient to exercise caution when using this drug, and in this he followed his mentor Pitcairne, who had been influenced by Willis's views on the matter.

139. J.C. Kramer, 'Opium Rampant: Medical Use, Misuse and Abuse in Britain and the West in the 17th and 18th Centuries', *The British Journal of Addiction to Alcohol and Other Drugs,* 74 (1979), 377–89.

140. See G. Young, *Treatise on Opium, Founded Upon Practical Observations,* 1st edn (London, 1753), vi; A.-H. Maehle, 'Pharmacological Experimentation with Opium in the Eighteenth Century', in R. Porter and M. Teich (eds), *Drugs and Narcotics in History* (Cambridge: Cambridge University Press, 1995), 52–76. Maehle points out that serious pharmacological research into the effects of opium did not start until after 1742, when Charles Alston, Professor of Botany and Materia Medica at the University of Edinburgh, published a series of experiments within a general dissertation on the drug. As a result of these experiments, Alston disputed the theory of rarified blood

supported by George Young. By the mid-eighteenth century the 'nerve theory' of the effect of opium came to displace the rarefaction of blood.

141. Maehle, *op. cit.* (note 140), 52.

142. *Ibid.*

143. J. Jones, *Mysteries of Opium Reveal'd,* 2nd edn (London, 1701), 92–234. Maehle says that Jones was keen to list all of the positive effects of opium in order to discredit traditional seventeenth-century theories, which argued that opium acted by diminishing the animal spirits. He sought, instead, to substantiate his own theory, which consisted of pointing out that opium caused a 'pleasant sensation'. Maehle, *op. cit.* (note 140), 67. Kramer suggests that Jones's enthusiasm for opium was 'so unbounded and his explanations of the ill effects so thoroughly rationalised that one suspects he may himself have been addicted' (380). Kramer, *op. cit.* (note 139).

144. Kramer, *op. cit.* (note 139), 385.

145. J. Wesley, *An Extract from Dr Cadogan's Dissertation on the Gout and all Chronic Diseases,* 1st edn (London, 1774).

146. Wesley, *op. cit.* (note 1), xv.

147. Cule, *op. cit.* (note 14), 46.

148. *Ibid.,* 44.

149. Wesley, *op. cit.* (note 1), xvii.

150. *Ibid.,* xviii.

151. This letter was written in response to Molyneux in 1692 when the latter sought recourse to Locke's opinion on a book written by Richard Norton about the fever. Locke believed Norton's work was full of speculation and demonstrated his contempt for it in the letter, which is cited in full by Dewhurst, *op. cit.* (note 37), 309.

152. S.J. Rogal, 'Pills for the Poor: John Wesley's *Primitive Physick*', *Yale Journal of Biology and Medicine,* 51 (1978), 81–90.

153. Wesley, *op. cit.* (note 34), Vol. I, 17.

154. J. Wesley, *What is Man?* (1788), in A.C. Outler (ed.), *The Bicentennial Edition of the Works of John Wesley* (Nashville: Abingdon Press, 1984-), Vol. IV (1987), 20–27: 21, n. 7.

155. Wesley, *op. cit.* (note 34), Vol. I, 12.

156. For Boerhaave's syncretic approach see G.A. Lindeboom, *Herman Boerhaave: The Man and His Work* (London: Methuen, 1968).

157. Quoted in G.S. Plaut, 'Dr Fothergill and Eighteenth-Century Medicine', *Journal of Medical Biography,* 7 (1999), 192–6: 192.

158. Cited by Kaplan, *op. cit.* (note 28), 226.

159. Young, *op. cit* (note 140), 10. Belief that there were varying reactions to specific medicines, depending upon the patient's constitution, was common in eighteenth-century medical practice. A person used to a rich lifestyle needed to be treated differently from those patients from the lower classes.

Moreover, it was assumed that a remedy given at the wrong stage during an illness could produce disastrous effects. Tissot points this out in the 'Preface' to his tract, F.B. Lee (trans.) *An Essay on the Disorders of People of Fashion* (London, 1771): 'The cure of a disorder varies and depends on many exigencies and circumstances. It may be considered as a machine composed of many parts; if they do not agree, if there is not a perfect harmony in all their movements, the effect must necessarily fail,' xvi.

160. Rogal, *op. cit.* (note 152), 87.
161. Porter, 'The Eighteenth Century', *op. cit.* (note 12), 425.
162. Rogal, *op. cit.* (note 152), 87.
163. Jordanova, *op. cit.* (note 18), 4.
164. This section has been published as an article. See D. Madden, 'Contemporary Reaction to John Wesley's *Primitive Physic*: Or, the Case of William Hawes Examined', *Social History of Medicine,* 17 (2004), 365–78.
165. Tyerman, *op. cit.* (note 6), Vol. I, 564.
166. Rousseau, *op. cit.* (note 15), 249.
167. For the full discussion of this see, *ibid.*, 250.
168. A.M. Lyles, *Methodism Mocked: The Satiric Reaction to Methodism in the Eighteenth Century* (London: Epworth Press, 1960); M.V. De Porte, *Nightmares and Hobbyhorses: Swift, Sterne and Augustan Ideas of Madness* (San Marino, CA: The Huntingdon Library, 1974), 40.
169. W. Warburton, *The Doctrine of Grace,* 1st edn (London, 1763), 137–44, 200–12.
170. Rousseau, *op. cit.* (note 15), 250.
171. Quoted in Tyerman, *op. cit.* (note 6), Vol. I, 563.
172. *Ibid.*, 564.
173. Tyerman, *op. cit.* (note 6), i. 564.
174. W. Hawes, *An Examination of the Rev. Mr John Wesley's Primitive Physic,* 2nd edn (London, 1780), n.p.
175. *Ibid.*, 82.
176. Wesley, *op. cit.* (note 1), xvi.
177. Hawes, *op. cit.* (note 174), 13.
178. *Ibid.*, 70.
179. Quoted in Dewhurst, *op. cit.* (note 97), 148.
180. Hawes, *op. cit.* (note 174), 20.
181. *Ibid.*, 83.
182. *Ibid.*, 64–5.
183. *Ibid.*, 64.
184. *Ibid.*, 65.
185. *Ibid.*, 65–6.
186. *Ibid.*, 66.
187. Quoted by Wesley in his letter 'To the Printer of the Gazetteer', Wesley, *op.*

    cit. (note 3), Vol. VI, 202–3 (25 January 1776).
188. *Ibid.*
189. Wesley, *op. cit.* (note 1), 84.
190. See Wesley, *op. cit.* (note 3), Vol. VIII, 69.
191. It was the Paracelsians who had developed the notion that poisons could be transformed into wondrous medicines, and that poison contained its own antidote. Kaplan observes that this was the starting point for Boyle's investigations. Kaplan, *op. cit.* (note 28), 108.
192. Mead, *op. cit.* (note 132), 109.
193. Cited by Hawes, *op. cit.* (note 174), 67.
194. Cited by Hawes, *op. cit.* (note 174), 67.
195. Wesley, *op. cit.* (note 3), Vol. VI, 225–6.
196. Wesley, *op. cit.* (note 1), xviii.
197. Hawes, *op cit.* (note 174), 21.
198. P. Bertucci, 'Revealing Sparks: John Wesley and the Religious Utility of Electrical Healing', *British Journal for the History of Science*, 39 (2006), 341–62: 350; J.C.D. Clark, *English Society 1688–1832* (Cambridge: Cambridge University Press, 1985), 239.

4

Preserving Health,
or a Few Plain and Easy Rules

Observe all the time the greatest exactness in your regimen or manner of living. Abstain from all mixed, all high-seasoned food. Use plain diet, easy of digestion; and this as sparingly as you can, consistent with ease and strength. Drink only water, if it agrees with your stomach; if not, good clear, small beer. Use as much exercise daily in the open air, as you can without weariness. Sup at six or seven, on the lightest food: go to bed early, and rise betimes. To persevere with steadiness in this course, is often more than half the cure. Above all, add to the rest, (for it is not labour lost) that old fashionable medicine, Prayer. And have faith in God who *killeth and maketh alive, who bringeth down to the grave, and bringeth up.*

John Wesley, 'The Preface', *Primitive Physic*

It is easier to preserve than recover health, to prevent than to cure diseases.

George Cheyne, *An Essay of Health and Long Life*[1]

Regimen and the non-naturals

Commitment to a constant regimen or 'Rules for Health' achieved harmony, and harmony was the resolution of contradictory forces. It was the golden mean in life, hence Wesley's injunction to 'observe all the time the greatest exactness in your regimen or manner of living'.[2] By some quirk of historical fate, Wesley's rule for living here paralleled that of the ancient Methodists; a sect of physicians under Nero so-called because of their insistence on a specific method of diet and exercise in the treatment of illness.

The resolution of contradictory forces involved harmonising mind, body and spirit. The positive pursuit of health, hygiene and temperance via regimen went beyond medicine and extended into the spiritual realm of morality, virtue, healing, purity and wholeness. This was something that Cheyne had been keen to stress in the 'Preface' to his *An Essay of Health and Long Life*.

155

The infinitely wise author of Nature has so contrived things, that the most remarkable rules of preserving life and health are moral duties commanded us...[3]

Regimen and temperance were moral duties, and Cheyne asked the reader to consider the example of those early eastern Christians who lived on very little food while maintaining a temperate lifestyle. He makes this same point in his *An Essay on Regimen, Together with Five Discourses, Medical, Moral, and Philosophical*, the subtitle of which indicated that the work contained *moral*, as well as medical and philosophical lessons:

[T]here is no possibility of happiness here or hereafter, without purity of heart and life; and that the true reason of the present darkness, both in Providence and Revelation, is the difficulty of recovering this purity of heart and life, to its utmost perfection....[4]

Those who 'wantonly' transgress the 'self-evident rules of health' were guilty of:

[A] degree of self-murder... and consequently the greatest crime he can commit against the *author* of his being; as it is slighting and despising the noblest gift he could bestow upon him....[5]

'Slighting' and 'despising' the 'noblest gift' had moral *and* physical consequences for the body, which could bring innumerable agonies. Men needed to control the gratification of their appetites, passions and desires in order to 'enjoy a greater measure of health than they do....'[6]

Of crucial importance in *Primitive Physic* is its recommendation of an exact manner of living or sensible regimen. Emphasising *preventative* strategies was how Wesley, like Cheyne, sought to increase awareness about health and hygiene in a way that was cost-effective and safe. This consisted of a sparing diet supplemented by copious amounts of fresh water and as much exercise as possible, preferably in the open country air. Cold bathing was an essential part of Wesley's regimen, but another major aspect of preserving health was for individuals to keep clean their clothes, houses and furniture. Following a Priestley-esque mode of pneumatic chemistry, Wesley identified the malodorous effect of poorly ventilated houses, hospitals and gaols.

The six non-naturals consisted of air, diet, sleep, exercise, evacuations or obstructions and the passions. Avoidance of excess in the non-naturals increased longevity, and Wesley constantly preached the importance of avoiding all extremes in food, drink and the passions. Cheyne argued that the non-naturals are so called:

[P]ossibly because that in their preternatural state they are eminently injurious to human constitutions; or more probably because tho' they be necessary to the substance of man, yet in respect of him, they may be considered as external, or different from the internal causes that produce diseases.[7]

The non-naturals did not depend on man's nature but profoundly affected his body.[8] In *Primitive Physic* Wesley does not explicitly refer to the term, but the 'Plain, easy Rules' adapted from Cheyne's *Essay* cover the six non-naturals and provide the reader with an essential guide to good health and life.[9] The non-naturals are also covered in the injunction given by Wesley, cited at the beginning of this chapter.

Regimen or regulation of the non-naturals was, according to Antoinette Emch-Dériaz, 'the most potent arm of medicine' until the twentieth century when the discovery of antibiotics left it moribund.[10] The non-naturals had been used since antiquity to treat patients, primarily because physicians recognised that knowledge of the body's constitution was out of reach. Regimen or preventative medicine was the best that could be achieved to keep patients healthy.[11] The founding text for regimen and control of the non-naturals, or what James C. Riley calls 'environmental medicine', was a text from the fifth-century BC 'Hippocratic Corpus', *Airs, Waters, Places*.[12] At its simplest level, it recommended the following points needed to be taken into account when assessing any given illness: north (cold) and south (hot) winds, which were equally unhealthy, could create specific diseases; rapid variations in climate or change of season could bring about epidemics; the potentially lethal nature of marshy areas and stagnant pools of water. A miasmatic (airborne) account of disease was used to explain how and why large groups of people were struck down by a particular illness at the same time. It was thought that water should be drawn from high hills, though the location and direction of those springs was also of crucial significance. Rain water, when clear and sweet, was especially efficacious, but also potentially dangerous due to the fact that it could become foul very quickly.[13]

Physicians of the seventeenth and eighteenth centuries continued to make use of the Hippocratic Corpus, and although Sydenham pioneered the application of quinine for malaria, he utilised the Hippocratic Corpus to advocate the 'cooling' regime of fresh air, exercise and water-drinking.[14] Dewhurst, in fact, notes that Sydenham frequently abandoned drugs altogether, preferring instead to prescribe regimen and purgative waters.[15] The Hippocratic Corpus interested Sydenham because of its emphasis upon clinical observation. This inspired him to build up disease-histories, which he broke down into 'species'.[16] He utilised this to observe how particular diseases and epidemics correlated with specific seasons in the year – referred to as 'epidemic constitutions'.[17] Dr John Arbuthnot, fellow of the Royal Society and 'Physician Extraordinary' to Queen Anne, praised Hippocrates as the physician *par excellance*, because he had 'observed with great assiduity the effects of air in the oeconomy of diseases'.[18] Sydenham, however, comes a close second for Arbuthnot, and it was the 'English Hippocrates' who, 'endowed with the genius' of that ancient physician, 'left us Epidemicks wrote upon the model of those of *Hippocrates*, containing the history of acute diseases as depending upon the constitution of the season'.[19] Arbuthnot's ideas were closely allied to those of Cheyne, who had stated in his *An Essay of Health and Long Life* that: 'the air with its different qualities can alter and quite vitiate the whole texture of the blood and animal juices....'[20] The way in which eighteenth-century physicians made use of the Hippocratic Corpus found its most interesting expression in *A Mechanical Account of the Non-Naturals* (1708), which was written by Dr Jeremiah Wainewright, who believed that seasonal change was the main cause of disease.

Increased anatomical knowledge and clinical expertise during the eighteenth century meant that physicians had a larger range of treatments which could be brought to bear on disease, but a healthy regimen remained the most effective means of staving off illness. This was certainly observed and noted by Wesley in the *Compendium*:

> It can scarce be conceived, after all that has been said and wrote on almost every subject, how very little is known to this day, concerning the causes of diseases. In most cases the most skilful physicians acknowledge that they have nothing but conjectures to offer.[21]

A number of other medical practitioners thought this was the case, preferring instead to endorse the classical indictment: patient *'heal thyself'*. Regimen was one way of doing so. Following in the footsteps of his mentor, Sydenham, Dover prescribed the cooling regime, especially when treating the smallpox, while Dr Wainewright set out to prove in *A Mechanical Account of the Non-Naturals* that a 'judicious' application of the non-naturals not only confirmed health, but could actually restore it:

> And that in many cases they will prove more efficacious than the most celebrated drug... I have cured of such distempers as would not yield to any medicine.[22]

Buchan suggested that while nature could cure some diseases, nothing would cure others – in the latter case, regimen could at least offer some sort of relief.[23] Those who paid attention to regimen, he argued, would 'seldom need a physician'; those who did not would 'seldom enjoy health'.[24]

A rise in literacy levels, combined with an atmosphere conducive to self-improvement and enlightenment, meant that every man could potentially be his own physician and, as Emch-Dériaz has shown, more people were able to understand the use and application of regimen and non-naturals.[25] Patients began to feel confident about taking charge of their own health, but Cheyne, Wesley, Buchan and, in the Swiss context, Tissot, were all concerned that when it came to the issue of regimen, 'ignorance' still prevailed.[26] This ignorance was widespread and spanned the social spectrum. Cheyne lamented the fact in the 'Preface' to *An Essay of Health and Long Life*:

> I have indeed long and often observed, with great pity and regret, many very learned, ingenious, and even religious persons, who being weak and tender… have suffered to the last extremity of a due regimen of diet, and other general directions of health, who had good sense enough to understand the force and necessity of such rules, valued health sufficiently, and despised sensual gratifications… as to be able and willing to abstain from every thing hurtful, deny themselves anything their appetites craved, and to conform to any rules for a tolerable degree of health, ease and freedom of spirits; and yet being ignorant how to conduct themselves from what to abstain and what to use, they have suffered… to mortal agonies.[27]

Buchan makes much the same observation in *Domestic Medicine* when he points out that the 'generality of people lay too much stress upon medicine', instead of placing emphasis on regimen. They needed to put more trust in their own endeavours: 'It is always, however, in the power of the patient, or of those about him, to do as much towards his recovery as can be effected by the physician.'[28] As long as patients were careful and paid due regard when implementing a regimen, there was no reason why they could not take matters into their own hands: regimen was based on nature and consistent with common sense.[29]

The system of non-naturals continued to be deeply appealing to eighteenth-century physicians, even the most 'rational', due to the fact that it carried a weight of tradition and was ideally suited to contemporary circumstances. Emch-Dériaz points out that the non-naturals was a body of knowledge which could be entrusted to lay practitioners; this was not the case for the active, 'heroic', treatments: bleeding, purging and emetics.[30] The non-naturals and regimen were both preventative and curative, with the added benefit that, as a system of health, it could be easily assimilated into ordinary, everyday life.[31] C.J. Lawrence argues that concern with regimen and hygiene was 'vigorously reborn' as a health movement during the eighteenth century. Awareness of the need for public health prompted campaigns for better hygiene in towns and on the streets.

John Bellers, the Quaker, wrote numerous works about the health of towns, emphasising population density as a factor in the propagation of disease.[32] He recommended installing a constant water supply to towns, municipal street-cleaning, refuse collection and a tighter regulation of noxious trades.[33] In fact, Dorothy Porter argues, the eighteenth-century campaign to avoid disease was led by philanthropists, and we can see how these 'improving' initiatives drew on the principle of practical piety. Eighteenth-century investigators came to associate dirt with disease, and the philanthropist, John Howard, who examined the state of gaols and hospitals in Britain and on the Continent, was convinced that filthy conditions, combined with enclosed contaminated areas, led to lethal illnesses such as gaol fever (typhus).[34] Methodists also vigorously campaigned for better conditions in gaols and Wesley actually wrote and commented on the deplorable state of prisons, which he regarded as being a national disgrace. Remarking on Ludgate and Newgate he states:

> What a scene appears as soon as you enter! The very place strikes horror into your soul. How dark and dreary! How unhealthy and unclean! How void of all that minister comfort![35]

A profusion of health and hygiene-related literature aimed at the individual was part of a utopian hope that widespread education could improve the health of community and nation. This was linked to concern about depopulation – an anxiety that, in retrospect, was misplaced.[36] Wesley, like Buchan and Tissot, believed that regimen and self-medication could empower the poor to take care of their own health while simultaneously removing the dangerous influence of unscrupulous medical practitioners. In keeping with this principle, Wesley sets down the following statement of intention in *Primitive Physic*:

> For the sake of those who desire, through the blessing of God, to retain the health which they have recovered, I have added a few Plain easy Rules, chiefly transcribed from Dr. *Cheyne*.[37]

Using the chapter headings listed in Cheyne's *An Essay of Health and Long Life*, Wesley divided them into numbered sub-sections or simple rules in the 'Preface' to *Primitive Physic*. This chapter will examine each sub-section by way of assessing exactly what the system of non-naturals and regimen meant to Wesley and how this was linked to the context of eighteenth-century environmental medicine and hygiene.

Air: wide interfused, embracing round this florid earth

Whatever shapes of death,
Shook from the hideous chambers of the globe,
Swarm thro' the shudd'ring air: whatever plagues
Or meagre famine breeds, or with slow wings
Rise from the putrid watry element,
The damp waste forest, motionless and rank,
That smothers earth and all the breathless winds....

Dr John Armstrong, *The Art of Preserving Health* (1744)[38]

We have noted already the way in which Wesley sought to show how it was man's rebellion against the sovereign that led to heaven and earth conspiring 'to punish the rebels' who had sinned 'against their Creator'.[39] If the sun and moon 'shed unwholesome influences' from above, and the earth exhaled 'poisonous damps' from beneath, the air surrounding 'us on every side' was 'replete with shafts of death'.[40] Wesley explicates the eschatological consequences of the Fall, but the language he uses to explain this is posited in terms of a physical phenomenon, which could also be accounted for by corpuscularian philosophy. The air, 'replete with shafts of death', was a carrier of effluvial particles. Noxious subterranean fumes were exhaled from the earth's 'poisonous damps' and belched up into the air. This could produce fatal diseases for those who inhaled the fumes, and it was Boyle who had argued that plagues and epidemic diseases were the most likely result of 'subterraneal effluvia'. The earth's interior contained its own heat and the subterraneal effluvia were the vaporous products of a chemical reaction.[41] Both Boyle and Locke had shown that those who inhaled 'aerial emanations' could become seriously ill. In May 1666, Locke communicated to Boyle the outcome of his investigations into the condition of lead mines, where the occupational hazard of 'fire damp' was ever present. Locke provided a first-hand account:

> Sometimes the damps catch them... and then, if they cannot get out soon enough, they fall into a swoon, and die in it, if they are not speedily got out; and as soon as they have them above ground, they dig a hole in the earth, and there put their faces, and cover them close up with turfs, and this the surest remedy they have yet found to recover them....[42]

In *Primitive Physic,* Wesley suggested that those exposed to lead or other noxious fumes should cover their mouths with heavy masks or 'mufflers' so that they 'may be in a good measure preserved from the poisonous fumes that surround them'.[43]

161

Supported by the work of Boyle, Sydenham and Locke, Wesley fused corpuscularian ideas with a belief in the divine author of nature. In so doing, he was able to create a holistic model of corpuscular activity, which could explain function and malfunction in both divine and physical terms.[44] With regard to disease, the effluvial action could insinuate itself into the body's pores and chemically alter its dynamics.[45] Air, Wesley states in his sermon *What is Man?*, is imbibed through the body's pores and 'continually taken into the habit'.[46] In addition to this chemical reaction, atmospheric pressure and temperature impacted upon the body.[47] According to Riley, Boyle's contribution here left an enduring legacy over eighteenth-century concepts of health and hygiene, but also in terms of seeing the environment as a site of disease and cure.[48] The importance of Boyle's work was largely due to the fact that corpuscular theory regarded agents of disease as being chemically distinct particles. Those distinct properties, contained in the air, could provide a plausible explanation for miasmatic illnesses.[49] The neo-Hippocratic medical meteorology, elaborated by Boyle, Sydenham and Locke, was aided during the Georgian period by those tools emblematic of seventeenth-century science: the barometer and air-pump.

By the time Wesley was writing *Primitive Physic*, eighteenth-century practitioners used mechanical explanations to show how particular atmospheric conditions in the air contributed to disease and illness. For example, cold moist air brought on asthma, pleurisies and rheumaticism, while dry hot air induced fevers and cholera. 'Rarefied' dense air, such as that in low valleys or high hills, was believed to be a contributory factor in diseases like consumption, asthma, the dropsie, agues (intermitting fevers) and hypochondria. 'Rarefied' air destroyed the elasticity of the body's solids and made the blood 'viscous'. 'Viscous' blood was less fluid and thus unable to pass through the capillaries easily.[50] When using this medical model, physicians and astute lay medics could 'foretell any considerable change of season' by noting bodily pain: blood is more rarefied against wet weather, while high winds would 'forcibly press the sensible membranes whereby pains will be felt'.[51] Physicians believed that too much heat could rarefy the blood, 'putting in motion the humors of our bodies' and 'relaxing solid parts'. This made the fibres weak. Heat dissipated the watery parts of the blood and made the humors 'thick'. Conversely, exposure to cold climes toughened fibres to such an extent, that they became tense, thus creating spasmodic contractions. Cold air obstructed perspiration, constricted the solids and congealed the fluids. Fibres that were too lax or constricted created obstructions and Georgian medics thought that the 'obstruction' brought about innumerable illnesses.

Depending on 'gravity, elasticity, moisture, dryness, heat or coldness', the air could be 'baneful' or 'benign'.[52] According to Cheyne's *A New Theory of*

Continual Fevers, one possible cause for this disease was 'a severe cold wind suddenly blowing....'[53] In the case of consumptions and other 'chronic' conditions (asthma, ague, dropsie, hypochondria), the right quality of air was absolutely critical. For consumption, Wainewright argued that a change of air did 'more than any medicine whatsoever'.[54] In the case of an asthmatic:

> A dry air best agrees... he is free from his fits in frosty weather if it be not too severe. Rain when it does fall does not much affect him, but the preceding vapours do; damp houses, fenny grounds, high winds and storms, mightily offend him... any kind of smoke is offensive... in summer the fits are both more frequent, and severe than in winter.[55]

Marshy areas were the worst possible locations which produced a range of serious diseases, such as malaria, known in the eighteenth century as the 'ague' or 'intermittent fever':

> But on the marshy plains that Lincoln spreads
> Build not, nor rest too long thy wand'ring feet.
> For on a rustic throne of dewy turf,
> With baneful fogs her aching temples bound,
> Quartana there presides: a meagre Fiend
> Begot by Eurus, when his brutal force
> Compress'd the slothful Naiad of the Fens.[56]

It was from the marshy grounds that 'eternal vapours' rose, bringing with it 'fev'rish blasts' and 'copious sweats'.[57]

From the mid-eighteenth century, air was subjected to chemical analysis in the work of Joseph Priestley and Joseph Black. Much of this work built upon the experiments of Stephen Hales, who had shown that air could be fixed in solid bodies. Hales, whom Wesley greatly esteemed, espoused mechanical explanations and conducted many experiments in physiology. He managed to reconcile this with deeply held pious beliefs, and he became an exemplary figure for Wesley. It was Hales who invented an artificial ventilator to increase circulation and inject 'fresh' air into the stale atmospheres of prisons, ships and hospitals.[58] It was thought that this type of ventilation mitigated malodorous atmospheres by producing a beneficial effect on airborne diseases, such as diptheria, influenza, measles, tuberculosis and pneumonia – the latter of which was a major killer in the period.[59]

Priestley and Black proved that atmospheric air was a mixture of airs or gases that contained different properties: only one-fifth of the air was fit to support life, whilst the remaining four-fifths extinguished it. The former was referred to by Priestley as 'eminently respirable air' – later identified by Antoine Laurent Lavoisier as oxygen.[60] The following passage taken from

163

Wesley's sermon *What is Man?* should be quoted at length because in it he is obviously referring to oxygen:

> In order to the continuence of... circulation a considerable quantity of *air* is necessary. And this is continually taken into the habit by an engine [the lungs] fitted for that very purpose. But as a particle of ethereal *fire* is connected with every particle of air (and a particle of water too), so both air, water, and fire are received into the lungs together, where the fire is separated from the air and water, both of which are continually thrown out, while the fire extracted from them is received into and mingled with the blood... is not the primary use of the lungs to administer fire to the body, which is continually extracted from the air by that curious fire-pump? By inspiration it takes in the air, water, and fire together. In its numerous cells (commonly called air-vessels) it detaches the fire from the air and water. This then mixes with the blood, as every air-vessel has a blood-vessel connected with it; and as soon as the fire is extracted from it the air and water are thrown out by expiration. Without this spring of life, this vital fire, there could be no circulation of the blood; consequently no motion of any of the fluids... therefore no muscular motion.[61]

This passage is interesting in that we can see how Wesley uses the language of primal elements and mechanical philosophy to reach conclusions arrived at by pneumatic chemistry. This is no polished scientific treatise, nor is it intended to be. Wesley's musings here on the 'vital fire' or oxygen have found their place in the rather unexpected context of a sermon. Pneumatic chemistry identified 'vital fire' in the air, and Hannaway sees how a direct outcome of this development was the invention of Priestley's eudiometer – an instrument designed to measure air quality.[62] This instrument could give a quantitative measurement of the 'respirable' part of air and was used to determine healthy or unhealthy atmospheres in those contaminated environments previously investigated by Hales.[63]

Priestley's experiments with the eudiometer were of interest to Wesley, although *Primitive Physic* incorporated both miasmatic and contagionist practical applications. This can be seen in the advice Wesley gives when treating the patient with a fever:

> 337. (To prevent catching an infectious fever do not breathe near the face of the sick person, neither swallow your spittle whilst in the room. Infection seizes the stomach first).[64]

Wesley's advice here is indicative of the fact that both miasmatic and contagionist theories overlapped during the period. It was Arbuthnot, in fact, who had complicated Sydenham's conception of infection by suggesting that nothing 'accounts more clearly for epidemical diseases seizing human creatures inhabiting the same tract of earth, who have nothing in common that affects them, except air'.[65] Until the development of germ theory in the nineteenth century this was the best that physicians and scientists could do. Stench implied miasmatic disease and stench-ridden areas included fetid sites such as cesspools, drains, rubbish dumps, marshy areas, ditches, dunghills and graveyards. It was commonly believed that living near these sites, combined with neglecting to ventilate enclosed spaces, could bring on serious illness. Hence, Armstrong advised the reader to:

> Fly the rank city, shun its turbid air;
> Breathe not the chaos of eternal smoke
> And volatile corruption, from the dead,
> The dying, sickening, and the living world
> Exhal'd to sully heaven's dome
> With dim mortality.[66]

Buchan instructed his readers to avoid living near graveyards, citing eastern countries by way of example:

> In most eastern countries it was customary to bury the dead at some distance from any town. As this practice obtained among the Jews, the Greeks, and also the Romans, it is strange that the Western parts of Europe should not have followed their example in a custom so truly laudable.[67]

The advice given by Armstrong and Buchan is illustrative of the fact that environmental medicine during this period moved away from the fatalistic attitude of antiquity. A range of methods was recommended to mitigate the worst conditions of airs, waters and places. Buchan suggested that the streets in large towns be 'open and wide' so that air would have a 'current through them'.[68] As Riley notes, the environment came to be seen as something that could be controlled and manipulated: 'drainage, the elimination of standing waters identified with heavy morbidity and mortality; lavation, the cleansing of streets and public areas; ventilation; the creation of air circulation in closed quarters' were innovations designed to combat disease wrought by insanitary conditions.[69] Where it was not possible to clear fetid sites, chemical treatments with lemon, vinegar or hydrochloric acid were recommended.[70] Despite the fact that many lives could be claimed by the deathly vapours rising 'from the putrid watry element', individuals could take some action to lessen its worst effects. Along with correcting soil, drying up sources of 'watry exhalation' and retrenching bogs, patients could regularly take a 'liquid balm' or 'smooth dilated chyle' to dissipate viscous blood.

Wesley certainly believed that particular measures could be taken to counter the hostile environment. This might very well be carried out by families unable to move from inauspicious areas or who did not live in houses with 'lofty ceilings' and 'ample rooms'. Indeed, this is precisely why the 'plain' and simple rules set out in the 'Preface' to *Primitive Physic* were so appealing: they were ideally suited for every circumstance. Under his 'Easy Rules', sub-section one dealt with the non-natural air:

1. *The air* we breathe is of great consequence to our health. Those who have been long abroad in Easterly or Northerly winds, should drink some thin and warm Liquor before going to bed, or a draught of toast and water.

2. Tender people should have those who lie with them, or are much about them, found sweet and healthy.

3. Every one that would preserve health, should be as clean and sweet as possible in their houses, clothes and furniture.[71]

Wesley advises those exposed to Armstrong's 'baleful East withers', which 'sourly checks the fancy of the year', as well as others living in the 'sprightly North', to take a liquid balm or 'draught of toast and water'. This cooling regime kept the blood free from obstructions which caused fevers.[72] Arbuthnot, too, praised the use of such liquors for treating inflammatory disorders, citing Hippocrates as the authority here, in his *An Essay Concerning the Nature of Aliments* (1731). Dr John Huxham argued in his *An Essay on Fevers and their Various Kinds* (1750) that most forms of this illness, which were linked to the climate, were the result of 'rigid' fibres and dense 'viscid blood'.[73] In this, but also by virtue of the fact that he drew his medical information from personal observations, Huxham was a follower of Sydenham. He was also keen to incorporate new medical findings and sought recourse to the mechanistic language of his old tutor, Boerhaave.

In keeping with neo-Hippocratic thinking, Wesley believed that a number of fevers, including ardent, inflammatory and intermitting fevers (the ague), could be prevented by a cooling regime. 'Warm' liquor, such as barley water, warm lemonade or gruel, came under the cooling and moistening regime. Warm, thin drinks were most appropriate in this context and advocated by Huxham in his *Essay*: 'Cooling, thin, diluting liquors are necessary to supply the continual waste of the lymph and serum, and to keep the whole mass in a due degree of fluxility'.[74] This could prevent obstructions. Behind Wesley's seemingly simple rule, we can thus see a logic that was perfectly compatible with contemporary medical theory and practice.

'Rules' 2 and 3 are concerned with the same issues surrounding hygiene. However, Rule 2 expresses this in the language of contagion or infection, whereas Rule 3 is miasmatic in its approach. In *An Essay of Health and Long Life*, Cheyne had already suggested the necessity of keeping houses clean and well ventilated.[75] Wesley endorsed this by including it in *Primitive Physic*, but in his 'Introduction' to *Advice* he also praised Tissot for warning against leaving patients in rooms with 'foul air'.[76] Tissot, in fact, believed that poorly ventilated studies could account for the increased levels of apoplexy amongst scholars and the literati – apoplexy was a stroke. Buchan was convinced that 'free circulation' and ventilation was of crucial importance in terms of both preventing and treating illness. When treating the sick, no medicine 'was so beneficial' as fresh air.[77] Cleanliness was also vitally important, and this included keeping clean a person's clothing, bed linen and surrounding floor areas. If it was not possible to open a window due to living near a fetid site, the sprinkling of vinegar and lemon juice was recommended by way of keeping rooms fresh and bacteria at bay.

Fresh, clean air or a change of environment could be the best possible remedy for those suffering from poor health or diseases like fever and consumption. Wesley was a firm advocate of this remedy and frequently recommended it in his letters to friends, preachers and followers. In a letter to his close friend, Ann Bolton, who was suffering from poor health, Wesley commends the efficacy of exercise and clear air: 'You must not leave off riding if you would have tolerable health. Nothing is so good for you as exercise and change of air.'[78]

Similarly, to John Valton, one of his preachers at Purfleet, Wesley makes the following suggestion for his 'bilious fever':

My Dear Brother,

You would do well to take a cup of decoction of nettles every morning and to observe what food agrees with you best. Inure yourself to the open air by going into it more or less every day when it does not rain.[79]

Imbibed through the pores, clean air diffused life and vigour through the 'tracts', channels and fibres of the body. In so doing, it could confound, or at least mitigate, sickness and pain. Furthermore, like Robert Burton, who pointed out in his *The Anatomy of Melancholy* (1621) that clean air cheered the spirits and cleared the mind, Wesley thought that fresh air had a discernable impact upon an individual's mental health.[80]

Ironically, the phrase, 'cleanliness is next to Godliness', is often associated with Wesley, even though it can only be traced to one sermon – that *On Dress* (1786).[81] This proverb, in fact, was well used even before Wesley's time, but its usage came into common currency via Methodism.[82] It is true to say that hygiene was of the utmost importance to Wesley. He was obsessed with the ideals of *Hygeia*, the goddess of health, and this obsession was duly imparted to his Methodist followers. Wesley's fixation with hygiene can be seen in the letter he sent to one of his preachers, Richard Steel, in April 1769. This letter was subsequently printed in the *Arminian Magazine* in 1784. Wesley tells the preacher that his instructions on the issue of cleanliness are essential: 'if you forget them, you will be a sufferer and so will the people; if you observe them, it will be good for you both':

> Be cleanly. In this let the Methodists take pattern by the Quakers. Avoid all nastiness, dirt, slovenliness, both in your person, clothes, house, and all about you. Do not stink above ground. This is a bad fruit of laziness; use all diligence to be clean, as one says,

> 'Let thy mind's sweetness have its operation
> Upon thy person, clothes and habitation'

> Whatever clothes you have, let them be whole; no rents, no tatters, no rags. These are a scandal to either man or woman, being another fruit of vile laziness. Mend your clothes, or I shall never expect you to mend your lives. Let none ever see a ragged Methodist.

> Clean yourselves of lice. These are a proof of uncleanness and laziness: take pains in this. Do not cut off your hair, but clean it and keep it clean.

> Cure yourself and your family of the itch… to let this run from year to year proves both sloth and uncleanness. Away with it at once….[83]

Wesley's approach here, as elsewhere, involved a belief that the maintenance of a pure spirit necessitated a clean body; that 'wholeness' of being is reflected in the state of one's garments and hygiene in general. Yet the prolegomena to this was an on-going practical concern, and Wesley alerts his followers to the means by which this could be achieved. The daily routine entailed in preserving body, home and clothing lies in the practical instructions given to Richard Steel, and here, it could be argued, Wesley's role in guiding and transforming communities had its most enduring legacy.

Diet: bread or the herb of the field

But other ills th' ambiguous feast pursue,
Besides provoking the lascivious taste.
Such various foods, th' harmless each alone,
Each other violate; and oft we see
What strife is brew'd, and what pernicious bane,
From combinations of innoxious things.

Dr John Armstrong, *The Art of Preserving Health.*

A regulated, frugal and 'cooling' diet was, in tandem with careful attendance to the other non-naturals, the surest way to guarantee health and long life. The greatest benefit to mankind, argued Cheyne, was a 'low', 'cool' and 'thinning' regimen of water, milk, seeds and vegetables with a small amount of animal food, primarily because this could:

> Keep the *stretched* and extended bowels and blood vessels, always fuller and plumper, and in their natural *tension*... and consequently will make the secretions more plentifully, and all the functions more natural, and easier....[84]

In his *An Essay on Regimen*, Cheyne devises four 'orders' and degrees for the regimen of diet:

> 1. The common diet or regime of a 'reasonable' proportion of animal food and fermented liquor. This was suited to every climate and country.

> 2. Diet of plain, fresh animal food (white meat, not red) once a day without fermented liquor (only fresh water). This was the 'trimming diet'.

> 3. Diet without animal food and consisting of milk, seeds, fruit and vegetables.

> 4. A total milk and seed diet only.[85]

All of the above diets were interchangeable and depended on individual circumstances. Arbuthnot was keen to point out in his *An Essay Concerning the Nature of Aliments* that a constant adherence to one type of diet was not advisable and he argued that drawing up general rules about diet, without due regard to different constitutions, was absurd.[86] Cheyne, though, adopted a total milk diet for some years by way of controlling his obesity, and in *The English Malady* this experience is presented as the 'Case of the Author'. Using himself by way of example, Cheyne pointed to the danger of poor diet and stated that high living had contributed to his weight – Cheyne was thirty-two stone. Despite this, Cheyne suggested that it was wise for a person in good health to adopt diet number one or the 'common regimen'.

The advice Wesley gives in *Primitive Physic* under the 'Rules' in subsection two dealing specifically with diet, is that the reader conform to Cheyne's 'common regime':

> 1. The great rule of *eating and drinking*, is to suit the quality and quantity of the food to the strength of our digestion; to take always such a sort and such a measure of food, as sits light and easy on the stomach.
>
> 2. All pickled, or smoaked, or salted food, and all high-seasoned is unwholesome.
>
> 3. Nothing conduces more to health, than abstinence and plain food, with due labour.
>
> 4. For studious persons, about eight ounces of animal food, and twelve of vegetable in twenty-four hours is sufficient.
>
> 5. Water is the wholesomest of all drinks; quickens the appetite, and strengthens the digestion most.
>
> 6. Strong, and more especially, spirituous liquors, are a certain, though slow, poison.
>
> 7. Experience shews, there is very seldom any danger in leaving them off all at once.
>
> 8. Strong liquors do not prevent the mischiefs of a surfeit, nor carry it off so safely as water.
>
> 9. Malt liquors (except clear, small beer, or small ale, of due age) are exceedingly hurtful to tender persons.
>
> 10. Coffee and tea are extremely hurtful to persons who have weak nerves.

The influence of Cheyne's *An Essay of Health and Long Life* is particularly evident in this series of 'Rules' where some points are quoted verbatim. It is therefore necessary to examine other textual evidence to see how vitally important regimen was to Wesley on his own account.

Wesley attributed much of his robust health to having applied the tenets of Cheyne's *An Essay of Health and Long Life* after reading it as a student. He made the following remarks concerning the *Essay* in a letter to this mother, written in 1724:

> I suppose you have seen the famous Dr. Cheyne's *Book of Health and Long Life*, which is, as he says he expected, very much cried down by the

170

physicians, though he says they need not be afraid of his weak endeavours while the world, the flesh, and the devil are on the other side of the question. He refers almost everything to temperance and exercise, and supports most things he says with physical reasons. He entirely condemns anything salt or high-seasoned, as also pork, fish, and stall-fed cattle; and recommends for drink two pints of water and one of wine in twenty-four hours, with eight ounces of animal and twelve of vegetable food in the same time... [it is] chiefly directed to studious and sedentary persons.[87]

He followed Cheyne's advice during his stay in Georgia, where it was used to aid his practical piety. Here, Wesley gave up meat and wine, opting instead to confine himself to one type of food, which was mainly a diet of vegetables with some rice and cereal.[88] On returning to England, Wesley resumed his former meat-eating habits, with the exception of a two-year period when he became a vegetarian and teetotaller because Cheyne had suggested that this was the only way to be 'free from fevers'.[89]

Wesley's diet had always been uncompromisingly 'plain' and simple, largely because his mother had inculcated the importance of regimen from early childhood. Susannah Wesley described the daily routine at Epworth rectory as her children were growing up:

> The children were always put in a regular method of living, in such things as they were capable of, from their birth... As soon as they were grown pretty strong, they were confined to three meals a day... Drinking or eating between meals was never allowed, unless in case of sickness, which seldom happened. Nor were they suffered to go into the kitchen to ask any thing of the servants, when they were at meat; if it was known they did, they were certainly beat, and the servants severely reprimanded.[90]

Evidence that Wesley valued an austere pattern for living, which he carried with him into adulthood, can be seen in the instructions he gives in the letter (cited in the last section) to the preacher Richard Steel in 1769:

> If you regard your health, touch no supper but a little milk or water gruel. This will entirely by the blessing of God secure you from nervous disorders; especially if you rise early every morning...

> Use no tobacco unless prescribed by a physician. It is an uncleanly and unwholesome self-indulgence; and the more customary it is the more resolutely should you break off from every degree of that evil custom.

> Use no snuff unless prescribed by a physician...

> Touch no dram. It is liquid fire. It is a sure slow poison. It saps the springs of life....[91]

171

His mother's influence can also be seen very clearly in his sermon *On the Education of Children* (1783), where the Lockean advice he gives almost duplicates his own childhood:

> A wise and truly kind parent will take the utmost care not to cherish in her children the desires of the flesh, their natural propensity to seek happiness in gratifying their outward senses. With this view she will suffer them to taste no food but milk till they are weaned (which a thousand experiments show is most safely and easily done at the end of the seventh month). And then accustom them to the most simple food, chiefly vegetables. She may inure them to taste only the one food, besides bread at dinner, and constantly to breakfast and sup on milk, either cold or heated, but not boiled... she need never, until they are at least nine or ten years old, let them know the taste of tea, or use any other drink at meals but water or small beer. And they will never desire to taste either meat or drink between meals... if fruit, comfits, or anything of the kind be given them, let them not touch it but at meals.[92]

Wesley's injunction to utilise a light, cooling diet is backed up by the work of Cheyne but harks back to his own childhood. The advice given here has something of a Victorian ring to it and looks forward to those prescriptions given by middle-class evangelical and philanthropist reformers who sought to 'educate' working-class mothers and thus 'improve' their conditions.

Wesley recommended, both for himself and others, a plain and light diet, which was supplemented by fresh water and an avoidance of tobacco and hard liquor. His view on the use of tobacco mirrored his cautionary advice on taking opium and again, he found himself amongst a small number: many physicians regarded tobacco as a panacea in medicine.[93] Generally speaking, Wesley believed that the best rule was to avoid all extremes, adopting instead the *via media* of moderation. If lengthy fasting was to be avoided, moderation also included being mindful about the quantity of food taken and, like Tissot, Wesley praised light suppers. To many physicians this was simply common sense and Wainewright argued that a person in good health should leave the table with some appetite left: 'if either the body or mind be less fit for action after eating, than before... he hath exceeded in the quantity'.[94]

Diet, it was believed, could dramatically alter the body's mechanics. The right diet was therefore crucial in terms of preservation of health and cure of disease.[95] According to Cheyne, secretions flowed from the fluids, not the solids, and food immediately acted upon those fluids, which were then saturated and transubstantiated into the solids. Fluids were readily acted upon and changed into different qualities; hence, the effect of diet was immediate and tangible.[96] Cheyne set out to explain this process, which he called the 'doctrine of nutrition', in his *An Essay on the True Nature and Due Method of Treating the Gout* (1722):

> Food received into the stomach, is there reduced to a milky substance: the finer part of which being separated by the lacteals, and sent by a large duct into the axillary vein, returning into the left ventricle, of the heart, is thence derived into the lungs: they send it into the right ventricle, and from thence it is squeezed through the arteries over the whole system of solids… hence it is easy to observe how many alterations food and medicines must undergo, and what a length of way they have to pass over before they can reach the fibres, which are constituent parts of all the solids.[97]

Wesley's sermon *On the Fall of Man* explicates this process and echoes that put forward by Cheyne:

> It is well known, the human body when it comes into the world consists of innumerable membranes, exquisitely thin, that are filled with circulating fluids, to which the solid parts bear a very small proportion. Into the tubes composed of these membranes nourishment must be continually infused; otherwise life cannot continue, but will come to an end almost as soon as it is begun. And suppose this nourishment to be liquid, which as it flows through those fine canals continually enlarges them in all their dimensions, yet it contains innumerable solid particles, which continually adhere to the inner surface of the vessels through which they flow; so that in the same proportion as any vessel is enlarged it is stiffened also. Thus the body grows firmer as it grows larger, from infancy to manhood.[98]

The juices or fluids circulating the tubes needed to be kept healthy, sweet and light.[99] The secret to good health was a correct diet because, argues Arbuthnot, this could keep 'the fluids in due proportion to the capacity and strength of the channels through which they pass'.[100] Here, Artbuthnot repeated Cheyne's instruction that the blood ought to be kept thin and fluid. Cheyne also argued that the '*primae viae*, or the *alimentary tube*, is, as it were, a common sewer' and could therefore become 'fouled or cleaned in the various manners, and with great facility'.[101] The right diet could keep the blood thin and the body's tubes clear, and this is why so many physicians, including Cheyne, insisted that regimen was the most 'infallible antidote for all the obstinate diseases of the body' and mind.[102]

Buchan argued that although diet may not cure disease as speedily as medicine, its effect was longer lasting. He pointed out that a moist diet would 'relax' the solids and render the body 'feeble', while one that was too dry would make the solids 'rigid' and humors viscid.[103] On this basis, medicine could seldom succeed in curing diseases 'where a proper regimen' was neglected. Yet there was no reason why regimen should be neglected as control of one's diet was within the reach of ordinary patients.[104] In a letter to a Methodist preacher suffering from an illness that is left unspecified, Wesley makes the following remarks, which emphasise the importance of regimen and diet:

> My Dear Brother,
>
> Medicines, I think, will be of no service to you, unless it were a course of tarwater. But very probably a change of air might be of service… Your diet in the meantime should be chiefly milk and vegetables; of which I judge turnips, potatoes and apples to be best….[105]

Food needed to be treated with respect because it had the capacity to chemically affect the blood, solids and fibres.[106]

This explains Cheyne's, and Wesley's, admonishment to avoid highly seasoned food. Rich food contained too many minerals and had a corrosive effect on the body's passages.[107] Porter shows how Cheyne used the chemical analysis of Keill, Freind and Hales to make an analogy between natural science and the effect of rich food on the stomach. This, he posited in terms of underground sulphurous discharges and detonating volcanic activity.[108] Rich food clogged the tubes and produced all kinds of illness. Conversely, bad quality food was a problem continually faced by the poor who suffered as a result of 'unsound provisions'.[109] Buchan stated that this was a potential disaster, primarily because the labouring poor were of 'great importance to the state'.[110] Even bread, that universal and 'most nourishing' of all food, was subject to the unscrupulous practice of adulteration, and Buchan warned his reader against using contaminated bread products. In spite of its many shortcomings, the frugal and active life of a labourer was still preferable to that of the rich and inactive gentleman. Cheyne stated that the Irish and Scottish labourers' lifestyle was exemplary and suggested that their diet made the population 'fertile'.[111]

In his *An Essay on the Disorders of People of Fashion* (1770), Tissot is eager to draw the same conclusion as Cheyne. Tissot compared the tables of the 'great' with the diet of the industrious poor, the latter of which is idealised in the following passage:

> The coursest bread, porridge, which is often only bread soaked in boiling water and seasoned with a very little butter and salt, skimmed milk, butter milk… whey separated from both grease and curd, though rarely of all the milk; new cheese… with very little salt; vegetables, and those commonly the least savoury, such as radishes, beans, kidney beans, cabbages, beetroots,

lettuces, potatoes, leaks; some common fruits; rarely butchers meat, and sometimes bacon, which is only seasoned with a little salt, are almost the only things which compose the food of the labourer, attached to what is really advantageous to him, regardless of custom. His only foreign seasoning is pepper; he sometimes adds onions or in some countries garlick... his drink is generally water.[112]

Tissot is referring primarily to the context of Lausanne and there would have been substantial variations in diet amongst the labouring poor throughout Europe. Yet some of the ingredients recommended in *Primitive Physic* bear witness to the fact that Wesley would have recognised a commonality of elements between Tissot's description and the diet of labourers in England.[113]

Tissot argued that the labourer's diet prevented his stomach from becoming 'over-charged' with quantity. Mastication and digestion was a good deal easier because the simple and wholesome food taken in could fully nourish without curdling or corrupting – there was no sharp 'acidity' or 'fumes' that would disorder the stomach and bowels. The labourer's diet caused neither 'colics' nor 'costiveness' because it created a 'soft chyle', which passed through the body's vessels without irritating or 'rendering them feverish'.[114] By contrast, the food weighing down those tables belonging to the rich consisted of:

The most juicy meats, the highest flavoured game, the most delicate fishes stewed in the richest wines, and rendered inflammatory by the addition of aromatic spices; poultry, crawfish, and their sauce; meat gravies, variously extracted; eggs, trifles; the most savoury vegetables, the sharpest aromatics lavishly used; sweet-meats of all kinds, brought from all parts of the world; candies infinitely various; pastry, fries, creams, the strongest flavoured cheeses... brandy, in their most attractive forms, coffee, tea, and chocolate, are found upon their tables... it is easy to perceive the different effects of such opposite regimens.[115]

A diet such as this meant that a person constantly needed to 'excite the palate' and indulge in more than was needful. The moralistic strains in Tissot's medical essay are apparent and reminiscent of Cheyne.[116] Tissot argued that the stomach used to a rich lifestyle constantly struggled and battled against the disorders wrought by rich food:

The frothy chyle, as sharp and nourishing, communicates the tremor to the vessels; the rapidity of the pulse, some hours after such a meal, proves its effect... all the organs of secretion being inflamed; the functions are disordered, and the whole animal oeconomy thrown into confusion.[117]

The comparison Tissot made in his *Essay* served to show that the labourer's regimen was conducive to health, while that of the rich actively destroyed it. In his *An Essay on Regimen*, Cheyne also sought to demonstrate the destructive influence of rich food and sauces:

> Most people that enter on a low diet for health and spirits, entirely *counteract* and defeat its beneficial effects. I have known some men of *quality*, and *gentlemen of fortune*, who have been advised a low diet, have their vegetables of the highest and *rankest flavour*, dressed with *burnt butter, hot spices, aromatics, onions, eggs*, and *salt*; so that they were infinitely more deleterious and hurtful, than a moderate quantity of plain *animal* food once a day....[118]

Wesley firmly believed that a rich lifestyle and diet was deeply destructive and would no more have endorsed it any more than an ornate style of writing or dress. He opted instead for a plain, frugal diet, and this chimed in with a theological belief in the necessity of an ascetic lifestyle.

Temperance was an essential element when adopting the correct regimen and in *Domestic Medicine*, Buchan endorses Jean-Jacques Rousseau's observation that 'temperance and exercise are the two best physicians in the world'.[119] Temperance was regarded as the parent of health: if health depended on the equilibrium of fluids, fibres and solids in order for the body to function, it was the case that a disturbance of this would dramatically impair wellbeing. Alcohol was a disruptive and destructive influence:

> Intemperance, however, never fails to disorder the whole animal oeconomy; it hurts the digestion, relaxes the nerves, renders the secretions irregular, vitiates the humors, and occasions numberless diseases.[120]

Cheyne thought that alcohol should only be consumed under very exceptional circumstances:

> Strong liquors were never designed for common use: they were formerly kept (here in *England*) as other medicines are, in *Apothecaries shops* and prescribed by *physicians*, as they do *Diascordium* and *Venice Treacle*, to refresh the weary, to strengthen the *weak*, to give courage to the *faint-hearted* and raise the *low-spirited*....[121]

Liquor inflamed the membranes and *membranous tubuli* (the nerves), which Cheyne believed were the bodily organs of the intellectual operations: 'It is the *fire sulphur* and *volatile tartar* of fermented liquors, that inflame, corrugate and stimulate these membranes', 'this creates 'overwhelming distempers.[122] Tissot also disapproved of spirits, suggesting that they damaged cerebral function. He believed that drunkenness was a contributory factor in illnesses such as inflammations of the breast and pleurisy.[123]

Wesley did not advocate a complete ban on alcohol but suggested drinking 'clear, small beer' and wine in moderation. In fact, Wesley questioned Cadogan's views concerning wine, when the doctor condemned it outright in his *A Dissertation on the Gout* (1771):

> But why should Dr. Cadogan condemn wine *toto genere*, which is one of the noblest cordials in nature? Yet stranger, why should he condemn bread? Great whims belong to great men![124]

Wesley preached temperance with regard to fermented liquors but regarded spirits, especially gin, as thoroughly poisonous and the cause of many nervous disorders. His views on alcohol had common currency in England at the time; the healthy and industrious virtues of beer were frequently contrasted favourably to the deathly distress and madness produced by gin, as evidenced by Hogarth's *Beer Street* and *Gin Lane* (1751).

Not only did Wesley believe that wine, in moderation, was good for the constitution, but thought that clear beer was preferable to drinking tea. Remarkably, he identified the effect of caffeine and understood that it could produce unwanted side effects. He regarded tea as an expensive indulgence, but warned too that it was injurious to health. He thought that it was a slow poison for those with weak nerves, akin to spirits.[125] This was based on personal experience; he found that his hands shook after drinking tea. After making some enquiries in 1746, he discovered that others had experienced this same side effect.[126] During his initial enquiries, Wesley assumed that the people he questioned had been affected in this way by drinking hard liquor. After questioning them further, however, he was confirmed in his suspicion that tea was the cause of this disorder:

> I immediately remembered my own case, and easily gathered from many concerning circumstances, that it was the same with them. I considered, what an advantage would it be to these poor enfeebled people, if they would leave off what so manifestly impairs their health....[127]

In a letter to 'a Friend', dated 10 November 1748, Wesley argued that it would be better for 'poor enfeebled people' to leave off tea and opt for milky drinks or English herbal infusions instead:

> 1. Take half a pint of milk every morning, with a little bread, not boiled, but warmed only; a man in tolerable health might double the quantity. 2. If this is too heavy, add as much water, and boil it together, with a spoonful of oatmeal. 3. If this agrees not, try half a pint, or a little more, of water-gruel, neither thick nor thin; not sweetened... but with a very little butter, salt, and

bread. 4. If this disagrees, try sage, green balm, mint or pennyroyal tea, infusing only so much of the herb as to change the colour of the water. 5. Try two or three of these mixed in various proportions. 6. Try ten or twelve other English herbs. 7. Try foltron, a mixture of herbs to be had at many grocers', far healthier as well as cheaper than tea. 8. Try cocoa. If, after having tried each of these for a week or ten days, you find none of them agree with your constitution, then use (weak green) tea again; but at the same time know that your having used it so long has brought you near the chambers of death.[128]

Wesley realised that if this issue were to be taken seriously he would have to lead by example. He therefore decided to abstain from tea and advised other Methodists to do the same, recommending the consumption of herbal infusions instead. A consequence of this abstinence saw Wesley set up a weekly poor box, which collected the money saved from giving up tea. The Methodist Society did raise some money on the savings here, and this was used as 'lending stock', which offered relief to the destitute.[129] Some Methodists followed Wesley's example in giving up tea, although others objected to his prescriptive advice and refused to follow suit. The issue, in fact, remained controversial for some time. But Wesley was not alone in his claim about the detrimental effect of tea, and while many physicians talked up its medicinal value, an anonymous work entitled *An Essay on the Nature, Use and Abuse of Tea: In a Letter to a Lady. With an Account of its Mechanical Operation* (1722), compared tea with opium and blamed it for 'hypochondriack' disorders:

> Its operation is not less destructive to the animal oeconomy, than opium… that this drug is useful in physick, is what I can no means deny: But as a medicine, makes it very hurtful as a diet….[130]

Wesley also objected to coffee and believed that this drink weakened the digestion.[131] Tissot warned against the effect of tea and coffee, but reluctantly accepted their place in medicine.[132] Adopting a tone of medical moralism in *The Health of Scholars* (1769), Tissot argued that promoting tea and coffee had corrupted western Europe. He observed that coffee accelerated blood circulation:

> It is a foolish belief of many sick persons that their ailments are due to an excessive thickness of the blood. Owing to this fallacy, they drink the harmful beverage coffee… the repeated stimulation of the fibres of the stomach weakens them in the end… the nerves are stimulated, and become unduly sensitive; the energies are dissipated.[133]

The debate over tea and coffee continued to be controversial throughout the eighteenth century with many physicians putting together arguments that ran contrary to those of Tissot, Wesley and Cheyne. Dr Benjamin Moseley defended coffee, arguing that it thinned mucus and improved circulation.[134] Moseley wrote *A Treatise Concerning the Properties and Effects of Coffee* (1785), in which he stated that coffee was good for headaches, as well as providing the physician with a useful purgative:

> A dish of strong coffee without milk or sugar, taken frequently in the paroxysm of an asthma, abates the fit; and I have often known it to remove the fit entirely. Sir John Floyer who had been afflicted with the asthma from the seventeenth year of his age until he was upwards of fourscore, found no remedy in all his elaborate researches, until the latter part of his life, when he obtained it by coffee.[135]

In place of fermented liquors, tea and coffee, physicians like Cheyne and Tissot recommended drinking fresh water. Tissot stated that water was 'a drink nature had given to all nations', and was thus agreeable to all palates.[136] In his *An Essay on Regimen,* Cheyne maintained in 'Aphorism 17' that clear, pure water was the 'sole beverage' that can both procure and preserve health. It is 'the sole fluid that will pass through the smallest animal *tubes* without resistance'.[137] Water would prevent the blood from thickening into a viscid 'curd', which could create obstructions.[138] In turn, this staved off illnesses such as melancholy, low spirits, lunacy and madness.[139] Water was something of a universal remedy and so Wesley recommends it for the following conditions in *Primitive Physic*:

WATER DRINKING generally prevents:

Apoplexies, Asthmas, Convulsions, Gout, Hysteric Fits, Madness, Palsies, Stone, Trembling.

To this children should be used from their cradles.[140]

The efficacy of water bathing was also crucially significant to eighteenth-century medicine and is recommended for numerous diseases in Wesley's text – an aspect of regimen that will be examined in the next chapter.

The avoidance of rich, highly fermented food or drink and adoption of plain, simple, cooked food, supplemented with good quality water was the mantra preached by Cheyne, Wesley, Buchan and Tissot:

Is this for pleasure? Learn a juster taste;
And know that temperance is true luxury.[141]

Buchan argued that the highest degree of human wisdom consisted in 'regulating our appetites… so as to avoid all extremes. 'Tis that alone, which entitles us to the character of rational beings'.[142] But Wesley also sought to demonstrate that nature delighted in simplicity and that the greatest comfort could be found in limitation. In this, man's identification with the natural world was an expression of his highest, rational and moral capabilities.

Sleep and exercise: sleep early, rise early

In study some protract the silent hours
Which others consecrate to mirth and wine;
And sleep till noon, and hardly live till night.

Begin with gentle toils; and, as your nerves
Grow firm, to hardier by just steps aspire.
The prudent, even in every moderate walk,
At first but saunter; and by slow degrees
Increase their pace.

Dr John Armstrong, *The Art of Preserving Health*

Phillip W. Ott has remarked that Wesley addressed the issue of sleep with the zeal of an evangel.[143] This was certainly true and the way in which Wesley dealt with the non-natural of sleep in his sermon, *On Redeeming the Time* (1782), shows how he saw the body, mind and soul as being inextricably linked. Here, spiritual and physical health are fused together and their relationship to temperance explicitly stated. In Wesley's discussion of sleep, the importance of health is identified as being an act of discipline but, he argues, this subject has been 'exceedingly little considered, even by pious men':

> Many that have been eminently conscientious in other respects have not been so in this. They seemed to think it an indifferent thing whether they slept more or less, and never saw it in the true point of view, as an important branch of Christian temperance.[144]

The 'fashionable intemperance' of oversleeping, he insists, directly hurts the soul by sowing the seeds of desire and inflaming man's 'natural appetites'.[145] Taking a Marcarian stance on this, Wesley sees oversleeping as a sin, which lends itself readily to other sins. In his letter to Richard Steel, Wesley advises the preacher to inform Methodist followers that they: 'Be active, be diligent; avoid all laziness, sloth, indolence. Fly from every degree, every appearance of it; else you will never be more than half a Christian.'[146]

Too much sleep hurts the soul, but it also has a detrimental physical effect that can hurt man's 'substance':

> The not redeeming all the time you can from sleep, the spending more time therein than your constitution necessarily requires, in the second place, *hurts*

your health. Nothing can be more certain than this, though it is not commonly observed. It is not commonly observed because the evil steals on you by slow and insensible degrees. In this gradual and almost imperceptible manner it lays the foundation of many diseases. It is the chief, real (though unsuspected) cause of all nervous diseases in particular... By *soaking* (as it is emphatically called) so long between warm sheets the flesh is, as it were, parboiled, and becomes soft and flabby. The nerves in the meantime are quite unstrung, and all the train of melancholy symptoms – faintness, tremors, lowness of spirits (so-called) – come on, till life itself is a burden.[147]

Once again, Wesley uses the language of mechanical philosophy to explain the physical effect of languishing in bed for longer than necessary. In his *A Mechanical Account of the Non-Naturals,* Wainewright argued that too much sleep 'relaxed' the body's 'solid' parts and Wesley pursues this same line of argumentation in his *Thoughts on Nervous Disorders* (1784), where he theorises that 'while we sleep all the springs of nature are unbent'.[148] If we sleep longer than is needful the springs become more relaxed and grow weaker. The reason why nervous disorders are so prevalent, Wesley argues, is due to the fact that people lie longer in bed and do not feel obliged to rise at 4am. Relaxed 'solids' also brought about physical conditions such as 'weakness of sight', which could be traced to the intemperate habit of oversleeping.[149]

In *Primitive Physic,* Wesley sets out two simple 'Rules' in subsection three dealing with the non-natural of sleep:

1. Tender persons should eat very light suppers; and that two or three hours before going to bed.

2. They ought constantly to go to bed about nine, and rise at four or five.

'Rule' 1 is extrapolated from Cheyne's advice not to go to bed on a full stomach, but Wesley's second instruction differs slightly than that recommended by the doctor who suggested going to bed at 10pm and rising at 6am.[150] Wesley repeatedly attributed his own robust health to the fact that he abided by these rules, which he makes clear in his sermon *On Redeeming the Time.*

If anyone desires to know exactly what quantity of sleep his own constitution requires, he may very easily make the experiment which I made about sixty years ago. I then waked every night about twelve or one, and lay awake for some time. I readily concluded that this arose from my lying longer in bed than nature required. To be satisfied I procured an alarum, which waked me the next morning at seven (near an hour earlier than I rose the day before), yet I lay awake again at night. The second morning I rose at six; but notwithstanding this I lay awake the second night. The third morning I rose at five; but nevertheless I lay awake the third night. The fourth morning I rose at four (as, by the grace of God, I have done ever since); and lay awake no more… by the same experiment, rising earlier and earlier every morning, may anyone find how much sleep he really wants.[151]

On the whole, Wesley thought that 'healthy men' needed 'little above six hours' sleep' while 'healthy women' a 'little above seven', though he did admit that those whose spirits were exhausted by 'hard or long-continued labour' needed more than this. Like Tissot, Wesley knew that fatiguing labour could lead to illnesses such as quinsies, pleurisies and fluxes. Regarding his own requirements, Wesley declared that: 'I myself want six hours and a half, and I cannot subsist with less'.[152]

The nexus between body, mind, spirit and sleep was something that Wesley was keen to explicate in a letter to his niece Sarah, daughter of Charles, in July 1781:

All are intemperate in sleep who sleep more than nature requires; and how much it does require is easily known. There is, indeed, no universal rule, none that will suit all constitutions… but what ill consequence is there of lying longer in bed – suppose nine hours in four-and-twenty?

1. It hurts the body. Whether you sleep or no… it as it were soddens and parboils the flesh, and sows the seeds of numerous diseases… faintness, lowness of spirits, nervous headaches, and consequently weakness of sight, sometimes terminating in total blindness.

2. It hurts the mind, it weakens the understanding. It blunts the imagination. It weakens the memory. It dulls all the nobler affections. It takes off the edge of the soul, impairs its vigour and firmness, and infuses a wrong softness, quite inconsistent with the character of a good soldier of Jesus Christ. It grieves the Holy Spirit of God, and prevents, or at least lessens, those blessed influences which tend to make you not almost but altogether a Christian.[153]

This letter is crucially important for two reasons. Firstly, we can see that the way in which Wesley divides the issue of sleep into the physical, mental and spiritual is indicative of his approach to health and healing generally. Secondly, and attendant to the first point, when taken as a whole, this letter is representative of Wesley's medical holism. The two points raised with his niece are separate issues, which are also intimately linked. But there is an implicit Anglican anxiety at root here too: like George Herbert, Wesley believed that every moment of the day should be given over to God. He insisted on rigorous discipline when it came to the issue of sleep, and training 'good soldiers' for Christ was what he hoped to achieve at the Kingswood school, set up in 1748 for young men who wished to prepare for the Christian ministry.[154] Here, the boys were expected to go to bed at 8pm and rise again at 4am.

The perfect antidote to excess sleep was exercise, another of Wesley's favourite mantras. Exercise released the 'ethereal fire', or animal spirits, which, when diffused through the body, enlivened it. Without exercise, he argued, 'we soon grow faint and languid', thus allowing nervous disorders to invade the body.[155] Wainewright insisted that the best way to counteract weak fibres – a result of too much sleep – was to take 'the cold bath', use a flesh brush, i.e. a dry brush to rub the skin vigorously, and adopt a regime of 'moderate exercise in the morning and evening'. This, he argued, should be combined with a 'sub-acid and sub-astringent diet'.[156] Some of the 'Rules' regarding exercise in subsection four of *Primitive Physic* also reflect Wainewright's views:

1. A due degree of *exercise* is indispensably necessary to health and long life.

2. Walking is the best exercise for those who can bear it; riding for those who can not. The open air, when the weather is fair, contributes much to the benefit of exercise.

3. We may strengthen any weak part of the body by constant exercise. Thus the lungs may be strengthened by… walking up an easy ascent; the digestion and the nerves, by riding; the arms and hams, by strongly rubbing them daily.

4. The studious ought to have stated times for exercise, at least two or three hours a day; the one half of this before dinner, the other before going to bed.

5. They should frequently shave, and frequently wash their feet.

6. Those who read or write much, should learn to do it standing; otherwise it will impair their health.

7. The fewer clothes any one uses, by day or night, the hardier he will be.

8. Exercise, first should be always on an empty stomach; secondly, should never be continued to weariness; thirdly, after it, we should take care to cool by degrees; otherwise we shall catch cold.

9. The flesh brush is a most useful exercise, especially to strengthen any part that is weak.

10. Cold-bathing is of great advantage to health: it prevents abundance of diseases. It promotes perspiration, helps the circulation of the blood, and

prevents the danger of catching cold. Tender people should pour water upon the head before they go in, and walk swiftly. To jump in with the head foremost, is to great a shock to nature.[157]

The passage is interesting in that it demonstrates the way in which contemporary medical theory underpins some of these seemingly simple or empirical sets of 'Rules'.

Before moving on to his more general observations about exercise, it is worth providing some explanation for Wesley's third point in 'Rule' 8 and his last comment in 'Rule' 10. That is, the importance of not exposing the body to extreme or sudden changes of temperature – in this case cold air or water. Wesley states in 'Rule' 10 that plunging into cold water was too great a shock to the system, and in 'Rule' 8 he insists upon the necessity of cooling 'by degrees'. Cold temperatures could constrict the fibres and make them rigid; hence it was essential that the individual acclimatise to cold water in a steady manner. Wainewright explained the effect of cold bathing on the body:

> We know by experience that cold contracts, and the more suddenly it is apply'd to our bodies, the more violently it operates… the contraction of the fibres is propagated throughout the whole body, upon which score all the humours in the body, must be propelled with greater force through the vessels in which they circulate; besides that the tensity of the fibres being greater, their vibration will both be quicker and stronger… so that the blood and spirits will… move more swiftly through the canals.[158]

Exposure to cold water – or air – was beneficial for some illnesses, such as rheumatism and nervous disorders, but was detrimental for others. Contracted and constricted fibres caused obstructions and, as Wesley points out, this could lead to such illnesses as the common cold.

On those general points and observations about exercise, Cheyne suggested that walking and riding were effectual and 'natural'. He argued that riding a coach should only be for the old and very young.[159] Wainewright explained that exercise in the cool air promoted digestion and strengthened the fibres whereby muscular motion was increased, which in turn lessened the quantity of viscid matter building up in the body.[160] Exercise, but especially walking and riding, was a 'grand medicine' repeatedly recommended by Wesley, who regarded it as particularly needful for those scholars confined to poorly ventilated rooms or libraries. This sedentary life, combined with excessive mental exertion, readily lent itself to nervous disorders and complaints. Wesley reformed Methodist circuits in 1790, making them larger in area, to ensure that preachers had to travel further on horseback. This, he thought, would positively contribute to their bodily health.[161] Sydenham believed that riding was enormously beneficial for many conditions and diseases such as biliary colic, but particularly for nervous and hypochondriac illnesses brought about by study: 'Riding is as good in a decline or in phthisis [tuberculosis] as in hypochondriasis. It has cured patients whom many medicines would have benefited as much as many words – and no more.'[162]

Wesley was convinced that his hardy constitution could be attributed to continual exercise and the fact that he travelled 'above four thousand miles in a year' on horseback – a point he eagerly restated in his journals and letters.[163] Wesley also advocated an indoor 'wooden horse' for exercise if bad weather or old age did not permit horse-riding.[164] He purchased a 'chamber-horse' for his house in London, which was a sturdier version of the 'wooden horse', and encouraged other members of his family to use it regularly.[165]

Wesley's letters are full of medical advice and instructions about how to keep the mind and body in a healthy state. Exercise was one way of achieving this and physical balance led to mental and spiritual equilibrium. Like Sydenham and Cheyne, Wesley was convinced that exercise in the cool, open air could mitigate and cure innumerable physical and psychological conditions. As the next section will show, keeping a tight rein on the cause of mental affliction could ensure that an individual enjoyed a healthy body and peace of mind. In fact, there was little point in applying medicine until the 'passions' were kept fully in check. Only then, would it be possible to keep acute and nervous disorders in abeyance.

The passions: this ruling power

The choice of aliment, the choice of air,
The use of toil and all external things,
Already sung; it now remains to trace
What good, what evil from ourselves proceeds:
And how the subtle Principle within
Inspires with health, or mines with strange decay
The passive Body.

Dr John Armstrong, *The Art of Preserving Health*

In common with physicians such as Cheyne, Tissot, Buchan and William Falconer, Wesley insisted that there was a close connection between physical, mental and spiritual health.[166] This did not lead to him conflating physical and spiritual health or spiritualising physical symptoms. Whilst the opening sections of 'The Preface' acknowledged man's post-lapsarian condition, this acknowledgement was perfectly in keeping with many other eighteenth-century medical manuals, and *Primitive Physic* offers nothing but practical solutions to physical symptoms in the main text. Moreover, Wesley's recommendation of prayer in 'The Preface', like that of Cheyne in *An Essay of Health and Long Life*, also contains a 'rationale'. The following injunction is 'Rule' 5 under subsection six, which deals with 'The Passions':

> The love of God, as it is the sovereign remedy of all miseries, so in particular it effectually prevents all the bodily disorders the passions introduce, by keeping the passions themselves within due bounds. And by the unspeakable joy and perfect calm, serenity, and tranquility it gives the mind, it becomes the most powerful of all the means of health and long life.[167]

The sentiment expressed here by Wesley has given rise to a great deal of confusion and has led to him being accused of spiritualising healing in a Puritanical fashion.

There is no doubt that Wesley, like Cheyne, believed in and commented on the curative powers of faith and prayer. Wesley's *Journal* is shot-through with statements endorsing this belief. However, what is striking about the passage from *Primitive Physic* is its rational basis. This 'Rule' is the very last piece of advice Wesley gives in 'The Preface' and in it he is not suggesting that prayer will overturn or cure physical diseases. Although his belief in the power of prayer is made explicit in the suggestion that the love of God is a 'sovereign remedy' for 'all miseries', this in its particulars is posited in terms of providing comfort and tranquillity to the mind. 'Keeping the passions' within 'due bounds' via prayer or faith could bring relief to a troubled individual, and this had a perceptible effect on the body. Wesley makes this clear in the rest of his 'Rules' concerning 'The Passions':

> 1. *The passions* have a greater influence on health, than most people are aware of.

> 2. All violent and sudden passions dispose to, or actually throw people into acute diseases.

> 3. The slow and lasting passions, such as grief and hopeless love, bring on chronical diseases.

> 4. Till the passion, which caused the disease is calmed, medicine is applied in vain.[168]

Re-reading 'Rule' 5 in the light of these rules means that it becomes easy to see how it fits into a more 'rational' mode of existence. Other physicians, such as Buchan, also promoted the power of prayer, faith and forgiveness. Buchan suggested that these qualities added 'to our own ease, health and felicity'.[169] Furthermore, 'true religion', as opposed to that which could evoke religious melancholy, inspired peace of mind.[170] Buchan was adamant that 'nothing tends so much to the health of the body as a constant tranquillity of mind'.[171]

The relationship between mind, body and soul, though tentative and implicit in 'The Preface' to *Primitive Physic*, is shown to be inviolable in Wesley's sermons, letters and journals. His oft-quoted journal entry for May 1759 demonstrates a holistic approach to healing, but also Wesley's impatience with medical orthodoxy:

> Reflecting today on the case of a poor woman who had continual pain in her stomach, I could not but remark the inexcusable negligence of most physicians in cases of this nature. They prescribe drug upon drug, without knowing a jot of the matter concerning the root of the disorder. And without knowing this, they cannot cure, though they can murder the patient. Whence came the woman's pain (which she would never have told had she never been questioned about it)? From fretting for the death of her son. And what availed medicines while the fretting continued? Why then, do not all physicians consider how far bodily disorders are caused or influenced by the mind, and in those cases which are utterly out of their sphere, call in the assistance of a minister....[172]

Wesley does not condemn physicians for failing to adopt a more holistic method in such cases, only for their reluctance to 'call in the assistance of a minister....' This is indicative of the fact that Wesley made a distinction between what was within the remit of medical orthodoxy and exactly what duties pertained to the clergy.[173] In those cases where a psychological or spiritual component came into play, Wesley considered himself wholly suited to the task of spiritual counsel: he was first and foremost a minister, though he was also in a position to dispense medicine in an orthodox manner when this was required.

What becomes apparent when reading Wesley's journal and letters is his ability to judge exactly which method was required. This he did on a case-by-case basis, switching from the mode of minister to physician as circumstances dictated. There are repeated instances of this in the *Journal*, where he judges each case on its own merits before deciding whether an individual is suffering from a physical, psychological or spiritual disorder. On those rare occasions in the early journals where Wesley is genuinely uncertain about the psychological or spiritual roots of an 'enthusiastic' episode, he makes no judgement, opting instead to report the incident factually and leaving it for his reader to decide. This can be seen in the following extract taken from his *Journal*, for January 1739, where he describes an encounter with a 'French prophet' – a woman of twenty-five.

187

The passage highlights Wesley's ambiguity on whether such episodes could be considered authentic:

> She leaned back on her chair, and seemed to have strong workings in her breast, with deep sighings intermixed. Her head, and hands, and, by turns, every part of her body, seemed also to be in a kind of convulsive motion. This continued about ten minutes, till… she began to speak (though the workings, sighings and contortions of her body, were so intermixed with her words, that she seldom spoke half a sentence together)… two or three of our company were much affected, and believed she spoke by the Spirit of God. But this was in no wise clear to me. The motion might be either hysterical or artificial… but I let the matter alone; knowing this, that 'if it be not of God, it will come to nought'.[174]

Despite the fact that Wesley worked from a holistic and theological perspective, and clearly believed in faith healing, he never became super-spiritual about sickness. Most of the time Wesley took a pragmatic approach, and this is evident in a journal entry for January 1779 where he gives an account of the time he visited a sick woman:

> I visited a young woman in such a terrible fit as I scarce ever saw before; and she was hardly out of one when she fell into another, so that it seemed she must soon lose her reason, if not her life; but Dr. Wilson in one or two days' time restored her to perfect health.[175]

Wesley was able to remain completely objective about sickness, even when he was asked to advise friends and family about particular diseases. Writing to his niece, Sarah, in March 1788 about the ill health of his brother Charles, Wesley made the following suggestions:

> My Dear Sally,

> When my appetite was entirely gone, so that all I could take at dinner was a roasted turnip, it was restored in a few days by riding out daily, after taking ten drops of elixir of vitriol in a glass of water. It is highly probable that this would have the same effect in my brother's case. But in the meantime I wish he would see Dr. Whitehead. I am persuaded that there is not such another physician in England; although (to confound human wisdom) he does not know how to cure his own wife.

> He must lie in bed as little as possible in the daytime; otherwise it will hinder his sleeping at night.

Now, Sally, tell your brothers from me that their tenderly respectful behaviour to their father… will be the best cordial for him under heaven. I know not but they may save his life thereby.[176]

This letter is particularly informative because Wesley advises treating the illness using a mixture of medicine and regimen – the latter of which includes keeping the passions under control and the mind free from worry. It is also interesting to note that Wesley has judged and assumed his brother's illness to be a purely physical matter to be dealt with in a fairly orthodox manner. Presumably, it is to his brother Charles, fellow Methodist founder, and in some ways even more deeply evangelical than John, that Wesley could have given nothing but spiritual counsel. The fact that he does not respond in this way is notable in itself.

The approach that Wesley takes with his friend Alexander Knox is somewhat different. Here, health is explained in the full-blooded theological and holistic language of 'inward and outward' health.[177] Furthermore, Wesley repeatedly offered Knox, who seemed to be labouring under some sort of psychological distress, both spiritual and medical counsel:

Dear Alleck,

[…] It will be a double blessing if you give yourself up to the Great Physician, that He may heal soul and body together. And unquestionably this is His design. He wants to give you and my dear Mrs. Knox both inward and outward health. And why not now? Surely all things are ready: believe, and receive the blessing. There can be no doubt but your bodily disorder greatly affects your mind. Be careful to prevent the disease by diet rather than physic. Look up, and wait for happy days![178]

Maddox has argued that Wesley was convinced that 'milder' forms of emotional stress or depression were 'authentic responses to spiritual realities'; particularly 'nervous lowness', which was God's way of indicating to an individual that they were not living as He would like them to be. By contrast, he also reminded followers that spiritual lowness was not always spiritual in essence and might reflect other diseases, fatigue or poverty.[179] Wesley assessed each individual's symptoms before deciding the origin of an illness, but even when he felt that a condition was spiritual in its basis, his letters usually recommend that the person apply regimen, medicine and faith. Ott thus notes that Wesley consistently underscored the interdependence of mind, body and soul. Here, he followed in the footsteps of Sydenham who believed that the mind could bring about substantial changes to the body.[180] Using the imagery and language of Cheyne's *An Essay of Health and Long Life*, but also *The English Malady*, Wesley argues in his

189

sermon, *The Fall of Man*, that although mind, body and soul were different substances, all were deeply interconnected. Thinking was not an 'act of pure spirit; but the act of spirit connected with the body, and play[ed] upon a set of material keys'.[181] Keeping to the analogy of musician in his sermon *Heavenly Treasure in Earthen Vessels* (1790), Wesley points out that

> If these instruments, by which the soul works, are disordered, the soul itself must be hindered in its operations. Let a musician be ever so skilful, he will make but poor music if his instrument be out of tune.[182]

When using the analogy of music Wesley alluded to Cheyne's *Essay*, but more specifically, *The English Malady*, where Cheyne had stated that

> The intelligent Principle, or Soul, resides somewhere in the Brain, where all the Nerves, or Instruments of Sensation terminate, like a *Musician* in a finely fram'd and well-tun'd Organ-Case; that these Nerves are like *Keys*, which, being struck on or touch'd, convey the Sound and Harmony to this sentient Principle, or *Musician*.[183]

According to Cheyne, emotional stress and intellectual fatigue weakened the nerves because body, mind and nerves were intimately connected.[184] Violent and sudden passions could stir up acute illnesses, while the 'slow and lasting passions' brought about chronic diseases. The general causes of nervous disorders, outlined in *The English Malady*, were:

1. Want or Excess of Humidity in the Solids.
2. Concretions of Salts.
3. The Interruption of Interception of the Vibrations of the Nerves by the Viscidity of the Juices.
4. The Weakness or Laxity of their Tone.[185]

The mind had a tangible effect on the body, but it was also the case that bodily disorder had a direct impact and a negative effect on the mind.[186] Hence, Cheyne argued, nervous disorders proceeded from glandular distempers (scrophulous or scorbutical) and 'knotted glands in the mesentery or guts'. A major contributory factor to nervous illness was 'a vitious liver or spleen'.[187] The cause of chronic nervous distempers were divided into three and attributed to:

1. A Sizyness or Viscidity in the Fluids.
2. A Sharpness or Corrosive Quality in the Fluids.
3. A Laxity or Want of due Tone in the Fibres or Nerves.[188]

Possessing a nervous illness in Georgian England was akin to owning a fashion accessory and Cheyne believed that England was suffering from an epidemic of such disorders. He linked this to the civilising processes of increased wealth and luxury, but also the particular climatic conditions in Britain, which made this a peculiarly *English* malady. This epidemic generated a great deal of literature, which expounded upon the various reasons for and ways to treat nervous disorders. For all of the literature generated, however, many physicians took a rather empirical stance on exactly how mind, body and soul interacted. Buchan acknowledged that the passions had tremendous influence on disease, but how the mind

> Acts upon matter, will in all probability, ever remain a secret. It is sufficient for us to know that there is established a reciprocal influence betwixt the mental and corporeal parts, and that whatever disorders the one, likewise effects the other.[189]

Buchan's position here is reminiscent of 'Proposition II' and subsequent 'Scholium' contained in Chapter VI, ('Of the Passions'), of Cheyne's *An Essay of Health and Long Life*:

> Proposition II. The union of these two principles [body and soul] in the compound... seems to consist in laws pre-established by the author of Nature, in the communications between bodies and spirits....

> Scholium. These laws of the actions of the soul on the body, and of the body upon the soul, are never known to us, but by their *effects*; as the laws of Nature in the actions of bodies upon one another, were first discovered by experiment and afterwards reduced into general propositions.[190]

Wesley, like Buchan, believed that anger hurried the blood and disordered the animal spirits and mind. William Falconer, an esteemed medic who had been elected physician to Bath General Hospital, argued in his *A Dissertation on the Influence of the Passions upon Disorders of the Body* (1772) that anger promoted perspiration and increased the pulse rate, which 'forced out some of the nervous juices'. This in turn produced a loss of strength: 'the sudden relaxation succeeding an overstrained exertion produces such a loss of tone, as the system cannot recover'.[191] This gave rise to acute diseases such as fever, epileptic fits, the iliac passion and even death. Contrary to the negative effect produced by anger, Falconer also suggested that it was a positive emotion, which had the potential to remove gout and palsy.[192]

Generally, it was best to avoid slow passions like resentment, fear, anxiety and grief, which led to chronic illness and had a wasting effect on the body. Fear and anxiety depressed the spirits, while sudden fear led to convulsive conditions. According to Falconer, fear rendered the pulse weak and this was why frightened individuals were usually pale and shivery. Fear gave rise to illnesses such as melancholy, apoplexy and insanity.[193] Yet Falconer also suggested that fear was a perfect remedy for conditions like haemorrhages and he made a rather 'unorthodox' recommendation to stop bleeding:

> A live toad, hung about the neck, is a noted remedy among the lower kind of people for a bleeding at the nose, and it is not improbable that the sentiments of aversion, dread and horror, impressed by such an odious contact, may act as a powerful sedative, and of course be serviceable in the disease by diminishing the force of circulation.[194]

As a member of the Royal College and Fellow of the Royal Society, Falconer's pedigree as a physician cannot be questioned. Yet one can imagine the sort of reaction Wesley would have received had he made such a suggestion in *Primitive Physic*.[195]

According to Buchan, grief was the most destructive of all the passions because its effect was permanent: 'it sinks deep into the mind' and generally proved fatal.[196] Wesley's castigation of the medical profession for neglecting to see that the 'poor woman… had continual pain in her stomach' because she was grieving for the death of her son might have been unfair. Clearly some physicians took disorders of the mind, such as grief, into account when making their diagnosis. Falconer, in fact, believed that grief was the most debilitating of all the passions; its protracted nature diminished bodily strength and perspiration (heat and circulation), which caused obstructions. Falconer, like Wesley, also pointed out that very few physicians paid attention to the relationship between mind, body and soul. In his *Dissertation* Falconer singles out Buchan for praise on the matter:

> Dr Buchan must indeed be excepted, as his directions expressly comprehend this article, and are, it must be acknowledged, very proper and judicious.[197]

Given Wesley's view that the passions should be kept within due bounds, it is even more ironic that he should have been dismissed as an 'enthusiastic' madman, responsible for encouraging those nervous disorders associated with religious extremism. Wesley, like many of his contemporaries, regarded the emotional excesses of religious convulsions, hysteria and ecstasies with suspicion. The more extraordinary claims of his followers were included in the *Journal*, but Rack makes two valuable and interesting points on this matter. The inclusion of 'enthusiastic' episodes in the *Journal* should be linked to Wesley's empiricist cast of mind: he accepted some of the claims as being true because he believed in the validity of individual testimony and common honesty. Related to this is Rack's second point. Wesley's *Journal*, he says, fits into that Puritan tradition in which journals and diaries are intended to be an inspirational aid to spiritual self-development.[198]

Wesley's sermon *On The Nature of Enthusiasm* made plain his distrust of the 'inward light' and he condemned this as a Quaker doctrine: 'Trust not in visions or dreams; in sudden impressions or strong impulses of any kind'.[199] He cautioned his hearers not to suppose that dreams and visions were directly from God and refused to admit to enthusiasm himself. Like Dr Johnson, Wesley genuinely feared the effect of real enthusiasm, which could potentially create a 'many-headed monster'.[200] Evidence of Wesley's dislike for excessive displays of emotion can be seen in his response to those 'enthusiastic' elements within the Methodist movement: action was swiftly taken to expel them from the societies. Furthermore, Wesley's demeanour in the presence of violent mobs, combined with his quiet, orderly lifestyle, and classical style of writing, belie descriptions of him as wild enthusiast – the *Calm* address and *Appeals* to men of reason are prime examples of his self-consciously measured style. This method grew out of a disciplined approach and it was his mode of existence.

It is easy to see why regimen and environmental medicine was so appealing to Wesley: it fitted into a Lockean epistemology and was compatible with the neo-Hippocratic writings of Sydenham, but also those of contemporary medical practitioners, such as Arthbuthnot.[201] It could very easily be combined with the mechanical philosophy of Boyle, Cheyne and Wainewright. More important, however, was the fact that Wesley could put the theory and method of regimen to theological and practical use. The moral and ascetic values attached to regimen by the Primitive Christians meant that Wesley was able to draw a direct parallel between physical and spiritual health as and when appropriate. In so doing, he provided his contemporaries with practical solutions to real and pressing problems while simultaneously offering them a glimpse of what could be attained when living the good and holy life.

An indication of how Wesley brought the physical and moral aspects of regimen together can be seen in the concrete example of the daily routine at Kingswood school. This regimen brought a pattern of moral instruction found in Locke's *Thoughts Concerning Education* (1693) together with neo-Hippocratic principles and the system of non-naturals. It was also reminiscent of Wesley's childhood at Epworth rectory. Underpinning the regimen at Kingswood was a pattern of early Christianity to which those seeking the common life of Christ should aspire and conform. Like Locke, Wesley believed that regimen could be used in a school environment in the same way as it was used to complement medicine. The purpose of regimen was educative and could teach individuals how to mitigate and correct the worst aspects of human nature. Wesley makes this clear when he cites an extract from William Law's *A Serious Call to a Devout and Holy Life* (1728) in his sermon *On the Education of Children*. The Lockean principles in Law's work are evident in the following passage:

> And as the only end of a physician is to restore nature to its own state, so the only end of education is to restore our rational nature to its proper state. Education therefore is to be considered as reason borrowed at second hand, which is, as far as it can, to supply the loss of original perfection. And as physic may justly be called the art of restoring health, so education should be considered in no other light than as the art of recovering to man his rational perfection.... And it is as reasonable to expect and require all this benefit from a Christian education as to require that physic should strengthen all that is right in our nature and remove all our diseases.[202]

The regimen at Kingswood was suitably austere, and the accommodation here was spartan. A typical day at the school would have seen the pupils undergoing the following regimen.[203] They rose and went to bed early. Between 4 and 5am, students were engaged in private reading and singing – the older boys used this time to meditate and pray. The time between 5 and 6am was spent working in the garden, walking or undertaking music practice, after which breakfast was served. Breakfast consisted of milk porridge or gruel. School hours started at 7am and the pupils spent the first part of the morning learning languages. From 9 to 11am elementary subjects, such as arithmetic and writing, were taken until it was time to take physical exercise or manual work.

At noon a very simple lunch was served, and here the menu ran to a fairly strict timetable: roast beef on Sunday, minced meat and apple dumplings on Monday, boiled mutton on Tuesday, vegetables with dumplings on Wednesday, boiled mutton or beef on Thursday and vegetables with dumplings on Friday. Bacon and vegetables were served on Saturday. Schmidt points out that fish was notably absent from this menu, though he does not say why this might be so.[204] Undoubtedly this was due to the fact that Cheyne had specifically informed the reader in his *An Essay of Health and Long Life* that fish and seafood were particularly difficult to digest, due to their 'salt element'.[205] Water was the only permitted drink and pupils were not allowed to eat or drink between meals. On Fridays, the pupils were encouraged to fast until 3pm, though this was not compulsory. School commenced again at 1pm with more language learning until 4pm. Other subjects were taught until 5pm, when private prayers began. Before supper at 6.30pm, a short period of time was given over to physical exercise. Supper was the lightest of meals, consisting of bread and butter with cheese. At 7pm, evening worship took place before bed at 8pm.

Regimen, or a few plain and easy rules, governed Kingswood as it had Wesley's life from early childhood. Regimen consisted of the golden rules that could lead to a happy and holy life. Small wonder that Wesley should write in such an animated fashion to his mother extolling the virtues of Cheyne's *Essay* in 1724. Cheyne's 'Rules' were immediately recognisable to him and he regarded it as an appropriate duty to extrapolate and include them in *Primitive Physic*. Regimen was Wesley's lifelong partner and he remarked in 1776, when seventy-three, that he was able to preach as well as he had at the age of twenty-three. This he attributed to regimen, which had been aided by the grace of God:

> What natural means has God used, to produce so wonderful an effect? 1. Continual exercise and change of air, by travelling above four thousand miles in a year. 2. Constant rising at four. 3. The ability, if ever I want, to sleep immediately. 4. Never losing a night's sleep in my life. 5. Two violent fevers and two deep consumptions. These, it is true, were rough medicines; but they were of admirable service, causing my flesh to come again as the flesh of a little child. May I add lastly, evenness of temper? I feel and grieve, but by the grace of God, I fret at nothing.[206]

Wesley complemented his use of regimen and the non-naturals with a cautious and empirically based approach to medicine. The way that he treated those illnesses which dogged eighteenth-century life, illnesses from which he himself suffered, is the subject of the next and final chapter.

Notes

1. J. Wesley, *Primitive Physic*, 24th edn (London, 1792), i; G. Cheyne, *An Essay of Health and Long Life*, 6th edn (London 1725), n.p. ('Contents Page').
2. Wesley, *ibid.*, xi.
3. Cheyne, *op. cit.* (note 1), 3.
4. G. Cheyne, *An Essay on Regimen, Together with Five Discourses, Medical, Moral, and Philosophical: Serving to Illustrate the Principles and Theory of Philosophical Medicine, and Point Out Some of its Moral Consequences,* 1st edn (London, 1740), vi.
5. Cheyne, *op. cit.* (note 1), 3.
6. *Ibid.,* 120.
7. *Ibid.,* 2.
8. A. Emch-Dériaz, 'The Non-Naturals Made Easy', in R. Porter (ed.), *The Popularization of Medicine 1650–1850* (London: Routledge, 1992), 134–59: 134.
9. Wesley, *op. cit.* (note 1), xi; P.W. Ott, 'Medicine as Metaphor: John Wesley on Therapy of the Soul', *Methodist History,* 33 (1995), 178–91: 187.

10. Emch-Dériaz, *op. cit.* (note 8), 134.

11. *Ibid.*, 135.

12. J.C. Riley, *The Eighteenth-Century Campaign to Avoid Disease* (London: Macmillan, 1987), 151; C. Hannaway, 'Environment and Miasmata', in W.F. Bynum and R. Porter (eds), *Companion Encyclopedia of the History of Medicine*, 2 vols. (London: Routledge, 1993), Vol. I, 292–308.

13. Hannaway argues that this Hippocratic concept of an atmospheric constitution continued to be used until the discovery of germ theory in the nineteenth century. Hannaway, *op. cit.* (note 12), Vol. I, 293–4.

14. J.C. Kramer, 'Opium Rampant: Medical Use, Misuse, and Abuse in Britain and the West in the Seventeenth and Eighteenth Centuries', *British Journal of Addiction to Alcohol and Other Drugs,* 74 (1979), 377–89: 382. Quinine had no cooling, heating or purging action.

15. K. Dewhurst, *Dr Thomas Sydenham (1624–1689): His Life and Original Writings* (London: Wellcome Historical Medical Library, 1966), 59.

16. *Ibid.*, 60.

17. Sydenham studied the London epidemics between 1661 and 1675. In this time he identified five periods: (i) 1661–4, (ii) 1665–6, (iii) 1667–9 (iv) 1670–72 (v) 1673–5. Each of these periods was characterised by an 'epidemic constitution': (i) intermittent fever and continued fever, (ii) plague, (iii) smallpox and variolous fever, (iv) dysentery, causing cholera and diarrhoea, (v) influenza. For a full explication of this see Dewhurst, *op. cit.* (note 15), 60.

18. J. Arbuthnot, *An Essay Concerning the Effects of Air on Human Bodies,* 1st edn (London, 1733), vii.

19. *Ibid.*, viii.

20. Cheyne, *op. cit.* (note 1), 3.

21. J. Wesley, *A Survey of the Wisdom of God in the Creation: Or, A Compendium of Natural Philosophy,* 5 vols, 3rd edn (London, 1763), Vol. I, 85.

22. J. Wainewright, *A Mechanical Account of the Non-Naturals: Being a Brief Explication of the Changes Made in Humane Bodies by Air, Diet, together with an Enquiry into the Nature and Use of the Baths,* 1st edn (London, 1708), n.p. ('Preface').

23. W. Buchan, *Domestic Medicine: Or, A Treatise on the Prevention and Cure of Diseases by Regimen and Simple Medicines,* 2nd edn (London, 1772); R. Porter, 'Spreading Medical Enlightenment: The Popularization of Medicine in Georgian England, and its Paradoxes', in R. Porter (ed.), *The Popularization of Medicine, 1650–1850* (London: Routledge, 1992), 215–31: 220.

24. Buchan, *op. cit.* (note 23), viii.

25. Emch-Dériaz, *op. cit.* (note 8), 137. Emch-Dériaz points to the fact that Tissot graduated in 1749 from the Montpellier School, where the neo-

Hippocratic influence was very strong.

26. Buchan's *Domestic Medicine* was part of this educative process. Lawrence shows that, like Wesley, Buchan owed a debt of gratitude to Cheyne, but that Buchan's 'handling of the same material fifty years later showed a distinct shift of emphasis from Cheyne's more traditional account' (25). Cheyne's *Essay* was divided into the headings of non-naturals, whilst Buchan made no explicit reference to them. Furthermore, argues Lawerence, Buchan introduced a 'strong social', as well as individual element. Buchan also provided detailed descriptions of diseases. For a full discussion, see C.J. Lawrence, 'William Buchan: Medicine Laid Open', *Medical History*, 19 (1975), 20–35.

27. Cheyne, *op. cit.* (note 1), v–vi.

28. Buchan, *op. cit* (note 23), ix.

29. *Ibid.*, ix.

30. Emch-Dériaz, *op. cit.* (note 8), 143.

31. *Ibid.*

32. D. Porter, 'Public Health', in W.F. Bynum and R. Porter (eds), *Companion Encyclopedia of the History of Medicine*, 2 vols (London: Routledge, 1993), Vol. II, 1231–61: 1235.

33. *Ibid.*, 1235.

34. James Lind and John Pringle campaigned for better conditions on ships and in army camps. *Ibid.*, 1236.

35. J. Wesley, *A Farther Appeal to Men of Reason and Religion* (1743), in G.R. Cragg (ed.) *The Bicentennial Edition of the Works of John Wesley. The Appeals,* (Nashville: Abingdon Press, 1989), 95–202: 241. Cragg points out in note 2 on page 241 that Wesley was familiar with John Howard's work, *The State of Prisons in England and Wales* (1777), which provided an accurate depiction of the prisons. Wesley was an 'indefatigable prison visitor' who knew at first hand the conditions he described.

36. Riley points to the fact that between 1670 and 1750 the crude death rate in Europe began to decline: 'falling from a range of 25 to 40 per 1,000 per annum to less than 10 per 1,000 in the... twentieth century'. This decline, he argues, is one of the most powerful factors behind modern population growth and is a noteworthy feature of history. Possible explanations for this growth are problematic and controversial but include nutritional advances, medical improvements such as smallpox inoculation and increased awareness of health and hygiene. Riley, *op. cit.* (note 12), 151.

37. Wesley, *op. cit.* (note 1), xi.

38. J. Armstrong, *The Art of Preserving Health* (London, 1744), in *English Poetry Full-Text Database* [Windows CD-ROM] (Cambridge: Chadwyck-Healey, 1993). All further quotations from this volume originate from this CD-ROM.

39. Wesley, *op. cit.* (note 1), iv.

40. *Ibid.*, iv.

41. B. Kaplan, *'Divulging of Useful Truths in Physic': The Medical Agenda of Robert Boyle* (Baltimore and London: John Hopkins Press, 1993), 108. Riley points out that Boyle's theory was vague in as much as it merged with Hippocratic miasmatic theories; those advocating environmental medicine wrote indeterminately about 'exhalations' and 'emanations'. Riley, *op. cit.* (note 12), 13.

42. Locke's letter, dated 5 May 1666, is published as part of R. Boyle's *General History of the Air* (London, 1692), 137–41: 138; K. Dewhurst, 'A Review of John Locke's Research in Social and Preventative Medicine', *Bulletin of the History of Medicine,* 36 (1962), 317–40: 318; see also, K. Dewhurst, 'An Oxford Medical Student's Notebook (1652–1659)', *Oxford Medical Gazette,* 2 (1959), 141–6.

43. Wesley, *op. cit.* (note 1), 41.

44. For an explication of Boyle's vision here, see Kaplan, *op. cit.* (note 41), 108.

45. *Ibid.*, 108–10. Kaplan makes the same point identified by Riley (see note 41 above) when she says that this notion was not original and had been handed down from antiquity: 'Aristotle himself had explained the formation of metals and minerals as a result of the congealing of vaporous and smoky exhalations deep in the earth… it is evident that in forming his ideas on environmental effects on health, Boyle borrowed much from earlier thought but extended it and placed it into a corpuscular framework. Hippocratic notions of the influence of climate and weather conditions on health are combined with Paracelsian notions of subterraneal chemical activity'. (110, 120).

46. J. Wesley, *What is Man?,* in A.C. Outler (ed.), *The Bicentennial Edition of the Works of John Wesley* (Nashville: Abingdon Press, 1984–), Vol IV, 20–7: 20.

47. Riley identifies a crucial distinction between Classical notions of this activity and those developed during the seventeenth and eighteenth centuries. In accordance with humoral theory, the ancients believed that the seeds of disease lay within the body, awaiting release. This release could occur as a result of external agents, such as the weather. Sydenham attempted to show that external agents, like air, provoked disease and upset internal bodily humors. This operated more forcefully than was traditionally allowed by the ancients: 'Later, as a more distinct environmentalist theory of disease aetiology developed, the air came to be seen as being by itself a sufficient cause for disease'. Thus, air no longer really constituted a non-natural as such, but environmental medicine retained it as a means of explaining large-group diseases and their avoidance. Riley, *op. cit.* (note 12), 15.

48. *Ibid.*

49. *Ibid.*

50. Wainewright, *op. cit.* (note 22), 63.

51. *Ibid.*

52. Armstrong, *op. cit.* (note 38).

53. G. Cheyne, *A New Theory of Continu'd Fevers,* 2nd edn (London, 1722), 26.

54. Wainewright, *op. cit.* (note 22), 58.

55. *Ibid.*, 16.

56. Armstrong, *op. cit.* (note 38).

57. *Ibid.* The malaria (literally meaning 'bad air') parasite was not discovered until 1880 and the role of the mosquito as vector not proved until later still. See Riley, *op. cit.* (note 12), 122.

58. S. Hales, *A Description of Ventilators,* 1st edn (London, 1743); S. Hales, *A Treatise on Ventilators,* 1st edn (London, 1758). Hales managed to get his invention fitted at the Savoy and Newgate Prisons and it has been said that this innovation reduced mortality rates in these places. Hales presented a paper in 1741 to the Royal Society about his ventilator. See F. Darwin, 'Hales, Stephen 1677–1761', in *Dictionary of National Biography* [Windows CD-ROM], (1890: Oxford University Press, 1995). Riley, however, argues that gaol fever would not have been reduced as a result of ventilation. This is due to the fact that gaol fever was transmitted by the faeces of body lice and vectors such as fleas. Hales's machine was a hand-operated bellows, later developed into a windmill device, which was installed into the prisons. Riley, *op. cit.* (note 12), 133, 107.

59. Riley, *op. cit.* (note 12), 132.

60. Hannaway, *op. cit.* (note 12), 305.

61. Wesley, *op. cit.* (note 46), 20–1.

62. Hannaway, *op. cit.* (note 12), 305.

63. *Ibid.*, 305. Hannaway shows how Jan Ingenhousz and Felice Fontana were the leading designers of eudiometers. She says that a failure of this instrument was its inability to measure significant differences in the respirability of the air in different locations.

64. Wesley, *op. cit.* (note 1), 59.

65. Cited by Riley, *op. cit.* (note 12), 22.

66. Armstrong, *op. cit.* (note 38).

67. Buchan, *op. cit.* (note 23), 93.

68. *Ibid.*

69. Riley, *op. cit.* (note 12), 30.

70. *Ibid.*, 98.

71. Wesley, *op. cit.* (note 1), xi–xii.

72. Armstrong, *op. cit.* (note 38).

73. J. Huxham, *An Essay on Fevers and their Various Kinds,* 1st edn (London, 1750), 40.

74. *Ibid.*, 8. Huxham also advocated, however, a 'warm, invigorating, attenuating

regimen' for the intermitting fever, which consisted of brandy, spirits and pepper (25).

75. Cheyne, *op. cit.* (note 1).

76. J. Wesley, *Advice with Respect to Health,* 4th edn (London, 1789), 4.

77. Buchan, *op. cit.* (note 23), 98.

78. J Wesley, *The Letters of the Rev. John Wesley A.M.,* J. Telford (ed.), 8 vols, (London: Epworth Press, 1931), v, 177.

79. *Ibid.,* vi, 307.

80. R. Burton, *The Anatomy of Melancholy,* H. Jackson (ed.), 3 vols (London: Dent, 1968), Vol. III, 178.

81. J. Wesley, *On Dress* (1786), in Outler, *op. cit.* (note 46), Vol. III, 248–59: 249.

82. A.W. Hill, *John Wesley Among the Physicians: A Study of Eighteenth-Century Medicine* (London: Epworth Press, 1958), 118. See Outler, *ibid.,* 249 n. 6.

83. In the *Arminian Magazine* it was addressed 'To Mr. S. at Armagh'. Telford suggests that 'Mr. S.' is Richard Steel, because this preacher was then based in Armagh. See Wesley, *op. cit.* (note 78), v, 133. Wesley's citation here is taken from George Herbert, though a slight modification of Herbert's stanza, the original being: 'Let thy mind's sweetness have its operation, upon thy body, clothes and habitation'. See G. Herbert, *The Temple: Sacred Poems and Private Ejaculations* (1633) (London: Nonesuch Press, 1927). This is also quoted in Wesley's Sermon *On Dress* (1786), see Wesley, *op. cit.* (note 81).

84. Cheyne, *op. cit.* (note 4), xxix. Cheyne did not advise a cool diet in all circumstances. 'Eruptive' or 'acute' cases of illness, such as fits of gout or a second fever when ill with smallpox, were to be aided by 'warmer' medicines. This is because nature needed to 'throw' morbidity 'outward'. In these cases a low and cool regimen was not be advised. *Idem.,* xix.

85. *Ibid.,* xxxv.

86. J. Arbuthnot, *An Essay Concerning the Nature of Aliments and the Choice of Them, According to the Different Constitutions of Human Bodies,* 4th edn (London, 1756), 98.

87. Wesley, *op. cit.* (note 78), Vol. I, 11. Telford points out that Cheyne was a pioneer of dietetics, citing a comment made by Arbuthnot in the 'Preface' to his *An Essay Concerning the Nature of Aliments,* that Cheyne's book 'produced... sects in the dietetick philosophy'. See Wesley. *op. cit.* (note 78), Vol. I, 11, n.1.

88. Pre-lapsarian humans were vegetarians and eating meat was another sign of man's fall. A. Guerrini, *Obesity and Depression in the Enlightenment: The Life and Times of George Cheyne* (Oklahoma: University of Oklahoma Press, 2000), 170.

89. Cited by L. Tyerman, *The Life and Times of the Rev. John Wesley, MA.,* 3 vols. (London, 1870–2), Vol. I, 117.

90. J. Wesley, *The Works of the Rev. John Wesley, A.M*, T. Jackson (ed.), 14 vols (London: Wesleyan Methodist Book-Room, 1831), Vol. I, 387–8; P.W. Ott, 'John Wesley on Health: A Word for Sensible Regimen', *Methodist History,* 18 (1979–80), 193–204: 199.

91. Wesley, *op. cit.* (note 78), Vol. V, 133–4.

92. J. Wesley, *On the Education of Children* (1783), in Outler, *op. cit.* (note 46), Vol. III, 347–60: 357–8.

93. Rudi Matthee, 'Exotic Substances: the Introduction and Global spread of Tobacco, Coffee, Cocoa, Tea and Distilled Liquor, sixteenth to eighteenth centuries', in R. Porter and M. Teich (eds), *Drugs and Narcotics in History* (Cambridge: Cambridge University Press, 1995), 24–53.

94. Wainewright, *op. cit.* (note 22), 159.

95. Arbuthnot, *op. cit.* (note 86); Buchan, *op. cit.* (note 23).

96. Cheyne, *op. cit.* (note 4), xxviii.

97. G. Cheyne, *An Essay on the True Nature and Due Method of Treating the Gout,* 6th edn (London, 1724), 87.

98. J. Wesley, *On the Fall of Man*, in Outler, *op. cit.* (note 46), Vol. II, 400–12: 409–10.

99. Cheyne, *op. cit.* (note 4), xii.

100. Arbuthnot, *op. cit.* (note 86), 91.

101. Cheyne, *op. cit.* (note 4), ii.

102. *Ibid.*, xv.

103. Buchan, *op. cit.* (note 23), 80.

104. *Ibid.*, 77, 172.

105. Wesley, *op. cit.* (note 78), Vol. VII, 151.

106. Cheyne, *op. cit.* (note 1); Cheyne, *op. cit.* (note 4); Wainewright, *op. cit.* (note 22).

107. R. Porter, 'Introduction', in *idem.* (ed.), *George Cheyne: The English Malady: or, A Treatise of Nervous Diseases of all Kinds (1733)* (Tavistock Classics in the History of Psychiatry), (London: Routledge, 1991), xxiii.

108. *Ibid.*, xxiii.

109. Buchan, *op. cit.* (note 23) 78.

110. *Ibid.*

111. Cheyne, *op. cit.* (note 97), 60.

112. S.A. Tissot, *An Essay on the Disorders of People of Fashion (1768),* F.B. Lee (trans), (London, 1771), 14.

113. Wesley makes reference to this in a letter, dated 12 November 1771, to one of his preachers, John Valton: 'Dr. Tissot wrote for Swiss constitutions: we must make allowances for English, which are generally less robust.' Wesley, *op. cit.* (note 78), Vol. V, 289.

114. Tissot, *op. cit.* (note 112), 16.

115. *Ibid.*, 14.

116. As has been already noted, Cheyne did compare the diet of the 'industrious', 'temperate' and 'labourious' favourably to that of the 'rich', 'lazy' and 'luxurious'. However, Porter points out that Cheyne regarded the lifestyle of the 'middling rank' as being best suited to the climate and conditions of England: 'Thus Cheyne hoped to civilise aristocratic consumption habits… the poor would be healthy through work; the rich would work at being healthy', Porter, *op. cit.* (note 107), xxxi.

117. Tissot, *op. cit.* (note 112), 17.

118. Cheyne, *op. cit.* (note 4), xlv.

119. Buchan, *op. cit.* (note 23), 116.

120. Buchan, *op. cit.* (note 23), 116.

121. Cited by Porter, *op. cit.* (note 107), xxiv.

122. Cheyne, *op. cit.* (note 4), xxv.

123. Emch-Dériaz, *op. cit.* (note 8), 146.

124. Quoted in Tyerman, *op. cit.* (note 89), Vol. II. 111.

125. Tyerman states that tea was sold for sixty shillings per pound until 1707, though by 1746 it was slightly cheaper. *Ibid.*, Vol. I, 521.

126. For a full discussion, see *ibid.*, Vol. I, 521–2.

127. Wesley, *op. cit.* (note 78), Vol. II, 162.

128. *Ibid.*, 162.

129. Tyerman, *op. cit.* (note 89), Vol. I, 522. Apparently, Dr Fothergill ordered Wesley to resume tea drinking.

130. Quoted in B.A. Weinberg and B.K. Bealer, *The World of Caffeine: The Science and Culture of the World's most Popular Drug* (London: Routledge, 2001), 114.

131. Emch-Dériaz, *op. cit.* (note 8), 145.

132. Weinberg and Bealer, *op. cit.* (note 130), 115.

133. Quoted in *ibid.*, 115. In his letter to 'a Friend', Wesley, in fact, argued that 'many eminent' physicians had declared that tea was 'prejudicial in several respects; that it gives rise to numberless disorders, particularly those of the nervous kind…. Wesley, *op. cit.* (note 78), Vol. II, 162.

134. Weinberg and Bealer, *op. cit.* (note 130), 116.

135. Quoted in Weinberg and Bealer, *op. cit.* (note 130), 117.

136. Emch-Dériaz, *op. cit.* (note 8), 146.

137. Cheyne, *op. cit.* (note 4), lxii.

138. *Ibid.*, xxv.

139. *Ibid.*

140. Wesley, *op. cit.* (note 1), 118.

141. Armstrong, *op. cit.* (note 38).

142. Buchan, *op. cit.* (note 23), 117.

143. Ott, *op. cit.* (note 90), 200.

144. J. Wesley, *On Redeeming the Time* (1782), in Outler, *op. cit.* (note 46), Vol. III, 322–32: 323.

145. *Ibid.*, 327.

146. Wesley, *op. cit.* (note 78), Vol. V, 133–4.

147. Wesley, *op. cit.* (note 144), Vol. III, 326–7.

148. Wainewright, *op. cit.* (note 22), 68; J. Wesley, *Thoughts on Nervous Disorders* (1784), in Jackson, *op. cit.* (note 90), Vol. XI, 515–20. Ott, *op. cit.* (note 90), 200.

149. Wesley, *op. cit.* (note 144), Vol. III, 327

150. Cheyne, *op. cit.* (note 4), lxvi.

151. Wesley, *op. cit.* (note 144), Vol. III, 325–6. Outler suggests that this was not as clear-cut as Wesley remembers. He argues that this is a 'conveniently oversimplified recollection' and that the early diaries show how Wesley was still experimenting with sleep patterns in 1729. It was in 1730 that he finally settled upon his regular waking hour of 4am. Outler also points out that Wesley fails to mention the fact that he took catnaps when it was convenient during the day. See Outler, *op. cit.* (note 46), Vol. III, 325 n. 7.

152. Wesley, *op. cit.* (note 144), Vol. III, 325.

153. Wesley, *op. cit.* (note 78), Vol. VIII, 75.

154. This school is not to be confused with that set up in 1738 by George Whitefield for the colliers' children, which was later taken over by Wesley. Rack shows that by 1749 there were four Methodist schools set up in the Kingswood area of Bristol: day schools for girls and boys, an orphan school for girls and the 'New House'. Despite the fact that the boys' school later became the place where itinerants sent their sons, the original design, Rack argues, was a school for the general public. The school would train children for the Christian ministry. For a full discussion of this see H.D. Rack, *Reasonable Enthusiast: John Wesley and the Rise of Methodism* (London: Epworth Press, 1992), 355.

155. Wesley, *op. cit.* (note 148), 517.

156. Wainewright, *op. cit.* (note 22), 68.

157. Wesley, *op. cit.* (note 1), xii–xiii.

158. Wainewright, *op. cit.* (note 22), 126–7.

159. Cheyne, *op. cit.* (note 1), 54.

160. Wainewright, *op. cit.* (note 22), 7.

161. Wesley, *op. cit.* (note 78), Vol. VIII, 206.

162. Quoted in Dewhurst, *op. cit.* (note 15), 54.

163. J. Wesley, *The Journal of the Rev. John Wesley, A.M.*, 4 vols (London: J. Kershaw, 1827), Vol. IV, 77.

164. R. Maddox, 'A Heritage Reclaimed: John Wesley on Holistic Health and Healing', in M.E.M. Moore (ed.), *A Living Tradition* (Nashville: Kingswood Books, forthcoming).

165. *Ibid.*
166. Emch-Dériaz, *op. cit.* (note 8), 145.
167. Wesley, *op. cit.* (note 1), xiv. This sentiment is repeated in 'The Preface' to his *Advice*. 'I have only to add (what would not be fashionable for a physician to believe, much less to maintain) that as God is the sovereign disposer of all things, and particularly life and death, I earnestly advise everyone, together with all his other medicine, to use that medicine of medicines, prayer. Dr. Tissot himself will give leave to think this, an universal medicine. At the same time that we use all the means which reason and experience can dictate....' Wesley, *op. cit.* (note 76), viii.
168. Wesley, *op. cit.* (note 1), xiv.
169. Buchan, *op. cit.* (note 23) 140.
170. *Ibid.*, 149.
171. *Ibid.*, 140.
172. Wesley, *op. cit.* (note 163), Vol. IV, 313 (1 May 1759).
173. Though Wesley did believe that the best physicians could only ever be 'experienced Christians', *ibid.*
174. *Ibid.*, Vol. I, 166.
175. *Ibid.*, Vol. IV, 138.
176. Wesley, *op. cit.* (note 78), Vol. VIII, 45.
177. *Ibid.*, Vol. VI, 327.
178. *Ibid.*, 327–8.
179. Maddox, *op. cit.* (note 164).
180. Ott, *op. cit.* (note 90), 196; *idem, op. cit.* (note 9); P.W. Ott, 'John Wesley on Health as Wholeness', *Journal of Religion and Health,* 30 (1991), 43–57.
181. Wesley, *op. cit.* (note 98), ii. 406.
182. Wesley, *Heavenly Treasure in Earthen Vessels* (1790), in Outler, *op. cit.* (note 46), Vol. IV, 161–7: 165; Ott, *op. cit.* (note 90), 196.
183. Cheyne, *op. cit.* (note 107), 5.
184. Porter, *op. cit.* (note 107).
185. Cheyne, *op. cit.* (note 107), xviii.
186. Porter argues that Cheyne was not really disposed to the view that psychological diseases existed independently in their own right, and that the root of such conditions lay within the body itself: 'agonies of mind were expressions of more basic physical sickness. There was no disturbance of consciousness without a prior somatic disorder'. See Porter, *op. cit.* (note 107), xxxiv.
187. Cheyne, *op. cit.* (note 107), xxviii.
188. *Ibid.*, xvii.
189. Buchan, *op. cit.* (note 23), 139.
190. Cheyne, *op. cit.* (note 1), 75.
191. W. Falconer, *A Dissertation on the Influence of the Passions upon the Disorders*

of the Body, 2nd edn (London, 1791), 9–10.

192. *Ibid.,* 13.

193. *Ibid.,* 15.

194. *Ibid.,* 51.

195. During his undergraduate days at Oxford, Wesley used to strip and plunge into the River Thames by way of arresting (through shock) a violent nose bleed. See W.J. Turrell, *John Wesley: Physician and Electrotherapist* (Oxford: Blackwell, 1938), 17.

196. Buchan, *op. cit.* (note 23), 148.

197. Falconer, *op. cit.* (note 191), 32. Falconer cites the following from *Domestic Medicine*: 'The mind of the patient ought not only to be kept easy, but soothed and comforted with hopes of a speedy recovery. Nothing is more hurtful in low fevers of this kind, than presenting to the patient's imagination gloomy or frightful ideas. These of themselves often occasion nervous fevers, and it is not to be doubted that they will likewise aggravate them'. See *idem.,* 32n.

198. Rack, *op. cit.* (note 154), 386, 421.

199. J. Wesley, *On The Nature of Enthusiasm* (1750), in Outler, *op. cit.* (note 46), Vol. II, 44–60: 49.

200. *Ibid.,* 58; M.R. Ryder, 'Avoiding the "Many-Headed Monster": Wesley and Johnson on Enthusiasm', *Methodist History,* 23 (1985), 214–22.

201. W.F. Bynum, 'Health, Disease and Medical Care', in G. Rousseau and R. Porter (eds), *The Ferment of Knowledge: Studies in the Historiography of Eighteenth-Century Science* (Cambridge: Cambridge University Press, 1980), 211–54.

202. William Law cited by J. Wesley, *On the Education of Children,* in Outler, *op. cit.* (note 46), Vol. III, 348–9.

203. M. Schmidt, *John Wesley: A Theological Biography,* N.P. Goldhawk (trans.), 2 vols (London: Epworth Press, 1985), Vol. II, 181.

204. *Ibid.*

205. Cheyne, *op. cit.* (note 1), 10.

206. Wesley, *op. cit.* (note 163), Vol. IV, 77.

PART II

PRIMITIVE PHYSIC:
'A COLLECTION OF RECEIPTS'

5

Primitive Physic:
Cheap, Safe and Natural Medicine for Health and Long Life

At the request of many persons, I have... added plain definitions of most distempers: not indeed accurate or philosophical definitions, but such as are suited to men of ordinary capacities, and as may just enable them, in common simple cases, to distinguish one disease from another. In uncommon or complicated diseases, where life is more immediately in danger, I again advise every man, without delay to apply to a Physician that fears God.

John Wesley, 'Postscript' to the 1755 edition of *Primitive Physic*

When the structure or disposition of the parts of the body is so disturbed and disordered, that the natural operations are no longer performed, or not in the manner they ought: This is a *preternatural state* of the body, otherwise termed as a disease.

The diseases of the *fluids* lie chiefly in the blood, when it is either too thick and sizy, whereby its motion becomes too languid and slow, whence spring diseases owing to obstruction: or too thin. From the former cause arises leprosies, schirrhis, lethargies, melancholy, hysteric affections. And if at the same time it... abound in acid salts, the sharp points of these tear the tender fibres and occasion the scurvy, Kings-Evil, consumption; with a whole train of painful distempers.

John Wesley, *A Survey of the Wisdom of God in the Creation: Or A Compendium of Natural Philosophy*

The blood, the fountain whence the spirits flow,
The generous stream that waters every part,
And motion, vigour, and warm life conveys
To every particle that moves or lives;
This vital fluid, thro' unnumber'd tubes
Pour'd by the heart, and to the heart again
Refunded; scourg'd for ever round and round.

Dr John Armstrong, *The Art of Preserving Health*[1]

209

Perfect health and good spirits depended chiefly on the 'easy' play of animal functions via correct digestion, respiration, perspiration, circulation, muscular motion and secretions.[2] The body's solids, fibres and fluids needed to be in a state of equilibrium. Avoiding disease meant ensuring that the blood was not 'sizy', thick or viscous, although, as Wesley points out in the passage above, neither should it be too thin or watery. With regard to proper digestion and perspiration, Wesley makes the following observations in 'The Preface' under his 'Rules' for regimen, subsection five:

> 1. Costiveness cannot long consist with health. Therefore care should be taken to remove it at the beginning; and when it is removed, to prevent its return, by a soft, cool, open diet.

> 2. Obstructed perspiration (vulgarly called catching cold) is one great source of diseases. Whenever there appears the least sign of this, let it be removed by gentle sweats.[3]

We have noted already how health of the body and mind could be regulated through these 'Rules'. But sickness and disease, as is made clear by Wesley in the passage given at the beginning of the chapter, results when the structure of the body is disturbed and disordered. 'Obstructions' stop the blood from making its full circle, which can lessen or increase its volume and upset the 'natural operations'. For this 'preternatural' state, medicine is required or, in the words of Cheyne, medicine could right the 'disorder'd machine'.[4] In *Primitive Physic,* Wesley sought to show how physic could be used to right the 'disorder'd machine' but, more importantly, that medicine was within the reach of men with 'ordinary capacities'.

For 'Costiveness' (constipation), which was not removed by regimen, he made the following recommendations in the main text of *Primitive Physic*:

> 205. Or, breakfast twice a week or oftener, on *water-gruel with currants.* Tried.

> 207. Or, take daily two hours before dinner a small tea-cupful of *stewed prunes.*

> 209. Or, live upon *bread,* made of *wheat-flower* with all the *bran* in it.

> 210. Or, boil an ounce and a half of *tamarinds* in three pints of water to a quart. In this strained, when cold, infuse all night two drachms of *sena,* one drachm of *red rose-leaves,* drink a cup every morning – See Dr. *Tissot.*[5]

The above remedies form four possible solutions from quite a long list. This advice is straightforward and in keeping with a fairly uncomplicated disorder. The remedies presented here by Wesley were also recommended by other leading physicians, such as Buchan, Wainewright and Tissot, who advocated this type of 'kitchen-physic' for minor complaints. Similarly, with regards to 'Rule' 2 of Wesley's regimen regarding the common cold, it was believed that an 'obstructed perspiration' accounted for the illness. In this 'Rule', Wesley instructed the reader to use gentle sweats, though this directive could be aided by the remedy set out for 'A Cold' in the main text, which involved drinking a very hot draught (in bed).[6] Drinking a hot draught would promote gentle sweats, thereby removing the offending obstruction. What lies behind Wesley's 'simple' remedies, therefore, is a complex body of medical knowledge that regarded the human frame as a system of hydraulics, which needed to protect itself against 'obstructions'.

By way of further illustrating this, we shall examine here a subset of illnesses and diseases that were commonly experienced during the eighteenth century – those specifically referred to time and again by Wesley in his letters and journals. What should become apparent is the 'syncretic' and practical method Wesley adopted when utilising a range of medical approaches. Moreover, we will see too, how articles changed over time in various editions of *Primitive Physic*, particularly after Hawes's criticism of the 16th edition in 1774. A brief explication of Wesley's incorporation of electrical therapy will illustrate how electricity, like regimen, was used to draw parallels between physical and spiritual health.

'A collection of receipts'

St Anthony's Fire

The name of this disease referred to St Anthony the Great, a third-century hermit and founder of Christian ascetic monasticism, though it can also be connected to the twelfth-century saint, St Anthony of Padua, who was renowned for restoring the insane to health.[7] This disease, which dominated Europe between 900 and 1700, was characterised by an inflammation or 'fire' of the skin that usually affected the face or legs and which could also be gangrenous. Wesley described it as such in a footnote in *Primitive Physic*:

> *St. Anthony's Fire* is a fever attended with a red and painful swelling, full of pimples, which afterwards turn into *small blisters*, on the face or some other part of the body. The sooner the eruption… the less danger. Let your diet be only *Water-Gruel*, or *Barley-Broth*, with roasted Apples.[8]

It was commonly believed that 'extremes' in temperature, the passions and excessive drinking brought on this disease. Hot temperatures relaxed the fibres and overheated the blood, making it coagulated, while extreme cold constricted the fibres and suppressed perspiration – both lax and constricted fibres produced obstructions. It is now known that the actual cause of this disease was due to being poisoned by ingesting the ergot fungus, which grew on rye.[9]

St Anthony's Fire included fever-like symptoms, with delirium, swelling and pustules (on the third or fourth day). Eyes could become so swollen that they were unable to open and the disease often progressed to such an extent that the patient suffered an inflammation of the brain. In the case of the latter, physicians recommended bleeding, and Wesley also believed that bleeding was 'necessary' once the disease 'attacks the head'.[10] He suggested gentle purges for when St Anthony's Fire inflamed the brain: '31. Or, take two or three gentle purges – no acute fever bears repeated purges better than this, especially when it affects the head.'[11]

Cautious bleeding and gentle purging could reduce the attendant inflammatory fever that overheated the blood and brain. Both Tissot and Buchan recommended bleeding and gentle purging in tandem with the patient bathing his legs in warm water.[12] Unusually, for a staunch defender of cold bathing, Wesley approved of this treatment in *Primitive Physic*, which he sees as being particularly soothing for St Anthony's Fire:

> 34. Bathing the feet and legs in *warm water* is serviceable, and often relieves the patient much – in Scotland the common people cover the part with a linen cloth covered with meal.[13]

A 'cool' regimen and 'slender' diet were the most appropriate for this disease and, as can be seen in the above-cited footnote relating to this condition, Wesley suggested a light diet of broth and gruel. This cooling, diluting diet, which could keep the blood light, is reflected in the following remedies:

> 29. Take a glass of *tar-water* warm in bed, every hour, washing the part with the same.
>
> 30. Or, take a decoction of *elder leaves*, as a sweat.
>
> 32. Or, if the pulse be low, and the spirits sunk, nourishing broths… may be given *to advantage.*
>
> 33. Or, let three drachms of *nitre* be dissolved in as much *elder-flower tea*, as the patient can drink in twenty-four hours.[14]

An elder-flower infusion is listed as a cooling draught for this disease in Buchan's *Domestic Medicine*.[15] Rather usefully, Wesley provides his reader with instructions on exactly how to make tar-water:

Tar-water is made thus – put a gallon of cold water to a quart of Norway tar. Stir them together with a flat stick for five or six minutes. After it has stood covered for three days, pour off the water clear, bottle and cork it.[16]

Meat, fish, spicy food and strong liquors were to be avoided due to the fact that they had a detrimental effect on the blood by making it 'sharp', 'acidic' or overheated. In *Examination*, Hawes objected to Wesley's prescription of tar-water for the 'erisipetalous' inflammation on this basis – though Hawes also castigated Wesley for the cooling remedies suggested for St Anthony's Fire.[17] Buchan strongly steered his reader away from blistering 'plaisters' and oily ointments on the grounds that they would heat and 'obstruct' rather than promote discharge of the pustules, characteristic of this disease.[18] Wesley's remedies in *Primitive Physic* echo Buchan's emphasis on regimen but also on the issue of topical remedies when he states that 'dressing the inflammation with greasy ointments, salves, &. is very improper'.[19] In general, emphasis was placed on regimen rather than physic for this particular condition and, indeed, Buchan argued that much mischief could be done here by using medicine. Wesley's cooling regimen for this illness was therefore completely in keeping with the applications used by contemporary physicians.

An apoplexy

This medical term comes from the Greek *apoplēxia* (*apoplēssein*, meaning to disable by a stroke).[20] In a footnote Wesley describes its symptoms:

An *Apoplexy* is, a total loss of all sense, and voluntary motion, commonly attended with a strong pulse, hard breathing and snorting.[21]

There were two types of apoplexy: sanguine and serous. According to Buchan it was caused by a compression of the brain, 'occasioned by an effusion of blood or a collection of watery humours'. Sanguine apoplexy pertained to an effusion of blood (increased blood circulation towards the brain), while serous apoplexy related to 'watery humours' (reduction of blood to the brain).[22] In *Primitive Physic*, Wesley outlines the differences:

There is a wide difference between the *Sanguineous* and *Serous Apoplexy;* the latter is often followed by a palsy – the former is distinguished by the countenance of appearing florid; the face swelled or puffed up; and the blood vessels, especially about the neck and temples, are turgid; the pulse beats strong; the eyes are prominent and fixed; and the breathing is difficult, and performed with a snorting. This invades more suddenly than the Serous Apoplexy. Use large bleedings from the arm, or neck; bathe the feet in warm water; cupping the back of the head, with deep scarification. The garters should be tied very tight to lessen the motion of the blood from the lower extremities... in the *Serous Apoplexy*, the pulse is not so strong, the countenance is less florid, and not attended with so great a difficulty in breathing. *This Apoplexy is generally preceded by an unusual heaviness, giddiness, and drowsiness.*[23]

It was believed that this condition attacked sedentary individuals who indulged in a rich diet. Other triggers involved intense periods of study, violent passions, the suppression of urine and evacuations, extreme temperatures – rapid cooling of the body when it was hot, or exposure to extreme cold. Highly seasoned food and hot baths could also occasion an attack of apoplexy.

In the case of sanguine apoplexy it was necessary to take every method to lessen the force of circulation towards the head. For this and with apoplectic conditions generally, the patient needed to be kept 'easy and cool'.[24] Diluting liquors (tartar) and 'cooling purges' (senna) were the best way of remedying the condition. Regimen consisted of guarding against the passions, avoiding extreme temperatures and taking exercise.[25] By way of prevention, Wesley suggested drinking water and cold bathing. This suggestion was criticised by Hawes, who argued that cold bathing could actually bring on a fit of apoplexy.[26] It was generally agreed that extreme temperatures should be avoided, but Wesley advocated cold bathing as a preventative measure. He might have avoided Hawes's criticism if he had confined this suggestion to those diseases prevented by 'Cold-Bathing', which are listed at the end of *Primitive Physic* under this heading.

In general, Wesley prescribed cooling liquors and purges with a light cool diet for the apoplexy. Hence, he states that: 'A *Seton* in the neck, with low diet, has often prevented a relapse – see Extract from Dr. *Tissot*, page 53.'[27] A 'seton' was a length of material that was placed below the skin, with the end protruding. It was used to promote drainage or absorb fluid. Wesley regarded this condition with the seriousness it warranted and also admonished the reader to send for 'a good Physician immediately' after the fit had occurred.[28] This mitigates Hawes's accusation that he meddled with remedies for serious illnesses when he should have instructed the reader to apply for medical assistance.[29] There are two other interesting points to note about Wesley's treatment of apoplexy in *Primitive Physic*. The first is his advice to use '*Emetic Tartar*' to vomit a patient suffering from serous apoplexy. In the case of sanguine apoplexy, it was inadvisable to vomit a patient due to the fact that vomiting increased blood circulation to the head. Conversely, when treating a bout of serous apoplexy, where the illness involved a *reduction* of blood to the head, bleeding was not necessary because the pulse was weak and a vomit would serve to increase circulation. Wesley's advice to use an emetic tartar vomit was based on sound medical grounds. He provided his own recipe for the emetic tartar vomit at the end of *Primitive Physic*, where he gives a range of suggested usages:

> The emetic tartar is best calculated for removing acidity, bile and putrid matter in the stomach. In the beginning of some nervous and putrid fevers, where the pulse is weak, and the stomach loaded with sour, fetid, yellow or green matter, there is, perhaps, no medicine equal to it.[30]

The second interesting point concerns Wesley's recommending 'large bleedings' and 'cupping on the back of the head, with deep scarification'. This recommendation had been modified from that given in the first edition of *Primitive Physic* – and repeated up until the sixteenth edition – where Wesley advised the patient to 'fix a cupping glass, without scarifying, to the nape of the neck....'[31] Wesley completely changed his position on the issue of scarification (superficial incisions to the skin) and altered this remedy accordingly. There is no doubt that this about-change was directly linked to the following criticism made by Hawes in his *Examination*:

> One of Mr. Wesley's shining qualities, is the adroitness with which he renders a good remedy inefficacious... here the cupping glasses recommended are very proper; but the directing them to be applied without scarifying, is in the highest degree absurd. By the scarifying, the blood vessels would have been unloaded of their contents, and the pressure upon the brain taken off.[32]

On the method of 'cupping' *without* scarification, Wesley had followed Boyle's *Medicinal Experiments,* but in light of the criticism made by Hawes he decided to investigate the matter before concluding that the doctor's observation was correct.[33] In this we can see how Wesley acted to make fairly radical alterations to his receipts in light of better techniques or more advanced medical evidence.

A consumption

This was a wasting disease, now commonly known to be tuberculosis. It was also referred to as phthisis or pulmonalis.[34] Like the 'fever', a great deal of literature was generated by this condition, which killed thousands every year. In *Domestic Medicine,* Buchan stated that:

> Dr. Arbuthnot observes, that in his time consumptions made up above one-tenth part of the bills of mortality in and about London. There is reason to believe they have rather increased since.[35]

Susan Juster has wryly remarked that consumption seems to have been the 'archetypal' disease for eighteenth-century evangelicals:

> Almost without exception, itinerant preachers feared at one time or another that they were dying of the disease, a fear that, for some became a reality... as consumption heated up the economic sphere, the disease whose name it shared grew to dominate health concerns among doctors and laity alike.[36]

She notes that cultural historians like to point to the tangled etymological roots of the term 'consumption', which in Britain denoted an emerging capitalist economy and overcrowded unsanitary living conditions.[37]

Clark Lawlor and Akihito Suzuki have also seen how consumption presents an interesting paradox in the cultural meanings of disease; although it was a major killer in the eighteenth century, its romantic allure was noted by contemporaries.[38] This 'aestheticisation' of consumption allowed it to function as a disease of the 'Self', formulated as a 'powerful cultural device of self-fashioning'.[39] Moreover, though a major killer, Lawlor and Suzuki see how patients sought to find something positive in consumption and even in the death of this disease, epitomised in the oft-cited deathbed scenes of consumptive patients, who are usually depicted as being calm and dignified. This conceptualisation contrasted markedly with that of physicians, who noted the way in which this disease corroded the body via putrid blood and ulcerous pus.[40] Here, consumption was framed in the language of 'medical horror and visceral disgust'.[41] Both evangelicals and physicians conjured up images of an overheated body 'becoming consumed from within by disease':

> In physiological terms, consumption is the inverse of sanctification: blood leaks into and clogs the lungs, contaminating, rather than purging the body... as they slid into what they feared was a 'consumptive' state, evangelicals felt their bodily and spiritual powers leached away.[42]

Given Juster's analysis here of contamination and purging in this context, it is interesting to note that the physician Blackmore offered a range of purgatives and vomits to his patients in his *A Treatise of Consumptions and other Distempers* (1725). Ironically, perhaps, *Primitive Physic* does not offer one single purge, though undoubtedly it is Wesley's treatment of this disease that provides the most intriguing points of contact with and difference from contemporary methods. The sheer range of physicians Wesley draws on in *Primitive Physic* when setting out his remedies for consumption is impressive. Only Tissot and Dover are cited directly, but it is clear that Wesley utilised the work of Radcliffe, Blackmore, Wainewright, Buchan and Fothergill.

Physicians attributed numerous causes to this disease, including excessive eating and drinking, internal distempers, and hereditary factors.[43] Blackmore suggested that 'immoderate evacuations' or diarrhoea, were a key factor because it 'defrauded the blood' of much needed 'materials'.[44] Buchan believed that other diseases brought on consumptions by 'vitiating the humours'. The conditions that were potentially accountable for this were scurvy, scrofula (also known as The King's Evil), asthma, smallpox, measles and venereal disease.[45] The list of causal factors for this illness was endless, but it included:

Unwholesome, stagnant air

Fumes from metals or minerals (those working in hazardous occupations such as miners and ironworkers susceptible to this illness)

Dampness (air, houses, beds, clothes)

Extreme change in temperature

Diet of 'sharp' and aromatic foods (which can inflame the blood)

Lack of exercise

Profuse sweating (especially from the feet)

Obstructed perspiration

Menstrual 'flux' (over-bleeding during menstrual cycle)

Nose-bleeds

Haemorrhoids

Infection from those with the disease

Intense study

Violent passions (or other intense emotions that affected the mind)[46]

Buchan argued that intense study of abstruse arts and sciences contributed to the consumption. Coming from a physician who declared in his 'Preface' that *Domestic Medicine* sought to utilise an empirical, common sense approach to physic, perhaps this was intended as a pointed remark.[47] Undoubtedly, the reason for so many causal factors being attributed to this disease was due to the fact that physicians conflated the deaths caused by other lingering and wasting illnesses with those of consumption.

Most physicians argued that consumption was hereditary and incurable. Blackmore thought this to be the case and offered his reader palliative care to reduce the severity of the symptoms.[48] Buchan stated that the disease was owing to an 'hereditary taint; in which case it is generally incurable'.[49] There is no evidence to suggest that Wesley thought the disease was hereditary. He differed too from other physicians in his belief that consumption could be cured, and in this respect *Primitive Physic* sought to offer hope to those suffering from a severely intractable disease. In fact, Wesley thought that providing hope to patients was a powerful aid to recovery in itself, but it was commonly acknowledged that melancholy sped up and increased the symptoms of consumption. Buchan argued that the patient's mind needed to be kept 'easy' and 'cheerful' for this reason.[50] Symptoms for consumptive illnesses covered the following:

Coughing up blood

Catarrh

Rapid or hard pulse

Vomiting

Pain in the breast

Unquenchable thirst

Fever

Excessive urination (which is discoloured)

Swollen feet and legs (which indicated that death was near)[51]

Regimen included clean air and exercise – for exercise, it was preferable to go horseback riding. The cold bath was recommended by Wainewright, who believed that the way in which cold water contracted fibres and solid parts would '*attenuate* the fluid' brought on by this disease, and 'evacuate at due intervals' the viscous matter (catarrh) lodged in the glands:

> Therefore gentle emetics, mild stomachics, moderate exercise, especially by riding, according to Dr. Sydenham's observation, a clear dry air, the use of the *cold bath*, provided the patient stay but a little time at once, and the distemper far advanced… with a diet of *easy digestion*, will best answer out expectation in the cure of a beginning consumption.[52]

The first recommendation Wesley makes in *Primitive Physic* for 'A Consumption' is 'cold bathing', which he states has 'cured many deep consumptions: tried'.[53] Individuals also needed to avoid damp (climate, houses, clothes) and inflammatory food. A light diet of vegetables and milk was the most effective way to mitigate those worst aspects of consumption, and Buchan thought that eating shellfish was especially efficacious. *Primitive Physic* strongly suggests following a light diet consisting of cooling liquors: 'For diet, use *milk* and *apples*, or *water-gruel* made with fine flour. Drink *cyder-whey*, *barley-water* sharpened with *lemon-juice* or *apple-water*.'[54]

Buchan advised those suffering from consumption to confine themselves to a diet of vegetables and asses' milk, which he calculated 'lessened the acrimony of the humours'.[55] Radcliffe was also a firm believer in taking asses' milk (with candy sugar) for consumption – asses' milk was preferable to that of cows because it was easier to digest.[56] Wesley, like Buchan, endorsed using apples and citrus fruit, especially lemons, due to the fact that the acids contained in this fruit seemed to be particularly good for treating consumption: they cooled the blood and quenched thirst. Given the fact that most physicians endorsed and advocated a cooling regimen for consumption, it is strange that Hawes takes Wesley to task for suggesting it in *Primitive Physic*. Hawes stated that Wesley's assertion of it may be acceptable 'in the neighbourhood of Moorfields: but we believe the *veracity* of it is not sufficiently *established*....'[57] Many of Hawes's criticisms of *Primitive Physic* are medically unfounded by his own contemporary standards.

In terms of physic it was essential that 'crudities' and 'impure humours' were discharged either by vomiting or by ensuring that the patient take medicines which could evacuate the catarrh. For this, Blackmore's rather revolting suggestion involved the patient making a 'horse-dung' infusion to remove the consumptive phlegm.[58] Animal odours were advocated by Dr Thomas Beddoes, who believed that butchers were free from consumptive disorders because they absorbed animal vapours.[59] On this, Porter has seen how these remedies, along with Beddoes's bleak description of consumption, formed part of a sustained attack against the aestheticisation and culture of pleasure that was growing out of this disease.[60] According to Wainewright, medicines that relaxed the solids and fibres would thicken the fluid, which would then fill the stomach with a 'glutinous slime'. In turn, this weakened digestion and increased the patient's thirst.[61] Medicines that constricted the solids would render the humours more fluid, the fibres more tense and evacuate the phlegm 'with which the glands of the stomach and those about the mouth are stuffed'.[62] Wainewright, however, does not state exactly which medicines are most appropriate and the reader must assume he is referring to those of a cooling nature. Buchan argued that the cure of this disease resided chiefly in a proper regimen, though he does suggest cooling draughts and 'bitter' plant decoctions, such as ground-ivy, camomile and comfrey-root.[63]

Wesley's cooling draughts for consumption included water, spring water, water-gruel, skimmed milk and juice of watercress – watercress was used to treat inflammatory and intestinal disorders, especially the lungs. For food, he recommended nothing but a light diet of butter-milk 'churned' with 'white bread', milk and apples.[64] This light regimen was advocated by Fothergill in his *Remarks on the Cure of Consumptions*.

> When a cough begins… let the quantity of diet, especially solids be lessened; let the deficiency be made up with warm suppings. Barley-water, milk and water, thin gruel, the lightest broths… if there be much heat, or any pain in the breast, bleeding will be indispensably necessary… in respect to medicines, the most demulcent and cooling are indicated… [65]

Fothergill, a leading and fashionable physician who conducted a great deal of research into drugs, was well known for his work on the ulcerated or 'malignant' sore throat.[66] More importantly, Wesley, who was one of his patients, received treatment for the consumption from Fothergill. R. Hingston Fox, Fothergill's biographer, notes that under his care Wesley proved to be a rather difficult patient:

> [F]or he had strong views on his own treatment. In 1753 he showed signs of consumption – cough, pain, slow fever. Fothergill insisted on country air, horse-riding and rest from his incessant work. So he took coach for Lewisham, and that night wrote the well-known epitaph upon himself. Later he 'broke through the doctor's order' and fell to his writing again. In the next year he took spells of treatment at the Bristol Hot-Well by Fothergill's advice and seems to have recovered his lung trouble.[67]

Wesley may have ignored the doctor's advice to leave off work, but he nevertheless fully endorsed Fothergill's method for treating the consumption, and it was incorporated into *Primitive Physic*.

Ground-ivy or hyssop infusions were also suggested in *Primitive Physic*, the former, we have already noted, was used by Buchan and the latter was recommended by John Hill in his *The Family Herbal* for coughs and obstructions of the breast.[68] Hyssop has fever-reducing qualities and indeed, is still used in 'complementary' medicine today to alleviate bronchitis. In the eighteenth century it was used to treat inflammatory disorders. Due to its poisonous nature, ivy has a very powerful effect on the internal organs, blood circulation and heart. As such, it was used by Georgian physicians to treat many different diseases.[69]

Wesley prescribed a number of inhalations and vapourisations in *Primitive Physic* for relieving consumption. He suggested inhaling burning frankincense, steam of 'white rosin' and steamed 'spirit of vitriol', the latter of which was commended by Fothergill.[70] The following inhalation remedy given by Wesley in *Primitive Physic* provoked scathing criticism from Hawes:

> 184. Or, every morning cut up a little turf of fresh earth, and lying down, breathe into the hole for a quarter of an hour – I have known a deep consumption cured thus.[71]

On the face of it this might seem quite a strange prescription and indeed, Hawes describes it as such:

> Here is another of Mr. W.'s remedies for a consumption, which need only to be mentioned to excite the reader's risibility. It is a recipe indeed truly worthy of the acute genius of the author of *Primitive Physic...* Mr. W.'s prudence, or art, or effrontery, is superior to that of common quacks... but he should remember, that all the people of England are not votaries to implicit faith, however strongly it may actuate the hearers at the Foundry.[72]

Yet Wesley's direction here is not as eccentric as it appears, and had been put forward by Blackmore in his *A Treatise of Consumptions*: turf was considered valuable for treating this disease because of its sulphurous odour. Blackmore argued that sulphur was particularly useful and explained how the 'chymists' had styled it a 'balsam' for 'the lungs' and blood. Turf was remarkable because it 'eminently contributes to the cure of those that are obnoxious to that distemper'.[73]

Another of Wesley's seemingly bizarre prescriptions for this disease includes sucking a 'healthy woman' (nursing woman): '191. In the last stage, *suck a healthy woman* daily. This cured my Father.'[74] Again, this was something that was frequently recommended by other physicians and in his *Domestic Medicine* Buchan recalls how breast milk cured a patient suffering from a deep consumption:

> It is better if the patient can suck from the breast than to drink it afterwards. I knew a man who was reduced to such a degree of weakness in a consumption, as not to be able to turn himself in bed. His wife was at that time giving suck, and the child happening to die, he sucked her breasts, not with a view to reap any advantage from the milk, but to make her easy. Finding himself however greatly benefited from it, he continued to suck her till he became perfectly well, and is at present a strong and healthy man.[75]

This remedy continued to be used for consumption throughout the period. Although use of human and animal preparations declined during the eighteenth century, they did not disappear altogether. A number of leading physicians, such as Radcliffe, Blackmore, Cheyne and Buchan, continued to recommend ingredients like cow and horse dung, crabs' eyes and claws, crushed oyster shells, woodlice, millipedes and cobwebs in small doses. For chin and convulsive coughs Cheyne suggested the following:

> Take two or three handfuls of millipedes, drown them in sufficient quantity of white wine, then strongly express or squeeze out the juice. This given by spoonfuls (to which end it may be sweetened with sugar) will infallibly cure children's convulsive or chin coughs.[76]

221

This remedy was thought by Cheyne to be equally 'excellent' for the jaundice. Buchan also advised the patient to take woodlice or millipedes, infused in wine, for the whooping cough.[77] Despite the fact that *Primitive Physic* has often been regarded as a 'folksy', popular medical text, it does not recommend insects and, in general, very few animal ingredients are contained in the manual. Moreover, those that do appear can be traced to authoritative sources, such as Radcliffe, Cheyne and Buchan.

The dropsy

This condition refers to oedema, and the medical term 'dropsy' has now become obsolete. The word comes from the Greek, *hudrōps*, meaning watery.[78] In a footnote, Wesley defines it as being:

> A preternatural collection of water in the head, breast, belly, or all over the body. It is attended with a continuous thirst. The part swelled pits if you press it with your fingers. The urine is pale and little.[79]

The disease was divided into two types: anaseara (tumour, mainly in the legs) and ascites (tumour anywhere else in the body, including the abdomen).[80] As a condition, dropsy is particularly interesting because the discovery of its cause, and investigation into its cure, spans the eighteenth century, and shows how perceptions of both illness and treatment changed in a relatively short space of time.

J. Worth Estes sees how physicians were slow to understand heart disease because they regarded the heart as being absolutely essential to life. A breakthrough in treating dropsy came when physicians and medical students discovered that a person could have a diseased heart without actually dying.[81] Collating work undertaken in the area of physiology by Harvey and Marcello Malpighi, Raymond Vieussens conducted research in Montpellier which involved dissecting dropsical patients.[82] By 1705, he discovered that oedema could be attributed to a structural disease of the heart.[83] Dropsy was a result of the heart's weak propulsions, and obstructions to the right of it. Hence it was discovered that this disease, particularly when it affected the lungs and thorax, was cardiac in basis.

Boerhaave, however, believed that dropsical fluid resulted from defective veins, which released the watery substance into the body's tissue. He also thought that dropsy was a type of fever.[84] Many physicians accepted Boerhaave's interpretation and ascribed the illness to 'weakness' and 'laxity' of the fibres, which were unable to act with sufficient force. Other interpretations put forward included that of Stephen Hales who, on the basis of animal experimentation, argued that the dropsy was caused by a depreciation of red blood cells. The body would compensate for this lack by heating the blood to a feverish state, which resulted in dropsy – and here Hales's theory came close to that of Boerhaave.[85] It was not until 1785, when William Withering's influential text, *An Account of the Foxglove* received critical acclaim, that a major breakthrough was made in the treatment of dropsy.[86] Although the foxglove is highly poisonous, its active ingredient, digitalis, is still extracted for chemical compounds to treat heart disease and oedema today. During the eighteenth century it was used to increase urine production.

Estes rightly points out that experimentation and knowledge about exactly how this ingredient worked was still in its infancy. Withering noted that 'the pulse rate fell in patients whose symptoms were ameliorated by the new drug, [but] he did not recognise the drug's tonic effect on the heart.'[87]

It was not until 1813 that the full extent of digitalis and its effect on the heart became known. Despite this, Withering's analysis fitted in with prevailing theories about lax fibres, and it was believed that digitalis stimulated and strengthened the body's system.[88] Before Withering's discovery, most medical practitioners, including Wesley, thought that the disease resulted from lax fibres, suppressed perspiration and decreased motion of blood. Wainewright described it very much in these terms. The blood, he argues:

Grows every day more watery; for the laxity of the fibres being so very great, and the motion of the blood so slow, the complicated arteries of which the glands are composed, cannot be sufficiently distracted, and therefore will separate very little from the mass of blood: so that the quantity of serum will continually increase, and the motion of the blood being so slow, the fibrous parts will retire into the middle of the canals....[89]

Wainewright argued that other factors, which could trigger the consumption, also accounted for dropsy. Buchan ascribed to it the following causes:

Hereditary

Excessive drinking of spirits

Excessive bleeding and evacuations

Sudden stoppage of evacuations

Drinking cold draughts when the body is hot

Damp conditions[90]

He believed that illnesses, such as jaundice, agues, diarrhoea and even consumption, could bring on the dropsy. Symptoms involved water retention in the legs, ankles, throat and body. Other indications could be loss of appetite, excessive thirst and discoloured urine.

Given the fact that an overly 'watery diet' could both provoke and exacerbate this condition, regimen needed to be 'dry'; a dry diet, with aliment consisting of a 'heating' quality, such as roasted aromatic vegetables. Wesley's heating remedies included roasted juniper berries (infused to produce a liquid 'like coffee').[91] Cold bathing was an excellent way of making lax fibres rigid, and again Wesley advised taking the cold bath daily, after a purge.[92] Wainewright argued that the cure for dropsy involved strengthening relaxed fibres by way of rendering the humours more fluid, thus increasing the blood's motion. This would promote secretions of urine and sweat, which was key to resolving the disorder. Dry food, air and cold bathing were the essential components required in the regimen to treat dropsy.

Tonic drugs, as well as powerful diuretics, vomits and purges were also needed. Most of the receipts listed for dropsy in *Primitive Physic* consist of herbal medicines that were diuretics which could remove urine: laurel leaves (powdered), 'pellitory of the wall' (boiled, cooled and corked), 'butcher's broom' (decoction) and 'oak-boughs' (decoction).[93] Both Wainewright and Buchan suggested using tartar, jalap and sena for their diuretic and purgative qualities. These ingredients are included in a remedy put forward in *Primitive Physic*:

> 266. Or, take *sena, cream of tartar* and *jalap* half an ounce of each. Mix them and take a drachm every morning in broth. It usually cures in twenty days. This is nearly the same with Dr. *Ward's* powder....[94]

Buchan argued that tartar produced 'extraordinary' results, due to its diuretic effect. *Primitive Physic* also advises its reader to take dwarf elder tea, drinking a cupful after every discharge – Wesley stated that he had known dropsy to be cured by this method 'in twelve hours'.[95] Indeed, dwarf elder is a powerful diuretic with fever-reducing qualities. Recommended in Hill's *The Family Herbal*, it was commonly used as an infusion to treat dropsy, kidney disorders, rheumatic pain, colds and cough, though its poisonous quality when taken in large doses was an efficacious vomit. As a decoction it was effective for treating sore throats and toothache.[96]

Drawing on Boerhaave, Wesley believed that massaging the dropsy with 'sallad' oil twice a day could ease the swelling.[97] In later editions of *Primitive Physic,* he also suggested that the heat induced by electricity could overturn this disease. One final point of interest about Wesley's approach to treating the dropsy can be seen in the way he changed his attitude on the issue of fluid-intake. In the earlier editions of *Primitive Physic* Wesley directs the reader to: 'Abstain from all drink for thirty days. To ease your thirst hold often on your tongue, a thin small slice of toasted bread, dipt in brandy.'[98]

By the 23rd edition, Wesley's stance on this had radically shifted as a result of new medical evidence. In light of new developments he omitted the above statement, replacing it instead with the following observation:

> How amazingly little is yet known, even of the human body! Have not dropsical persons been continually advised to abstain from drink as much as possible? But how can we reconcile this with the following undeniable facts, published in the late *Medical Transactions*?[99]

Wesley goes on to cite three patient case studies, presented in the *Medical Transactions*, which proved the efficacy of taking a plentiful supply of fluids. Clearly, this change of attitude reflects the fact that Wesley kept up with all of the medical discoveries needed to make necessary changes to *Primitive Physic*.

A fever

This notoriously theory-laden disease generated a massive volume of literature in the eighteenth century.[100] It was Pitcairne, Cheyne and Boerhaave who dictated the terms here and Cheyne not only identified the internecine 'war on the subject of fevers', but suggested that the best way to deal with this war was to follow Pitcairne's example and provide an even more 'specious account' of the disease.[101]

Porter points out that 'fever' tended to be an umbrella-term in the eighteenth century: it covered both epidemic and individual febrile crises.[102] It was also broken down into specific types, which had different causes and triggers. The various types were identified by Huxham and presented in his *An Essay on Fevers*:

> Ardent and inflammatory fevers are naturally the effect of over-elastic and rigid fibres, and a very dense viscid blood; as the low and slow nervous kind are of a too lax state of vessels, and a weak thin blood – but there are several diseases, especially those arising from contagion, which are common to both.[103]

Primitive Physic lists various types of fevers and offers a range of cures. This is indicative of the fact that Wesley understood how each fever needed to be treated on its own account. The different fevers were arranged in the following order from the first edition onwards:

105. A Fever

106. A High Fever

107. An Intermitting Fever

108. A Fever with pains in the Limbs

109. A Rash Fever

110. A Slow Fever (nervous fever)

111. A Worm Fever (not listed in the first edition).

The 'hectic' and 'continual' fevers were included in the first edition but were subsequently omitted.

Conflicting interpretations of the fever and its appropriate treatment co-existed and often made unhappy bedfellows in the eighteenth century. By way of mitigating confusion and tension surrounding this disease, the physician William Cullen drew up a nosology, which dealt with those infectious illnesses associated with fevers. This, he set out in his *First Lines of the Practice of Physic* (1778–9) where infectious diseases came under the category of *Pyrexiae* (febrile).[104] Cullen's nosology gave a prominent role to contagion in the cause of fever and this was his way of imposing order on an issue riven by controversy – though it remained true that the disease, as Porter argues, assumed various forms, both contagious and miasmatic. It is worth quoting Porter in full on this point because he explicates the complicated nature of the various interpretations of fever in a succinct way:

> Conditions like smallpox with well defined symptoms and spread by contact were attributed to specific contagions. Intermediate between these and the diseases of locality... (typified by ague or intermittent fever, associated with the rotting vegetation of marshes) lay the 'doubtful' diseases, which were 'sometimes contagious and sometimes not'... the least defined pyrexiae were the continued fevers, divided mainly into typhus... and relapsing.[105]

We have noted how Sydenham, by making use of the Hippocratic Corpus, developed classifications of the fever, which relied on external factors (miasmatic).[106] Following on from this, eighteenth-century physicians, such as Arbuthnot and Huxham, investigated the relationship between air and fever epidemics.[107] Margaret DeLacy has shown that contagion theories also began to compete with those of miasma from the mid-century onwards. She identifies Fothergill's *An Account of the Sore Throat Attended with Ulcers* (1748) as a turning point in this development. This essay, she argues, described an epidemic of what was scarlet fever and attributed it to a specific contagion, 'a *miasma sui generis*'.[108]

Theories surrounding exactly what caused a fever and the best method of treatment were multiple and created much infighting amongst leading medical practitioners. There were, however, some points on which physicians could agree. An inflammatory fever, like a cold or pneumonia, which may or may not have been contagious, was characterised by a strong, hard pulse but no delirium. This was categorised by Cullen as *Synocha*. An inflammatory fever accompanied by delirium, Cullen labelled *Typhus*.[109] Porter shows that eighteenth-century physicians identified three stages in the fever:

1. Debility with relaxation (*atony*) of the arteries

2. Irritation

3. Hot stage – resulting from arterial spasm[110]

In terms of treating the fever, it was thought that an obstruction needed to be expelled from the body.[111] Unless the obstruction was removed, it was feared that the fever could 'turn in' on the patient and induce conditions favourable to more threatening illnesses.[112] In the main, physicians tended to follow methods set down by Cheyne and Boerhaave, both of whom ascribed the cause of fever to obstructions and advised treatment in terms of bleeding in the first instance. Cheyne argued that the 'General Proposition' of *all* fevers is 'the obstruction or dilation of (the complicated *nerve* and *artery*, the *excretory duct* and *conservatory* one, or rather all these; which, shall be afterward shewn make up) the *glands*....'[113]

This obstruction leads to the pulse feeling strong and hard because blood and the '*Liquidum Nervorum*' (nervous fluid) could not pass through the canals, nerves and fibres easily. This strong pulse caused a headache and:

> [A] burning heat... upon these accounts, 1. Because there is a greater quantity than ordinary running in the passable canals, there must be a greater motion than ordinary and consequently a greater heat. 2. Merely upon the account of the increased quantity (without considering the thereby produc'd greater velocity) there must be felt a greater heat....[114]

Internal heat therefore brought on an unquenchable thirst when running a fever.

Cheyne argued that the best way to treat this illness was to bleed (if pulse was strong), purge and sweat the patient in the first instance, although he also advised mercurial medicines by way of removing obstructions. With the exception of advocating mercurial medicine, this method is evident in *Primitive Physic* and Wesley makes the following direction at the beginning of his receipt for 'A Fever':

105. A Fever.

In the beginning of any fever, if the stomach is uneasy, vomit; if the bowels, purge: if the pulse be hard, full or strong, bleed.[115]

Cheyne's *New Theory* sought recourse to intricate language and mathematical formulations to demonstrate that all fevers were the result of obstructions or dilations of the glands. Purging, sweating, vomiting or bleeding had to be prescribed – in other words, bad matter had to be eliminated in some way. In Cheyne's work, the theory surrounding disease is postulated in a language that is medically and scientifically specified. Yet diagnosis itself remains traditional. When critics accuse Wesley of stripping Cheyne's work of its theory, this is exactly what they are referring to. The direction given in *Primitive Physic* to treat fever reveals that Wesley follows the same procedure as Cheyne: vomiting, purging and bleeding. Medical jargon is absent, but the relationship between disease and remedy is just as precisely set out, although Wesley inserted this direction in those later editions of *Primitive Physic*, following the 15th edition of 1772. Undoubtedly, he inserted this information on the basis of Hawes's criticism in *An Examination*:

Among all Mr. Wesley's remedies for fevers, *bleeding* is never once advised to lower the action of the vessels, which is exceedingly necessary when the pulse is hard, full and strong… nor does he once advise an *emetic* or a *purgative* at the beginning of fevers, although there may be symptoms indicating their use….[116]

Wesley was dissuaded in earlier editions from including the established method of bleeding a fever because he considered it to be dangerous, particularly when used over-liberally. On this point he was not alone: the physician John Millar believed that those deaths reported in the Mortality Bills relating to fever could be attributed to doctors over-bleeding their patients. Millar argued that as the Peruvian bark came to substitute bleeding for treating fever, so the number of deaths relating to this illness decreased.[117] We know already that Wesley had strong feelings on the issue of treating fevers with Bark. Despite the fact that he also regarded (excessive) bleeding with suspicion, this was preferable to the bark – particularly when Wesley himself had suffered such negative side effects when taking the Peruvian Bark for an ague. As is always the case in medical practice, it was a matter of balancing competing risks: recommending the bark was not an option but, as Hawes pointed out, running a fever represented much more of a mortal risk to patients than cautious bleeding. In light of this, Wesley calculated that it would be better to steer the patient towards bleeding, providing the pulse was 'hard, full or strong'.

It was taken for granted that physicians should bleed patients who were running a fever (when the pulse was full and strong). Here, medical practitioners, such as Huxham, followed a course already set down by Cheyne and Boerhaave. Huxham had completed his medical training as a student under Boerhaave's instruction at Leyden. In his *An Essay on Fevers*, he argued that the velocity of heat and pulse, occasioned by a febrile state, needed to be lessened by bleeding:

> By this means the red globules of the blood and *vis motrix* are lessened. By bleeding *ad deliquium*, as Galen, and some of the ancient physicians did in inflammatory fevers, the bloods motion almost quite ceases for a short time.[118]

The longer that bleeding was neglected, the more viscous and acrimonious the blood became. Huxham advised caution when bleeding and stated that the quantity of blood to be taken very much depended on the strength of an individual's pulse rate. Doctors needed to exercise caution and bleedings had to be taken little and often.[119]

The therapeutic value of bloodletting has been explored recently in a fascinating study undertaken by a Canadian physiologist, Norman Kasting.[120] Looking at a range of historical evidence in tandem with animal experimentation, Kasting concluded that bleeding had an effective antipyretic stimulus on patients. There were three major reasons for this: firstly, loss of blood reduced the body's temperature, thus drawing pressure away from the brain. A subsidiary result of this was that the patient could rest and sleep more easily, thus aiding recovery – all of which was duly noted by physicians spanning the early-Greek period to the mid-nineteenth century. Secondly, the loss of iron involved in reducing blood-levels meant that harmful bacteria feeding on this constituent could be lessened. Thirdly, loss of blood causes the pituitary gland to release hormones such as vasopressin, which stimulates the immune system.[121] Kasting therefore determined that bleeding had been beneficial to patients suffering from febrile illnesses and this explained its repeated use throughout the ages. Although particular physicians objected to its over-use, venesection remained the only viable option in terms of reducing the temperature associated with fever until the discovery of sodium salicylate in 1876, which was extracted from willow bark and manufactured as aspirin in 1899.[122]

Eighteenth-century physicians also believed that bleeding a patient made way for those thin, diluting liquors, which were 'necessary to supply the continual waste of the lymph and serum, and to keep the whole mass [of blood] in a due degree of fluxility'.[123] Huxham's directives here followed the diluting diet advocated by Cheyne and Boerhaave – though Huxham believed that drinking water for the fever was inadvisable, on the basis that it did not mix well with blood. He also thought that cooling too quickly during a fever was potentially dangerous. Instead, the physician needed to recommend sugary drinks, syrups and fruit cordials or juice.[124] Wesley advocated a cooling regimen and medicaments for the fever (particularly the intermitting fever) which included drinking warm lemonade, balm-tea, tar-water and water-gruel with honey. In fact, like Buchan, Wesley thought that regimen (fresh air, cooling diet, exercise) was preferable to physic. Water-drinking was central to Wesley's regimen in general, so he would not have agreed with Huxham's stance on its inefficacy when treating fevers. Indeed, water-drinking was recommended in the first edition of *Primitive Physic* for the fever and is retained in all subsequent editions: '352. Drink a pint or two of *cold water* lying down in bed: I never knew it to hurt'.[125]

The remedies put forward in *Primitive Physic* to alleviate, if not cure, the fever follow a fairly orthodox path in that they are concerned to reduce the body's temperature (bleeding) and clear the intestines (purging, vomiting, clysters) in order to make room for diluting liquors, which could remove obstructions. *Primitive Physic* only strays from this path in its recommendation of 'treacle plaisters', which were to be applied to the wrists, head and soles of feet. Cheyne considered 'outward applications' only useful in that they removed the accidental effects of fever – to appease the heat associated with fever – rather than the illness itself. In his adoption of the plaisters Wesley extracted from Tissot's *L'Avis*; the Swiss doctor recommended using sugary plasters to raise a sweat, but it was also an effective way of killing germs.[126]

Porter argues that very little could be done about the fever, particularly the epidemic kind. The best a physician could do was to support the patient and trust in 'the healing power of nature'.[127] There is no doubt that *Primitive Physic* sought to put its trust in nature, but it is clear that Wesley's method of treating the fever, like that of the consumption, formed part of a much bigger debate about disease and its possible cures. In the case of fever, debates were controversial and it is interesting to see the way in which Wesley negotiated his way through an issue which was fraught with tension and theory. On the whole, *Primitive Physic* advocated conventional treatments for the fever while simultaneously adding one or two flourishes that bear the mark of Wesley's strong medical opinions.

The gout in any limb

It is now known that this chronic complaint is induced by an excessive level of uric acid in the blood (hyperuricaemia), which creates a deposition of sodium urate in the joints and extremities.[128] It was regimen and dietetic therapies that were used to prevent, treat or control the gout, primarily because it was thought that rich food and alcohol created this condition.[129] This thinking is thoroughly epitomised by Buchan in *Domestic Medicine*:

> There is no disease which shows the imperfection of medicine, or sets the advantages of temperance and exercise in a stronger light than this. Few who pay a proper regard to these are troubled with the gout. This points out the true source from whence that malady originally sprung, viz. excess and *idleness*. It likewise shows us that the only safe and efficacious method of cure, or rather of prevention, must depend, not upon medicine, but on *temperance* and *activity*.[130]

Like nervous diseases, gout was associated with an indolent, rich and urban lifestyle, which meant that medical practitioners like Cheyne, Tissot, Buchan and Wesley took a moralistic stance on the issue – a view that reached full fruition in the controversial work written by Cadogan, *A Dissertation on the Gout, and all Chronic Diseases, Jointly Considered as Proceeding from the Same Causes*. Cadogan argued that the gout was a European illness, symptomatic of a highly civilised, luxurious lifestyle.[131]

Factors believed to contribute to the gout included:

Heredity

Acid liquors and salts (wine, tea, coffee, meat, fish and highly seasoned food)

Oily foods

Intense study

The passions

Obstructions

Perspiration

Wesley's complex stance on the cause of this chronic disease has already been identified. He took Cadogan to task in the introductory remarks to his *Extract from Dr Cadogan's Dissertation on the Gout and all Chronic Diseases* for denying the role heredity played in the illness.[132] Cadogan argued that if gout were hereditary, it would affect women and children. Yet Cheyne had suggested that women did not suffer from the gout because their fibres and solids were generally in a more 'relaxed' state, which meant that obstructions did not clog up the body's system so readily in the first instance. Cadogan insisted that, if hereditary, gout would be incurable – like scrofula and madness. He believed that the illness could be remedied by a mainly milk

231

diet. Cadogan's outright denial of heredity playing its part in this condition provoked a great deal of controversy and a number of physicians sought to challenge his work. Wesley believed that heredity was a significant factor in the disease but that a combination of regimen and medicine could mitigate, if not cure, the gout. In fact, he argued that very few of the 'chronic' distempers associated with the disease were truly hereditary, but stemmed rather from an intemperate and indolent lifestyle. This he makes clear in a journal entry, dated 9 September 1771:

> It is certainly true, that 'very few of them [Chronical Distempers] are properly hereditary'; that most of them spring either from indolence, or intemperance, or irregular passions.[133]

Unlike his contemporaries, Wesley did not take an either/or position on the issue but presented a range of possible 'cures' in *Primitive Physic*. In so doing, he sought to provide hope to those suffering from an 'inveterate' disease that could make life pretty miserable. Most physicians thought that gout was incurable; indeed, William Stukley argued that those afflicted with hereditary gout should give up trying to find a remedy and concentrate instead on relieving its symptoms.[134] Wesley, like Cadogan, believed that the gout could be cured:

> Regard not them who say, the Gout *ought not* to be cured. They mean, it *cannot*. I know it cannot by *their irregular prescriptions*. But I have known it cured in many cases, without any ill effects following.[135]

Cheyne argued that it was difficult to work out exactly what caused gout, but believed the 'gouty' person had smaller, narrower vessels, which were stiffer and more rigid.[136] The 'goutish' humour mixed with the blood, rendering it sizy, thus reducing circulation and creating obstructions.[137] Gout worked its way out of the body via the extremities because the smallest vessels were compressed in the joints and so susceptible to obstruction. Ironically, Cheyne argued that gouty persons were generally quite healthy; it was only their small, stiff vessels which gave rise to the complaint.[138] Given this, there was no universal cure for the problem, though a moderate diet could help:

> For unless a remedy could be found, which at once could change and new mould the solid parts of human bodies; alter the nature and qualities of animal and vegetable bodies; and destroy parts that are in their own nature fixed and permanent, it is impossible it should be certain and universal.[139]

Regimen was the only viable answer to effecting an alleviation, and Cheyne counselled those suffering from the gout that evacuations were particularly efficacious – the reason being that evacuation could dispel the salts and acids which aggravated the disease.[140] On this, Cheyne disagreed with Sydenham, who he described as an 'accurate observer of Nature' and most 'judicious practitioner', though mistaken on the issue of evacuations for treating the gout.

Due to the fact that gout rose out of an exorbitant collection of 'bitter and sour juices', evacuation and dilution were required in the very first instance.[141] Diluting drinks and infusions were essential, and Cheyne advocated drinking spring water, green tea, bitters and dwarf elder tea. For medicines, it was useful to take an infusion of bark. Mercurial vomits for the persistent gout was an active medicine that could break down bad matter and render the humours fluid, though 'spirit of vitriol' was also recommended by Cheyne. If the pain became unbearable the patient needed to take opium or hot baths.[142] *Domestic Medicine* differs very little from Cheyne's prescriptions, and diluting liquors, exercise, purges and active treatments, such as the bark, are cited as possible remedies. Buchan strongly advises the patient to bathe in warm water frequently, but insists too on the importance of blistering plaisters to draw the gouty humour out of the body.[143]

Wesley's remedies for the 'Gout in any Limb' are fully conversant with those presented by Cheyne and Buchan. He also suggests a treacle plaister: '378. Rub the part with *warm treacle*, and then bind on a flannel smeared therewith. Repeat this, if need be, once in twelve hours.'

He was convinced that this method would draw out the gouty humour and insisted that it had 'cured an inveterate Gout in thirty-six hours'.[144] Other treatments listed for the gout included a diluting drink (to reduce sour juices of the humour) and warm bathing to ease the pain:

> 379. Or, drink a pint of strong infusion of *elder-buds* dry or green, morning and evening. This has cured inveterate Gouts.

> 380. Or, at six in the evening, undress and wrap yourself in blankets. Then put your legs up to the knees in water, as hot as you can bear it. As it cools, let hot water be poured in, so as to keep you in a strong sweat till ten....[145]

Elder-bud was an especially efficient herb and Wesley's source here is unclear – it could well have been based on his own experience, or that of his mother, who also suffered from the condition. Elder-bud not only acted as a diuretic, but when infused as a tea had a tranquillising quality. This could well have eased the pain of a gouty swelling. As a final recommendation, Wesley points out that 'the very matter of the Gout is frequently destroyed by a steady use of *Mynficht's Elixir of Vitriol*'. Here, it is unlikely that he was simply following Cheyne's usage because this observation was added to later editions and is not included in the first.[146]

It is necessary to consider one final point on the issue of Wesley's treatment of the gout. This point was raised by Hawes in his *Examination*, where he aims fire at Wesley's remedy for 'Gout in the Foot or Hand', listed separately from the 'Gout in any Limb'. For 'Gout in the Foot or Hand' Wesley asks the patient to: '[377] Apply a raw lean *beef-steak*. Change it once in twelve hours, till cured. Tried.'[147]

It is not clear from which source Wesley derived this remedy. Despite Hawes's criticism, Wesley was keen to retain it in those editions following the *Examination* on the basis that, having been 'Tried' and tested, it had actually worked. The condemnation invoked by the remedy did not come directly from Hawes himself, but from the Calvinist minister, Augustus Toplady, with whom Wesley had been embroiled in numerous controversial theological debates. In a moment of sheer opportunism, Hawes uses Toplady's remarks to attack *Primitive Physic*:

> Instead of making any remarks of my own upon this curious remedy, I shall here take the liberty of transcribing what hath been said in relation to it by the Rev. Mr. Toplady. 'In Mr. Wesley's book of receipts, entitled *Primitive Physick,* he advises persons who have the gout in their feet and hands, to apply raw lean beef steaks to the part affected… somebody recommended this dangerous repellent to Dr. T. in the year 1764 or early in 1765. He tried the experiment; the gout was, in consequence, driven up to his stomach and head, and he died a few days after at *Bath*, where I happened to spend a considerable part of those years; and where at the very time of the Dean's death, I became acquainted with the particulars of that catastrophe. I am far from meaning to insinuate, because I do not know, that the person who persuaded Dr. T. to this fatal recourse derived the recipe immediately from Mr. Wesley's medical compilation. All I aver is, that the recipe itself is to be found there, which demonstrates the unskilful temerity, wherewith the compiler sets himself up as a physician of the body. Should his quack pamphlet come to another edition, 'tis to be hoped that the *beef steak* remedy will… be expunged from the list of receipts for the gout – 'tis, I acknowledge, an effectual cure: cut off a man's head, and he'll no more be annoyed by the toothache…'.[148]

Toplady goes on to state that the man who concerns himself in everything 'bids fair not to make a figure in anything' and accuses Wesley of this tendency.[149]

A number of important points have been raised here by Toplady's critique. Firstly, is the fact that this case had been relayed second-hand to

Toplady and might, for this reason, have been inaccurate. Secondly, even Toplady himself is forced to admit that the recipe used by 'Dr T.' may not have been derived from *Primitive Physic*. Thirdly, without knowing the particulars of how, exactly, the patient died, it is difficult to make any assessment. Clearly, this attack was not based on medical grounds, evidenced by Toplady's reference to Wesley's 'quack pamphlet'. Given that Toplady and Wesley's debates usually revolved around theological points of principle, it is obvious that the critique here was sectarian in basis.[150] The fact that Wesley neither removed nor amended the recipe attests to the fact that he understood this and dismissed it as such.

The King's Evil

This disease, also known as 'scrofula', is something that can only be defined historically – though it was not a term used by ancient physicians. The history of medicine scholar R.K. French explains that 'scrofula' is:

> [A] term about which there was some measure of consensus in the past, but one that has now been largely superseded by terms that indicate some form of tuberculosis.[151]

French points out that historians should not automatically assume that this condition was, in fact, tuberculosis. The name, 'King's Evil', was coined in the mediaeval period and came into being as a result of widespread belief that the King, possessed of divine rights, could cure this disease by touch. By the eighteenth century this belief had all but disappeared, though French observes that up until 1789, kings continued to 'touch' on the Continent.[152] Buchan observed that the vulgar were:

> [R]emarkably credulous with regard to the cure of scrofula, many of them believing in the virtue of the Royal touch, that of the seventh son… the truth is, we know but little either of the nature or cure of this disease, and where reason or medicines fail, superstition always comes in their place.[153]

Both terms, 'The King's Evil' and 'scrofula', continued to be used in their adjectival forms throughout the eighteenth century, though the disease was fraught with different theories and no cure was ever postulated.[154]

Physicians believed the illness to be hereditary, though not chronic or infectious.[155] Wesley provides a description of 'The King's Evil' in *Primitive Physic*:

> It commonly appears first, by the thickness of the lips; or a stubborn humour in the eyes; then come hard swellings in the neck chiefly: then running sores.[156]

Symptoms of this disease took the form of small 'knots' under the chin, around the neck and behind the ears. Eventually, this cluster of knots developed into one large tumour. Other symptoms involved swollen glands (armpits, groin area, feet and eyes). Internal swellings included the liver or spleen and the lungs might also become ulcerated. The causes of The King's Evil were attributed to 'vitiated' humours and extreme temperatures. Neglect of proper regimen, such as a lack of exercise, unwholesome air, damp and poor hygiene, was also thought to be contributory factors.[157]

Regimen (dry air, moderate exercise and cold bathing) was thus central to effecting prevention and cure, but Buchan also believed that this disease would cure itself. This was why, he argued, 'quack' remedies and those of 'old women' gained applause when they deserved none.[158] Medicines needed to be cooling and diluting, with very mild purgatives. *Primitive Physic* listed several cooling drinks and strongly endorsed cold bathing for The King's Evil. Undoubtedly, the most effective cooling drink advocated by Wesley was a 'strong decoction of *devil's bit*'.[159] This decoction was especially good for treating disorders of the lungs (ulcerated) and is listed as such by Hill in *The Family Herbal*.[160] Wesley also instructed the reader on how to prepare a 'diet' drink, used specifically for scorbutic sores, which could be both diuretic and purging. As a diuretic, the drink enabled the (internal) bad matter to be carried off safely, thus preventing it from corrupting the blood. However, like Buchan, Wesley counselled the patient to avoid using violent purges, as this could aggravate the disease.[161] The diet drink was also effective as an external application to treat the sores, which were often attendant to The King's Evil.[162] In his directives for treating The King's Evil, Wesley managed to encapsulate the best of what was currently available to patients.

Lunacy, raging madness, nervous disorders

Wesley's treatment of insanity has given rise to innumerable caricatures and confusions. Historians have often accused Wesley of conflating madness and demonic possession. Undoubtedly, they have not read the prescriptions for lunacy or madness in *Primitive Physic*, all of which tie-in with eighteenth-century medical practice. This caricature is based on the fact that, as a Christian, Wesley sought to distinguish organic or psychological symptoms of madness from those which were spiritual or diabolical in orientation: as a minister, he would have considered it vital to ensure that he was not resisting the world of spirits.[163]

It was often the case that Wesley expressed impatience with contemporary physicians who dismissed spiritual suffering as madness, and in his *Thoughts on Nervous Disorders* (1784) he makes a swingeing attack on this tendency:

When Physicians meet with disorders which they do not understand, they commonly term them nervous; a word that conveys to us no determinate idea, but is a good cover for learned ignorance. But these are often no natural disorder of the body, but the hand of God upon the soul, being a dull consciousness of the want of God, and the unsatisfactoriness of everything here below.[164]

Wesley was right to point to the fact that 'nervous disorders' was a term used to cover a multitude of illnesses and complaints. He makes this statement in the first paragraph of the tract on nervous disorders, but in the second paragraph he is keen to state that there are:

[N]ervous disorders which are purely natural. Many of these are concerned with other diseases, whether acute or chronical. Many are forerunners of various distempers, and many are consequences of them. But there are those which are not connected with others, being themselves a distinct, original distemper.[165]

Paul Laffey raises a crucially important issue when he argues that Wesley distinguished organic madness from religious experience in order to make a moral point:

His insistence that religion 'stands in direct opposition to madness of every kind' also signals a key point about his understanding of the difference between genuine madness... on the one hand, and the spiritual troubles and travails experienced by men and women, on the other... in pragmatic terms he indeed held insanity to be distinct from religious experience.[166]

This distinction has already been identified in Chapter 4, where the role Wesley ascribed to the 'passions' in causing disease was examined. Here, we saw how he assessed individuals on a case-by-case basis before deciding the best way to proceed in terms of regimen and physic. Even in circumstances where there was sufficient uncertainty about whether an 'episode' was organic or spiritual, Wesley usually prescribed a mixture of regimen, physic and prayer.

Wesley's *Journal* and letters reveal that he regarded some instances of insanity as symptoms of spiritual malaise, but it is important to highlight the ways in which he acknowledged genuine madness. In 1766, he made this clear when relating an incident that took place in Weardale:

A poor woman was brought to us who had been disordered several years, and was now raving mad. She cursed and blasphemed in a terrible manner, and could not stand or sit still for a moment. However, her husband constrained her to come to the place where I was going to preach; and he held her there by main strength, although she shrieked in a most dreadful manner; but in a quarter of an hour she left off shrieking, and sat motionless and silent, till she began crying to God, which she continued to do, almost without intermission, till we left her.[167]

Remarking on this passage, Laffey observes that Wesley is content to recognise the organic nature of this woman's madness, indicated by the fact that he does not attempt to draw her into prayer. Neither does he seek to provide moral or spiritual intervention.[168] This woman clearly needed medical, as opposed to purely spiritual, intervention and Wesley understood that not all instances of mental distress were diabolical.[169]

In common with many contemporary physicians, Wesley thought that genuine cases of madness were physical disorders and needed to be treated as such. Irregular blood circulation or hurried, agitated animal spirits gave rise to disordered thoughts or raging madness. Nervous disorders stemmed from an obstruction, relaxation or malfunction of the nerves, and although physicians like Willis, Sydenham and Cheyne dismissed the idea of hysterical symptoms arising from the womb, all agreed that women generally suffered more from hysteria. This was due to the fact that women's animal spirits, nerves and fibres were weaker.[170] All of the prescriptions given in *Primitive Physic* for 'Lunacy', 'Raging Madness' and 'Nervous Disorders' were designed to deal with bodily disorder:

151. *Lunacy*

468. Give decoction of *agrimony* four times a day:

469. Or, rub the head several times a day with *vinegar*, in which *ground-ivy leaves* have been infused:

470. Or, take daily an ounce of *distilled vinegar.*

471. Or, boil juice of *ground-ivy* with *sweet oil* and *white wine* into an ointment. Shave the head, anoint it therewith, and chafe it in warm every other day for three weeks. Bruise also the leaves and bind them on the head, and give three spoonfuls of the juice warm every morning. This generally cures melancholy. The juice alone, taken twice a day, will cure.

472. Or, *electrify.* Tried.

152. *Raging Madness*

473. Apply to the head, cloths dipt in *cold water.*

474. Or, set the patient with his head under a great *water-fall,* as long as his strength will bear: or, pour water on his head out of a tea-kettle:

238

475. Or, let him eat nothing but *apples* for a month:

476. Or nothing but *bread* and *milk*: Tried.

161. *Nervous Disorders*

502. When the nerves perform their office too languidly, A GOOD AIR is the first requisite. The patient also should rise early, and as soon as the dew is on the ground, walk: let his breakfast be *Mother of Thyme* tea… or the common *Garden Thyme*, if the former cannot be procured. When the nerves are too sensible, let the person breathe proper air. Let him eat veal, chicken or mutton. Vegetables should be eat sparingly; the most innocent is the French bean; and the best root, the turnip. Wine should be avoided carefully: so should all sauces. Sometimes he may breakfast upon a quarter of an ounce of *Valerian root* infused in hot water, to which he many add cream and sugar. Tea is not proper. When the person finds an uncommon oppression, let him take a large spoonful of the tincture of *Valerian root*.

503. But I am firmly persuaded, there is no remedy in nature, for nervous disorders of every kind, comparable to the proper and constant use of the *electrical machine*.[171]

In a footnote attached to 'Raging Madness' Wesley makes the following citation from Mead:

It is a sure rule that all madmen are cowards, and may be conquered by binding only, without beating. (Dr Mead). He also observes, that blistering the head does more harm than good. Keep the head close shaved, and frequently wash it with vinegar.[172]

Wesley's use of cold-water therapy and astringent remedies for raging madness corresponds to the advice set down by Mead – although most of the above remedies had been suggested in the 1st edition of *Primitive Physic*, and Wesley would not have been familiar at that point with this aspect of Mead's physic.[173] Other physicians used the cold-water treatment, and Tobias Smollet argued in his *An Essay on the External Use of Water* (1752) that it increased motion and circulation.[174] Water-therapy had, in fact, been advocated for centuries and continued to be widely used in the Georgian period, though from the mid-eigheenth century onwards electricity began to displace water treatments. His footnote drawing on Mead is striking in its emphasis on therapeutic solutions, as opposed to advocating punishment and beatings, and reflects the fact that a more 'humane' approach to madness was developing at this time. Eventually this would reach full fruition in the moral therapy and philanthropic endeavours of the Tuke family, who opened the York Retreat in 1796.[175]

In the case of nervous disorders, Buchan argued that they were the most difficult to treat. Nervous disorders were variable, with symptoms affecting individuals very differently. He therefore believed that the best remedy rested with regimen and, like Wesley, advocated early rising, fresh air, exercise and a nourishing diet. Like Cheyne, Buchan thought that a diluting diet to thin the fluids was best, but suggested the patient avoid anything that tended to 'relax or weaken' the body's fibres and nerves, such as tea, coffee and alcohol. This disease was largely due to a 'lax' state of fibres and it was necessary to restore tone and elasticity. Vigorous exercise such as riding was essential because it gave motion to the body without unduly fatiguing the patient, and fresh air generally 'braced' the body. Rising early, using the flesh brush and cold bathing all constricted lax fibres and were crucial elements to the regimen required for treating nervous disorders:

> Few things tend more to strengthen the nervous system than cold bathing. This practice, if duly persisted in, will, produce very extraordinary effects.[176]

It is clear that Wesley generally favoured regimen and believed it was an essential aid when curing this disease. He instructed the reader of *Thoughts on Nervous Disorders* to avoid the 'fashionable poison' of spirits and tea.[177] In *Primitive Physic,* Wesley strongly recommends cold bathing and electrical therapy for nervous disorders. In his direction of the patient to the Valerian root (infused or in tincture form) he follows advice set down by Hill, who had written a tract entitled *Valerian: Or, the Virtues of that Root in Nervous Disorders* (1758). Here, Hill had pointed out that this aromatic root was the 'sovereign medicine' for all nervous disorders and:

> [I]n particular exceeds all the remedies commonly used against that worst of headaches… it alone has cured epilepsies: and of late has been used very successfully in hysteric complaints; and in that terrible disorder the convulsive asthma. It alleviates pain in the manner of the more gentle opiates; and is found highly effectual in fits proceeding from the obstructions of the menses; not only taking off the symptoms but removing the cause…

It is interesting that Hill suggested this drug in place of opiates. Opiates were commonly used for treating nervous disorders and although Buchan asks his reader to use the drug sparingly, it is still listed amongst his list of remedies in *Domestic Medicine.* Given Wesley's general distrust of those 'Herculean' medicines, it was necessary to find a suitable alternative. Like Hill, he suggested taking valerian as a tincture and instructs his reader on how to do this:

> This tincture should be made thus: – cut to pieces six ounces of wild Valerian root, gathered in June, and fresh dried. Bruise it by a few strokes in a mortar,

that the pieces may be split, but it should not be beat into a powder: put this into a quart of strong white wine: cork the bottle and let it stand three weeks, shaking it every day; then press it out and filter the tincture through paper.[178]

A full-scale analysis of the changes that took place in the treatment of insanity and mental health lies well beyond the scope of this book and is anyway not entirely relevant to our concerns. Suffice it to say, at its simplest level, eighteenth-century physicians regarded troubled minds as indicative of bodily disorder. Cullen defined insanity as a neurological disorder and concurred with Locke's assumption that madness was a false association of ideas.[179] Madness was physical in its basis and so it could be managed by physic (bleeding, blistering, purging, tonic medicines or opium) or, more usually, by 'moral management'.[180] Here, madness was regarded as a psychological condition or 'defect' of the understanding, which could be corrected by the superior will, personality and insights of the 'mad-doctor'.[181] In many ways Wesley thoroughly endorsed contemporary views on madness and this is especially evident in his sermon on *The Nature of Enthusiasm* where he uses Lockean language to hypothesise a madness that stemmed from wrong ideas: 'a madman draws right conclusions, but from wrong premises. And so does an enthusiast'.[182] Yet Wesley was keen to discern whether symptoms presented as mad were actually psychological, as opposed to spiritual. Laffey summarises Wesley's position very well:

> Wesley was wholly a man of his age: he bowed to strict rationalism in his understanding of what insanity was and what it represented, even though he differed from many of his contemporaries in viewing much of what they regarded as madness as denominating spiritual or demonic strife instead.[183]

This stance explains Wesley's attitude to madhouses in general and Laffey points out that his missionary activity in Bedlam, amongst other institutions, arose from a concern, not with the genuinely insane, but with those inmates wrongly diagnosed – those who were really suffering from spiritual and not mental torment:

> Another of Dr. Monro's patients came to desire my advice. I found no reason to believe that she had been any otherwise mad than every one is, who is deeply convinced of sin; and I cannot doubt, but if she will trust in the living God, He will 'give medicine to heal her sickness'.[184]

Asylums were not inherently bad places and Wesley would not have taken a principled position against the existence of these institutions. Indeed, for those individuals who represented a danger, asylums offered a very convenient and effective remedy, even if their practices might be improved.[185] In fact, Wesley wrote in fairly glowing terms about St Luke's

Hospital, which was opened to rival Bedlam in 1751. His comments were recorded in a journal entry for 21 December 1762:

> I had an opportunity of looking over the register of St Luke's Hospital; and I was surprised to observe that three in four (at least) of those that are admitted receive a cure. I doubt this is not [*sic*] the case of any other lunatic hospital in Great Britain or Ireland.[186]

Laffey observes that Wesley had no problem with the 'secular' medical practices offered at St Luke's once he had satisfied himself that an individual was suffering from madness and not spiritual suffering:

> Wesley regarded genuine madness as that which betokened loss, degradation and absence: the lunatic was not wholly human... to Wesley insanity was to be stigmatised; to fail to do so would not have made sense within the theological perspective he championed. We must take seriously his proposal that 'religion... stands in direct opposition to madness of every kind'.[187]

He made his views on this matter crystal clear on numerous occasions but most notably in his *Appeals*, where it was carefully explicated with great rhetorical flourish:

> It is not strange, then, that some, while under strong impressions of grief or fear from a sense of the wrath of God, should for a season *forget* almost all things else, and scarce be able to answer a common question... [this] and whatever less common effects may sometimes accompany this conviction, are easily known from the natural distemper of madness, were it only by this one circumstance, that whenever the person convinced tastes the pardoning love of God they all vanish away in a moment.[188]

Proof of 'real' madness for Wesley lay in the fact that it was usually long-lasting and entrenched. It could only be managed and the condition of sufferers possibly improved by the long and painstaking work of secular physic. For those who were afflicted by the wages of God's wrath, His healing presence was much more immediate and real. Yet, in terms of practical approach, a firm distinction had to be drawn between the two phenomena and Wesley's conceptualisation of mental illness as such was thus considerably strengthened.

Smallpox

Before examining the general cure-all remedies of cold bathing and electricity set out in *Primitive Physic*, it is important to draw attention very briefly to Wesley's treatment of smallpox. As is commonly acknowledged by historians of medicine, the development of an inoculation for this disease stands out as one of the major achievements in eighteenth-century medical practice. Inoculation, which was first used in London in 1721, was a procedure that involved extracting matter from the pox of a smallpox sufferer and applying it onto an incision in the arm or leg of someone who did not yet have the disease. This preciptated a form of the disease to develop, though it was a good deal milder than that contracted randomly.[189] Sara Stidstone Gronim has observed that historians are often quick to cite instances in which eighteenth-century medical practitioners rejected the procedure, which is usually attributed to religious ethics or lack of access. These interpretations, she argues, overlook the fact that inoculation was seen to be unfamiliar and 'strange'. There was no obvious reason why smallpox contracted via inoculation would differ from that caught inadvertently. Furthermore, inoculation, an invention that entered the Atlantic world from the Ottoman Empire and West Africa, was thought to be 'exotic' and therefore believed to have little medical value.[190] It is thus necessary to understand why this treatment is not included in *Primitive Physic*.

In spite of the discovery of inoculation, the disease of smallpox continued to have a variety of treatments.[191] Many physicians were sceptical about the efficacy of inoculation due to its patchy success and the fact that its use was concentrated in the hands of Faculty members. Buchan believed that the reluctance of professional physicians in making inoculation more accessible to lay practitioners meant that the method became shrouded in secrecy.[192] He claimed that no specialist knowledge was required for the procedure of administering the inoculation and that it was simply a matter of 'common sense and prudence' when managing the operation. Lawrence undoubtedly exaggerates Wesley's distrust of the medical profession when he states that this non-professional practitioner 'saw the ritual of medicine as a deliberate conspiracy to keep healing out of the hands of the layman'. This may account, in part, for the fact that Wesley was not forthcoming in his praise for inoculation, though it is highly likely that he would have objected more generally to both its cost and inaccessibility.[193] Wesley was not opposed to the inoculation of adults but worried about using this treatment on children. This anxiety was expressed in a letter to George Merryweather, dated November 1766.[194] On the whole, Wesley was anxious about treating children in general and his lack of formal qualifications in medicine meant that he was careful not to stray into areas in which he felt out of his depth. *Primitive Physic* lists one or two articles suitable for children, such as whooping cough and colic, but tends to steer away from prescriptions for babies and children.

In place of inoculation, *Primitive Physic* prescribed Sydenham's cooling regimen, whilst also citing Huxham – the latter of which included bathing the patient's legs in warm water and ensuring that they were kept in clean bed linen.[195] This latter point about keeping the patient in clean, warm linen was controversial; many physicians believed that the stench and purulent matter caused by the pustules of smallpox were harmless if not curative. Lawrence also makes a valuable point when he says that regularly changing the bed linen would not have been a realistic option for the poor. Given that the procedure of inoculation was inaccessible to most of Wesley's readers, it is entirely appropriate that he found other ways and means of providing a 'cure' for this disease. Indeed, there is no doubt that Wesley would have regarded it as imperative to provide a viable alternative for what Buchan described as being a 'most contagious malady' – a disease very few escaped and which proved to be 'the scourge of Europe' during this time.[196]

Cold-bathing

The therapeutic use of water, both internal and external, obviously dates from antiquity – the Roman *balnea* provided a foundation for the study of bathing cures. Centuries of practical application foreshadowed Boyle's *The Natural Experimental History of Mineral Waters* (1684), which stimulated numerous eighteenth-century discussions on the matter.[197] J. Eklund describes balneotherapy in the Georgian period as a curious and semi-scientific discipline, which was not quite acceptable to the medical profession, no matter how many of its members prescribed it.[198]

The eighteenth-century fashion for spas cannot be fully understood without an understanding of the cool regimen. Controversy raged as to the source of their curative power and N. Coley points out that the four-element theory proved an adequate basis on which most theories rested for the greater part of the century.[199] Physicians debated over whether spas were effective cures for a number of diseases, including the bladder-stone and 'gravel', but these debates were often complex and fraught. Eighteenth-century physicians had a vested interest in perpetuating and promoting the curative value of spa waters. In spa towns, such as Bath, Bristol and Leamington, huge financial rewards attracted resident physicians who could inflate their professional reputations. By contrast, Methodists organised visits to 'minor' spas as an alternative to those fashionable resorts – although Wesley did visit Hotwells in 1754 after being advised by his physician, Fothergill, that this would cure his consumption.

Wesley recommended water for drinking, cold baths and cold-water applications for innumerable illnesses in *Primitive Physic*, some of which are listed at the end of the volume, under the general heading, 'Cold-Bathing'. Water also forms an essential ingredient in his preventative regimen generally: 'washing the head every morning in cold water, prevents the rheums, and cures coughs, old headaches and sore eyes'.[200] Cold-water therapy was included in his repertoire for treating mental afflictions, such as raging madness and nervous disorders: 'it frequently cures every nervous and every paralytic disorder'.[201] Wesley believed cold bathing to be a universal remedy, though he inserts one or two provisos to its recommendation:

> But in all cases where the nerves are obstructed, (such as are those marked thus*) you should go to bed immediately after, and sweat. 'Tis often necessary to use the *hot bath* a few days before you use the *cold*.[202]

Despite Hawes's criticism to the contrary, Wesley advised general rules of caution when using cold bathing as a treatment:

> 20. Or, use the *cold-bath*. (Unless you are of an advanced age, or extremely weak). But when you use this on any account whatever, it is proper,
>
> 1. To bleed or purge, before you begin:
>
> 2. To go in cool: to immerge at once, but not head-foremost; to stay in only two or three minutes, or less, at first:
>
> 3. Never to bathe on a full stomach:
>
> 4. To bathe twice or thrice a week at least, till you have bathed nine or ten times:
>
> 5. To sweat immediately after it (going to bed) in palsies, rickets, and all diseases wherein the nerves are obstructed:
>
> 6. You may use yourself to it, without any danger, by beginning in *May*, and at first plunging in, and coming out immediately. But many have begun in winter without any inconvenience.[203]

In terms of its internal application, Wesley believed that water-drinking could prevent a relapse of any disease.

Generally, Wesley distrusted hot-water bathing, though it is suggested for some illnesses, such as the gout, smallpox and St Anthony's Fire.[204] On the whole, he believed that hot bathing weakened the constitution. The following endorsement of it by Smollet would have been the very reason Wesley distrusted this treatment for fevers:

> In ancient times, as well as these days, it has been considered as part of luxury and pleasure; witness those magnificent baths of the Romans described by Pliny... the warm bath conduces the restoration of health by rendering rigid fibres more pliable and supple.[205]

Apart from treating those illnesses in which rigid fibres and nerves needed to be rendered more pliable, Wesley associated hot-water bathing with indolence, luxury and sexual pleasure. This view was compounded by works, such as *The Ancient Psychrolusia Revived: Or, An Essay to Prove Cold Bathing Safe and Useful* (1702), a text co-written by Edward Baynard and Sir John Floyer, but also John Hancoke's radical tract on cold water as a sovereign remedy, *Febrifugem Magnum* (1722). In common with Floyer, Wesley believed that cold bathing was best suited to the colder English climate. Wesley followed Floyer's line of thinking on a number of issues: Floyer had argued that hot bathing was for effeminate men, who also liked languishing in warm beds, smoking tobacco and consuming tea, coffee and chocolate. Both were committed to the idea that children should be dipped in cold water from an early age to prevent innumerable illnesses.[206] Dr Richard Russell's work outlining *The Use of Sea Water* (1750) is also cited with approval in Wesley's preface to *The Desideratum*.

Like Floyer, Wesley wished to identify the spiritual component in water. Floyer cited Scripture and Tertullian to prove that baptism by immersion in rivers was the general practice of Primitive Christians.[207] For this reason, water held a deeply religious and symbolic meaning for Wesley: 'water, which as it has a natural power of cleansing, is the more fit for its symbolic use… the washing of regeneration'.[208] Cleansing and salvation of the soul was conducted through 'living water' containing a divine spirit. Water was both spiritually and physically regenerating. Spiritually, it signified new birth and baptism into Christ's Church; physically it braced the fibres and strengthened the body. Small wonder, Wesley recommended it so liberally in the *Primitive Physic*.

Electrifying, in a proper manner

Wesley took an avid interest in the new scientific advances in electricity recorded by Benjamin Franklin, Richard Lovett and Joseph Priestley. In 1747, Wesley's journal records how he had gone to see electrical experiments and was deeply impressed:

> Who can comprehend how fire lives in water and passes through it more freely than through air? How flame issues from my finger, real flame, such as sets fire to spirits.[209]

He thoroughly endorsed the use of electricity as a means of healing, and in 1756 set up various surgeries in London and Bristol where 'electric treatment' was given using a 'frictional machine' – in 1756 Wesley reported that he had 'procured' an apparatus for the purpose. A portable electrical machine dating from this period, apparently designed by Wesley and made for him by one of the London makers, is preserved in the museum at his house in City Road.[210] Patients were treated at the Foundry in City Road, but also in Southwark, Seven Dials (near Charing Cross) and St Paul's.[211] Wesley

246

Figure 5.1

Electrical machine designed by John Wesley for the treatment of melancholia
Courtesy: Wellcome Library, London.

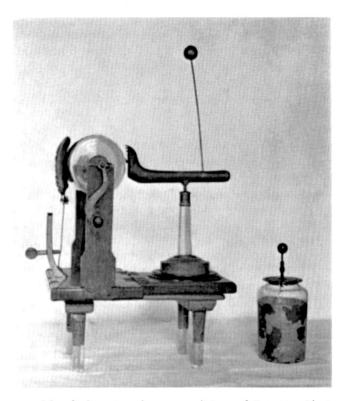

incorporated his findings in subsequent editions of *Primitive Physic*, and electrical therapy started to creep into his 'Collection of Receipts' from the mid-1750s . An explicit statement of this fact was outlined in the 'Postscript' for 1760:

> In [the] course of time I have likewise had occasion to collect several other Remedies, tried and tested by myself or others, which are inserted under their proper heads. Some of these I have found to be of uncommon virtue, equal to any of those which were before published: and one, I must aver from personal knowledge, grounded on a thousand experiments, to be far superior to all the other medicines I have known: I mean *Electricity*. I cannot but intreat all those who are well-wishers to Mankind, to make full proof of this.

Certainly it comes the nearest to an universal medicine, of any yet known in the world.[212]

After reading Franklin's *Experiments*, he tabulated, under nine headings, the sum of knowledge known about electricity. This was included in an anonymously written tract on electricity entitled, *The Desideratum: Or, Electricity Made Plain and Useful by a Lover of Mankind and Common Sense*. This work passed through five editions by 1781. Again, Wesley's conscious espousal of 'plain style' made clear a commitment to the empiric tradition of 'common sense'. As a 'lover of Mankind', *The Desideratum*, like *Primitive Physic*, represented Wesley's duty to man and God, and placed him squarely in the tradition of practical piety. This text he divided into two: 1. the experiments and theories of his day – made *plain*, and 2., his own practical applications of those experiments and theories (case studies) – made *useful*. His use of electricity as a curative method put him in a minority, and some physicians equated electrical therapy with mesmerism. Medics and scientists were slow to recognise the medical efficacy of electricity, and this was noted by Priestley in his *The History and Present State of Electricity, with Original Experiments* (1767). A notable exception, Priestley argued, was Richard Lovett who:

> [H]as been indefatigable in the application of electricity to a great variety of diseases. His success has been very considerable, and all the cases he has published seem to be well authenticated.[213]

In 1767, Middlesex Hospital seems to have acquired an electrical machine, whilst St Bartholomew's obtained one in 1777. William Hey, a friend of Priestley and surgeon to Leeds Infirmary, was asked by the Board to obtain one of Priestley's electrical machines in 1769. From 1778, a machine was in use at St Thomas's Hospital.[214] By the latter half of the century, medical electricity became increasingly fashionable and, as Bertucci notes, in spite of a distinctively diffident attitude amongst the medical establishment, a number of self-styled electricians made a living by attracting patients from either end of the social spectrum. The sheer volume of publications devoted to extolling the curative powers of medical electricity indicate that it extended its reach into more provincial areas. This proliferation prompted Tiberius Cavallo, a leading electrician at the Royal Society, to publish *An Essay on the Theory and Practice of Medical Electricity* (1780) – hitherto the Royal Society displayed a sceptical attitude towards the theory and practice of this subject.[215]

The association of Wesley's use of electricity with mesmerism was particularly unfortunate because it tended to compound contemporary suspicions of religious enthusiasm. To those objections raised against 'lay' experimenters, such as Lovett and Wesley, Priestley responded by stating that criticism would always be levelled against non-Faculty members because it was assumed that they were incapable of ascertaining a degree of accuracy:

> But, on the other hand, this very circumstance of their ignorance… supplies the strongest argument in favour of its innocence… if in such unskilful hands it has produced so much good, and so little harm; how much more good, and how much less harm would it probably have produced in more skilful hands.[216]

This sentiment was fully endorsed by Wesley in 'The Preface' to *The Desideratum*, where he stated that a degree of perfection could only be achieved when those 'Gentlemen of the Faculty' paid more 'regard to the interest of their neighbours than to their own'.[217] He condemned the attitude of orthodox practitioners and defended electrical therapy, not as a panacea, but as one of the best remedies available. This can be seen in his concluding remarks to *The Desideratum*:

> In some cases, where there was no hope of help, it will succeed beyond all expectations. In others, where we had the greatest hope, it will have no effect at all. Again, in some experiments, it helps at the very first, and promises a speedy cure: but presently the good effect ceases, and the patient is as he was before. On the contrary, in others it has no effect at first: it does no good, perhaps seems to do hurt. Yet all this time it is striking at the root of the disease, which in a while it totally removes. Frequent instances of the former we have in *paralysis*, of the latter in rheumatic cases.[218]

Wesley's experiments in electrical therapy were unsystematic and tentative, though they also fitted into a much wider debate about its many possible uses.[219] Adapting John Hedley Brooke's interpretative framework, in which he has noted 'religious utility' as being an important component of Enlightenment science, Bertucci has suggested that Wesley's electrical therapies were motivated by his concern as a High Church Tory. Wesley, she suggests, was responding to 'the High Church's preoccupation with loss of authority faced with the growing success of Newtonian experimental philosophy and its allegiance to Whig politics'. His interest in the 'subtil medium' was sparked, so to speak, once he realised that electrical experiments could be detached from their association with aristocratic entertainment and fostered instead to disseminate a politically and religiously instructive morality to Methodist followers. Indeed, according to Bertucci, it was this shift from those thrilling shows of electrical performance intended for a 'polite' audience, to the 'revealing sparks' of medical electricity which could be used for the poor, that first attracted Wesley's attention. This shift not only mirrored Wesley's Puritan distaste for the theatrical and, specifically, his 'ban on all manner of entertainment', it supplied him with the efficacious remedy of electricity. For Wesley this realisation entailed a 'revision of the morality of electrical experiment', which, now shorn of its decadent associations, could promote his 'method', or a 'way of life that would give the faithful the guidelines for proper behaviour and moral conduct and therefore prevent their going astray'. Just as the 'dreadful powers of electricity' could be controlled and conducted through a frictional machine, so Wesley believed that human passions, 'when tempered according to the dictates of Methodism' would bring about political obedience and social harmony.[220]

In her rush to say what she thinks is distinctive on the subject, Bertucci has taken me to task for 'unproblematically' including Wesley's electrical healing as part of his philanthropic concerns about health and hygiene.[221] A more sensitive and less caricatured reading of my work would certainly have removed any anxieties on this score whilst alerting Bertucci to the fact that I have consistently attempted to show how Wesley's medical activity, along with his enthusiasm for the advances in electricity recorded by Priestley, Lovett and Franklin were, indeed, deeply 'imbued with moral and religious purports'.[222] It is now sufficiently well known that 'eighteenth-century natural philosophy was characterised by the convergence of theological, moral and political issues'[223] – issues that have been explicitly and implicitly referred to in my published work. As an Anglican, Wesley's use of natural philosophy and empirical method is, in itself, suggestive of the fact that he was ready to protect revealed religion by fending off a deistic challenge to theological orthodoxy and, by implication, a subversive critique of High Church politics. For this reason it hardly needs to be said that obedience to God necessarily extended to obedience to King and country.

The raw material of Bertucci's research findings are extremely useful and most welcome for injecting life into a subject that has not received the precise scholarly attention that it deserves. Yet this fruitful research is mitigated by Bertucci's partisan stance, which sees Wesley as a calculating High Church ideologue. In this all-too-familiar story, Wesley is cast as a backward-looking theologian, whose 'insistence on the sense of awe towards divine power', provoked by electrical experiment, reminded followers that political and religious obedience to worldly authorities was the mark of all good Christians. Accordingly, Wesley's medical philanthropy was driven with the goal of this obedience uppermost in his mind. Wesley's 'sense of bewilderment' when witnessing experimental performances also fares badly when compared to the rationalist, progressive and improving philosophy of Priestley, which was borne out of his Dissenting theology. In place of awe and mystery, Priestley's search for truth led to a study of nature that nourished a healthy criticism of political and religious authorities.[224]

Bertucci's line of enquiry lacks the scent of authenticity, not least because it forms one part of a complicated narrative about Wesley's long vocation as Methodist leader. When faced with the urgent political crisis of the colonists' revolt in America, Wesley deferred to authority by preaching non-resistance and obedience to the Crown. We know already that Wesley frequently bowed to theological, political and medical authority when the need arose. Yet we should not forget that Methodism also violated Church authority and disrupted parish life with its innovations; field preaching, often undertaken by laymen and women, was bitterly denounced by Anglican divines. These innovations, with fresh emphasis placed on the 'New Birth' and 'Justification by Faith' meant that Wesley moved further from away theological orthodoxy. This was made worse by the fact that Methodists appeared to be beyond the reach of law because they did not need to register officially under the Toleration Act.

Despite Wesley's personal distaste for enthusiasm, the enthusiastic strains amongst Methodist followers threatened to further undermine conformity to the religious and political establishment. Conformity to the church was analogous to political obedience, but theological innovation masked sedition and subversion. Wesley's appeal to Anglican orthodoxy, combined with his claim that he 'lived and died in the Church of England', failed to convince most High Churchmen, who, until his overt political opposition to the American revolt, remained sceptical about this claim. Churchmen remained sceptical about Wesley's loyalty when plain facts suggested that Methodism threatened to create a schism. Emphasis upon particular strands of the Thirty-Nine Articles upset eighteenth-century canons; 'Justification by Faith' denigrated good works and could lead to antinomianism, whilst assurances of Perfection were closely associated with moral corruption.

If Wesley used natural philosophy and empiricism as an act of conformity, he also utilised these tools to steer a *via media* between religious and political disunity by way of arriving at a consensus in matters that were medical and scientific. Part of his distaste for having to deal with attacks from Hawes and Toplady was precisely because he detected the sectarian content of their complaints, which were medically unfounded. Moreover, as Bertucci points out herself more than once, contrary to other High Church theologians, such as John Freke or George Horne, Wesley did not attack electrical experiment, making it clear, in fact, that his findings were derived from a 'thousand experiments'.[225] Wesley's *The Desideratum*, like *Primitive Physic*, thus testifies to his eirenic approach in science and medicine in its 'heterogeneous range of sources which included both Promethean electricians such as Franklin, Wilson, Watson and Martin and the pietist

John Freke'.[226] Typically, he extracted what was useful and put it to practical effect.

His fascination with electricity was largely due to the fact that it was cheap and effective. He may have exaggerated its value when he called it a thousand medicines in one, but trial and error had shown Wesley that electricity worked successfully on a range of illnesses and he discovered remarkable results when treating nervous disorders. In his *The History and Present State of Electricity*, Priestley showed that electricity was thought to be the best treatment for palsy on the Continent.[227] He had observed that experiments conducted by Jean Jallabert, Professor of Experimental Philosophy and Mathematics in Geneva, showed electricity to work successfully on the palsy. Wesley's own experience, however, led him to believe that a long-standing palsy could not be healed by electricity and Priestley thus noted that:

> Mr. Wesley candidly says, he has not known any instance of the cure of an hemiplegia; and although many paralytics have been helped by electricity, he scarcely thinks that any palsy of a year's standing has been thoroughly cured by it.[228]

Wesley suggests using electricity for the palsy in *Primitive Physic* but is eager to affirm its general efficacy:

> Nor have I yet known one single instance, wherein it has done harm; so that I cannot but doubt the veracity of those who have affirmed the contrary. Dr. *De Haen* positively affirms, 'it can do no hurt in any case': that is, unless the shock be immoderately strong.

> The best method is to give fifty, or even a hundred small shocks, each time; but let them be so gentle as not to terrify the patient in the least.

> *Drawing sparks* removes those tumours on the eye-lids, called barley-corns, by exciting local inflammation, and promoting suppuration.[229]

He subjected himself to electrical therapy, most notably in 1765 after a riding accident.[230] Wesley's advice to administer many small shocks, as opposed to few great ones, followed that of Franklin, who only recommended the therapeutic use of electricity in conjunction with regimen and medicine.[231]

Wesley believed that electricity worked by removing obstructions and here was led by Lovett – a medical influence that was picked up on by Priestley:

> The Rev. Mr. J. Wesley has followed Mr. Lovett in the same useful course of medical electricity; and recommends the use of it to his numerous followers,

and to all people. Happy it is when an ascendancy over the minds of men is employed to purposes favourable to the increase of knowledge, and to the best interests of Mankind.[237]

Priestley has fully captured the motivating force behind all of Wesley's social endeavours. It is Wesley's ideas about electricity, in fact, which reveal best his comprehensive interpretation of nature and healing: electricity is a movement of *invisible* but *materially* effective spirit, and for him this division represented both the divine and natural. Using electricity demonstrated a disciplined commitment to healing and complemented the sensible regimen and natural remedies advocated in *Primitive Physic*.[233]

For somebody concerned with practical piety, the discovery of electricity was deeply significant. It seemed to provide evidence for the claim that fire was the soul and motivating force behind the universe. The significance of William Law over this aspect of Wesley's thinking here is obvious, but Law had also greatly impressed Cheyne, another pietist who regarded fire as the instrument of all motion. Electricity was the elementary fire of the ancients, the fulfilment of prophets, and the *materia subtilis* described by Descartes. It demonstrated the animating principle of the entire natural world and provided a crucial link between spirit and matter. Electrical healing revived animal spirits and removed physical obstructions. Here, Wesley made a parallel between electrical healing and spiritual regeneration through divine grace – spirit was the vital breath of the ancient Church. Electricity was therefore an invisible agency, analogous to the divine. Though strongly influenced by the pietistic ideas of Cheyne and Boerhaave, Wesley retained the traditional distinction between spirit and matter and would not have endorsed Priestley's collapsing of the matter–spirit duality.

Wesley believed that the air was 'universally impregnated' by fire, but identified what was later discovered to be oxygen, with Newton's ether and the electric charge of particles. Oxygen was identified by Priestley but discovered by Lavoisier during the 1770s:

> Electricity will probably soon be considered as the great vivifying principle
> of Nature by which she carries on most of her operations. It is a fifth element
> distinct from and of a superior nature to the other four.[234]

Wesley was not unduly concerned about the theoretical side of electricity and wanted only to reveal its practical application: 'if we aim at theory, we know nothing'.[235] Thus in 'The Preface' to *The Desideratum* he states that his work is:

Chiefly indebted to Mr. Franklin for the speculative part, and Mr. Lovett for the practical: tho' I cannot in everything subscribe to the sentiments of either one or the other.[236]

In December 1760, Wesley responded to a long series of questions in the *London Magazine*, which had raised general criticisms about his social and philanthropic endeavours. One of the questions was: 'Why do you meddle with electricity?' Unsurprisingly, the answer Wesley gave was: 'For the same reason as I published *Primitive Physic* – to do as much good as I can'.[237] In 1793, the London Electrical Dispensary, an institution for electrical treatment, was opened on the City Road. It has been suggested that the location of the dispensary was calculated to continue the electrical therapy, which had been initiated by Wesley.[238] Indeed, Bertucci, who notes that this institution was founded by his rival, Hawes, sees how the Dispensary was conceived to offer free electrical treatment for the poor.[239] Between the years 1793 and 1814, this Dispensary treated an average of three hundred patients per year. Given that Wesley had been at the forefront of such initiatives, this development would have pleased him a great deal.

Having analysed several principal diseases in this chapter, we have seen how Wesley culled from the best sources available when compiling *Primitive Physic*. He used these important medical and scientific advances, but had his own definite and well-informed ideas about putting them into practice – seen in his adoption of electrical treatment. Wesley did not seek to explain the *cause* of disease in *Primitive Physic* and focused instead on collecting empirically proven remedies that he believed to be effective. Each recipe was carefully calibrated and rigorously underpinned by contemporary medical practice. He did not worry about how his text fitted into one consistent theory of medicine because he was not an orthodox physician attempting to forge a medical career and cared little about pleasing established physicians of the Faculty. Having said this, it is clear that Wesley held firm to the prevailing mechanical theory of 'obstructions', espoused by the leading physicians, such as Cheyne and Boerhaave.

Trial and error were Wesley's judge and jury and in this he remained committed to that Baconian empirical tradition taken up by those members of the Oxford Philosophical Club which included Locke, Sydenham and Boyle. To anyone unfamiliar with medical practice in the period, the remedies set out in *Primitive Physic* may appear to be unthinkingly empirical, 'folksy', 'absurd' or even 'revolting'. Yet the remedies contained in *Primitive Physic* are easily located in their medical context and are recognisable to eighteenth-century 'professional', 'orthodox' physic. Even what seems to be the most ludicrous remedy, that which requires the patient to hold a 'live puppy on the belly' for the iliac passion, can be traced to the authoritative sources of Sydenham and Boerhaave. This remedy is often singled out by historians as being representative of the quack methods adopted by Wesley. Yet it too contained a rationale: 'accubitus' was a way of treating 'devitalising' patients and involved using a live animal or young person. Rousseau makes a valuable observation when he suggests that:

> However occult or charmed [Wesley's] methods seem to us, they were no more varied or superstitious than those of his best contemporaries, as one may see by comparing these recipes by those prescribed for similar illnesses in Robert James's *A Medical Dictionary* (1743–45).[240]

Some of the remedies prescribed in *Primitive Physic* are still useful, though, as an historian looking critically at Wesley's text, this anachronism is a breach of scholarly rules. Nevertheless, a diet of vegetables to prevent excess fat, the syringing of ears with warm water to remove hard wax, sucking on barley sugar to ease a tickling cough and eating of prunes or currants to relieve 'costiveness', are methods still routinely used today. Other 'sensible' remedies that were very much needed in Wesley's own day, however, included a recommendation to eat or drink the juice of citrus fruit for scurvy and gargling on salty water for rotten gums.

Significantly, the subject on which *Primitive Physic* is notably understated and ambivalent is venereal disease. Here, Wesley's text radically differs from that of other eighteenth-century medical volumes – popular or otherwise. Buchan, for example, decided that the only way to deal with the ubiquitous nature of sexually transmitted diseases was to address the issue in a bold and aggressive manner. By contrast, Wesley refrained from an explicitly campaigning stance, leaving prescriptions for sexual health to others. For venereal disease, listed as '*Lues Venerea*', he recommends that the patient take 'an ounce of quicksilver every morning' and a 'spoonful of *aqua sulphurata* in a glass of water, at five in the afternoon'. Wesley insists that this simple procedure cured a person 'when supposed to be at the point of death'. More astonishing, however, is the fact that this procedure had been carried out on someone 'who had been infected by a foul nurse, before she was a year old'. Wesley, who generally avoided prescribing medicines for children and babies, inserted a remedy for this disease specifically, he says, 'for the sake of such innocent sufferers'.[241]

The general principle of regimen, particularly when fostered in the religious and moral context of Methodism, would have been taken to imply sexual continence alongside a self-controlled lifestyle generally. This strategy for dealing with the intractable, but highly commercial and profitable problem of venereal disease is interesting because it is so atypical. For Wesley its cure lay, not in choosing from a plurality of medical responses or remedies, but in one simple rule of chastity, which could ward off something unholy. What I have attempted to show in this chapter, but in the book as a whole, is the necessity of uncovering and following the course of Wesley's treatments in *Primitive Physic* precisely. It is only by taking the time to do this that their rationale and consistency can be brought to light. As we have seen in the example of veneral disease, this also holds true for what is omitted in *Primitive Physic*. By placing *Primitive Physic* into its discursive cultural context and comparing it with a range of other contemporary medical practitioners it has thus been possible to turn Rousseau's observation into a proved demonstration.

Notes

1. J. Wesley, *Primitive Physic,* 5th edn (London, 1755), xvi. J. Wesley, *A Survey of the Wisdom of God in the Creation: Or, a Compendium of Natural Philosophy,* 5 vols, 3rd edn (London, 1763), Vol. I, 83–84; J. Armstrong, *The Art of Preserving Health* (London, 1744), in *English Poetry Full-Text Database* [Windows CD-ROM] (Cambridge: Chadwyck-Healey, 1993).

2. G. Cheyne, *An Essay on Regimen, Together with Five Discourses, Medical, Moral, and Philosophical: Serving to Illustrate the Principles and Theory of Philosophical Medicine, and Point Out Some of its Moral Consequences,* 1st edn (London, 1740), lx.

3. J. Wesley, *Primitive Physic,* 24th edn (London, 1792), xiii–xiv.

4. G. Cheyne, *A New Theory of Continu'd Fevers,* 2nd edn (London, 1722), 2.

5. Wesley, *op. cit.* (note 3), 44.

6. *Ibid.,* 38.

7. A.G. Carmichael, 'St Anthony's Fire', in K.F. Kiple (ed.), *The Cambridge World History of Human Disease* (Cambridge: Cambridge University Press, 1993), 989–90: 989.

8. Wesley, *op. cit.* (note 3), 23n*.

9. Carmichael, *op. cit.* (note 7), 989.

10. Wesley, *op. cit.* (note 3), 24.

11. *Ibid.*

12. S.A. Tissot, *L'Avis,* quoted in J, Wesley, *Advice with Respect to Health,* 4th edn (London, 1789), 104; W. Buchan, *Domestic Medicine: Or, A Treatise on the Prevention and Cure of Diseases by Regimen and Simple Medicines* (1769), 2nd edn (London, 1772), 320.

13. Wesley, *op. cit.* (note 3), 24.

14. *Ibid.*

15. Buchan, *op. cit.* (note 12), 315.

16. Wesley, *op. cit.* (note 3), 23.

17. W. Hawes, *An Examination of the Rev. Mr John Wesley's Primitive Physic,* 2nd edn (London, 1780), 15. Hawes argues that this hot, stimulating substance

would increase the inflammation and that 'turpentines' should not be given for inflammatory illnesses.

18. Buchan, *op. cit.* (note 12), 317.
19. Wesley, *op. cit.* (note 3), 24.
20. *Concise Oxford English Dictionary,* 10th edn (Oxford: Oxford University Press, 1999), s.v. 'Apoplexy'.
21. Wesley, *op. cit.* (note 3), 24n *.
22. Buchan, *op. cit.* (note 12), 519.
23. Wesley, *op. cit.* (note 3), 25.
24. Buchan, *op. cit.* (note 12), 520.
25. Tissot, *op. cit.* (note 12), 53; Buchan, *op. cit.* (note 12), 520; R. Boyle, *Medicinal Experiments: Or, A Collection of Choice and Safe Remedies For the Most Part Simple and Easily Prepared,* 4th edn (London, 1703), 93.
26. Hawes, *op. cit.* (note 17), 16.
27. Wesley, *op. cit.* (note 3), 25. A 'seton' was a length of material that was placed below the skin, with the end protruding. It was used to promote drainage or absorb fluid.
28. *Ibid.,* 24.
29. Hawes, *op. cit.* (note 17), 20. Hawes makes this criticism of *Primitive Physic* based on his reading of the 16th edition (1774), yet Wesley's recommendation that the patient apply for medical assistance was contained in earlier editions, including the 8th edition of 1759.
30. Wesley, *op. cit.* (note 3), 115.
31. J. Wesley, *Primitive Physic,* 1st edn (London, 1747), 29; *Primitive Physic,* 8th edn (Bristol, 1759), 33–4; *Primitive Physic,* 15th edn (London, 1772), 35–6; *Primitive Physic,* 16th edn (London, 1774), 35–6.
32. Hawes, *op. cit.* (note 17), 17.
33. See Boyle, *op. cit.* (note 25): 'Fix a cupping glass (without scarification) to the nape of the neck, and another to the shoulders….' (40). It is not clear exactly where Wesley got the information necessary to make the distinction between sanguine and serous apoplexy in the later editions of *Primitive Physic.* He obviously drew on Tissot and Buchan for some of the facts.
34. C. Lawlor and A. Suzuki, 'The Disease of the Self: Representing Consumption, 1700–1830', *Bulletin for the History of Medicine,* 74 (2000), 458–92: 494.
35. Buchan, *op. cit.* (note 12), 218. Fothergill, however, made the following announcement to the Medical Society in London, taken from vol. iv of 'Medical Observations and Inquiries' (n.d.): 'In this city the weekly bills are supposed to exhibit a tolerably exact account of those who die of the respective diseases mentioned in that list. But I am informed, that the article of consumptions includes generally all those who die of any lingering disease, and are much emaciated; by which the list is vastly enlarged beyond what it

ought to be [and] foreigners imagining that this disease is much more frequent amongst us, than in reality' (*Remarks on the Cure of Consumptions* [n.d.], in J. Elliot (ed.), *A Complete Collection of the Medical and Philosophical Works of John Fothergill* (London, 1781), 390–405: 391n.

36. S. Juster, 'Mystical Pregnancy and Holy Bleeding: Visionary Experience in Early Modern Britain and America', *William and Mary Quarterly,* 57 (2000), 249–88: 271.

37. *Ibid.*; see also R. Porter, 'Consumption: Disease of the Consumer Society?' in J. Brewer and R. Porter (eds.), *Consumption and The World of Goods* (London: Routledge, 1993), 58–81.

38. Lawlor and Suzuki, *op. cit.* (note 34), 460.

39. *Ibid.*

40. *Ibid.*, 462.

41. *Ibid.*, 463.

42. Juster, *op. cit.* (note 36), 272.

43. R. Blackmore, *A Treatise of Consumptions and other Distempers belonging to the Breast and Lungs,* 2nd edn (London, 1725); J. Wainewright, *A Mechanical Account of the Non-Naturals: Being a Brief Explication of the Changes Made in Humane Bodies by Air, Diet, together with an Enquiry into the Nature and Use of the Baths,* 1st edn (London, 1708).

44. Blackmore, *ibid.*, 1.

45. Buchan, *op. cit.* (note 12), 219.

46. Blackmore, *op. cit.* (note 43); Wainewright, *op. cit.* (note 43); Buchan, *op. cit.* (note 12), 219.

47. Buchan, *op. cit.* (note 12), 219.

48. Blackmore, *op. cit.* (note 43); Wainewright also argued that this disease was hereditary in Wainewright, *op. cit.* (note 43).

49. Buchan, *op. cit.* (note 12), 219–220.

50. *Ibid.*, 228.

51. Wainewright, *op. cit.* (note 43); Buchan, *op. cit.* (note 12); Fothergill, *op. cit.* (note 35).

52. Wainewright, *op. cit.* (note 43), 27.

53. Wesley, *op. cit.* (note 3), 41.

54. *Ibid.*, 43.

55. Buchan, *op. cit.* (note 12), 222.

56. J. Radcliffe, *Pharmacopaeia Radcliffeana: Or, Dr Radcliffe's Prescriptions, Faithfully Gathered from his Original Recipes,* 3rd edn (London, 1718), 13; Buchan, *op. cit.* (note 12), 226.

57. Hawes, *op. cit.* (note 17), 37–8.

58. Blackmore, *op. cit.* (note 43), 155.

59. Lawlor and Suzuki, *op. cit.* (note 34), 475. See also, R. Porter, *Doctor of Society: Thomas Beddoes and the Sick Trade in Late-Enlightenment England*

(London: Routledge, 1992).

60. Porter, *ibid.*, 106; Lawlor and Suzuki, *op. cit.* (note 34), 475.
61. Wainewright, *op. cit.* (note 43), 27.
62. *Ibid.*
63. Buchan, *op. cit.* (note 12), 230.
64. Wesley, *op. cit.* (note 3), 41–3.
65. Fothergill, *op. cit.* (note 35), 398.
66. Fothergill had undertaken his medical training at Edinburgh and was a Member of the College of Physicians. He was a Fellow of the Royal Society and Royal Society of Medicine in Paris. See R. Hingston Fox, *Dr John Fothergill and his Friends: Chapters in Eighteenth-Century Life* (Macmillan: London, 1919)
67. *Ibid.*, 44.
68. J. Hill, *The Family Herbal, or An Account of all those English Plants, which are Remarkable for their Virtues* (1st edn., London, 1755), 175.
69. A. Príhoda, *The Healing Powers of Nature* (Leicester: Blitz Editions, 1998), 90, 97.
70. Physicians believed that vitriol 'braced' the body and Wesley argued on a number of occasions that it was the best bracer available.
71. Wesley, *op. cit.* (note 3), 42.
72. Hawes, *op. cit.* (note 17), 38.
73. Blackmore, *op. cit.* (note 43), 57.
74. Wesley, *op. cit.* (note 3), 43.
75. Buchan, *op. cit.* (note 12)., 225.
76. Cheyne quoted in Anon., *The Family Guide to Health; Or, A Practice of Physic: In a Familiar Way,* 1st edn (London, 1767), 56.
77. Buchan, *op. cit.* (note 12), 362.
78. *Concise Oxford English Dictionary* (note 20), s.v. 'Dropsy'; J. Worth Estes, 'Dropsy', in Kiple, *op. cit.* (note 7), 689–96.
79. Wesley, *op. cit.* (note 3), 49.
80. Wainewright, *op. cit.* (note 43), 33.
81. Estes, *op. cit.* (note 78), 693.
82. *Ibid.*
83. *Ibid.* Estes points out that another medical student, Giovanni Mana Lancisi, from Rome, made the same discovery during this period.
84. *Ibid.*
85. *Ibid.*, 694.
86. *Ibid.*, 695.
87. *Ibid.*
88. *Ibid.*
89. Wainewright, *op. cit.* (note 43), 35.
90. Buchan, *op. cit.* (note 12), 477.

91. Wesley, *op. cit.* (note 3), 50.

92. *Ibid.*, 49.

93. *Ibid.*, 49–51. These herbals are also listed (alphabetically) in Hill's *The Family Herbal.*

94. *Ibid.*, 51.

95. *Ibid.*, 50.

96. Hill, *op. cit.* (note 68), 123.

97. Wesley, *op. cit.* (note 3), 49. Boerhaave was a firm advocate of using massage for a range of illnesses generally.

98. Wesley, 1st edn, *op. cit.* (note 31), 52.

99. Wesley, *op. cit.* (note 3), 51.

100. R. Porter, *The Greatest Benefit to Mankind: A Medical History of Humanity from Antiquity to the Present* (Harper Collins: London, 1997), 259.

101. G. Cheyne, *An Essay of Health and Long Life,* 6th edn (London 1725), Vol. II. Boerhaave argued that fevers arose from a friction between solids and fluids, compacted because of blockages in the vascular channels.

102. Porter, *op. cit.* (note 100), 259.

103. J. Huxham, *An Essay on Fevers and their Various Kinds* 1st edn (London, 1750), 40n.

104. Porter, *op. cit.* (note 100), 261.

105. *Ibid.*, 261.

106. M. DeLacy, 'The Conceptualization of Influenza in Eighteenth-Century Britain: Specificity and Contagion', *Bulletin of the History of Medicine,* 67 (1993), 74–118.

107. DeLacy points out that it was Huxham who introduced the term 'influenza' into English in his *An Essay on Fevers, ibid.*, 77.

108. *Ibid.*, 83.

109. Porter, *op. cit.* (note 100), 261.

110. *Ibid.*, 262.

111. This was the basis of Cheyne's *A New Theory,* in which he argued against those physicians who believed fever to be caused by 'morbifick matter', which mixed and circulated with the 'mass of blood'. Cheyne declared that this argument was nonsense because nothing could get into the mass of blood. This illness was due to to an obstruction in the glands and intestine. It was this obstruction in the glands that affected the quantity of the blood and '*Liquidum Nervorum*'. Cheyne, *op. cit.* (note 4), 34, 57, 88.

112. Porter, *op. cit.* (note 100), 260.

113. Cheyne, *op. cit.* (note 4), 11.

114. *Ibid.*, 17.

115. Wesley, *op. cit.* (note 3), 59.

116. Hawes, *op. cit.* (note 17), 44.

117. J.C. Riley, *The Eighteenth-Century Campaign to Avoid Disease* (London:

Macmillan, 1987), 86.

118. Huxham, *op. cit.* (note 103), 5.

119. *Ibid.*, 6–7.

120. N. Kasting, 'A Rationale for Centuries of Therapeutic Bloodletting: Antipyretic Therapy for Febrile Diseases', *Perspectives in Biology and Medicine,* 33 (1990), 509–16; see also, R. Root-Bernstein and M. Root-Bernstein, *Honey, Mud, Maggots and other Medical Marvels: The Science behind Folk Remedies and Old Wives' Tales* (London: Pan Books, 2000).

121. Kasting, *ibid.*, 510–12.

122. Matthew Baillie, physician and nephew of John Hunter criticised and denounced the practice of blood-letting in 1817.

123. Huxham, *op. cit.* (note 103), 7.

124. *Ibid.*, 8–9.

125. Wesley, *op. cit.* (note 3), 59.

126. *Ibid.*, 59. Much scientific research and analysis has been conducted into the effect of sugar, honey and treacle pastes when treating specific conditions. Burns, wounds, bedsores, ulcers, infectious trauma-related injuries and even internal complaints (through osmosis) have been found to respond well to sugar pastes, which act as an anti-bacterial, anti-septic. See R. Root-Bernstein and M. Root-Bernstein, *op. cit.* (note 120), 31–43.

127. Porter, *op. cit.* (note 100), 260.

128. R. Porter and G.S. Rousseau, *Gout: The Patrician Malady* (London: Yale University Press, 2000), 4.

129. Blackmore differed on the issue of alcohol in that he thought that wine was good for gouty conditions, *ibid.*, 4, 59.

130. Buchan, *op. cit.* (note 12), 484.

131. W. Cadogan, *A Dissertation on the Gout, and all Chronic Diseases, Jointly Considered as Proceeding from the Same Causes,* 9th edn (London, 1771), 20.

132. *Ibid.*, 19–22.

133. J. Wesley, *The Journal of the Rev. John Wesley, A.M.,* 4 vols (London: J. Kershaw, 1827), Vol. III, 429.

134. W. Stukley, *Of the Gout,* 1st edn (London, 1735), 6.

135. Wesley, *op. cit.* (note 3), 66n *.

136. G. Cheyne, *An Essay on the True Nature and Due Method of Treating the Gout,* 6th edn (London, 1724), 2.

137. *Ibid.*, 5.

138. *Ibid.*, 9.

139. *Ibid.*, 11.

140. *Ibid.*, 17.

141. *Ibid.*, 112.

142. *Ibid.*, 18–44.

143. Buchan, *op. cit.* (note 12), 489–91.

144. Wesley, *op. cit.* (note 3), 66.

145. *Ibid.*

146. *Ibid.* It is likely that he verified Cheyne's use of this against a number of other physicians.

147. *Ibid.*, 65

148. Rev. Toplady, quoted in Hawes, *op. cit.* (note 17), 56.

149. *Ibid.*

150. Wesley and Toplady had been engaged in a sometimes bitter debate over Predestination in 1739.

151. R.K. French, 'Scrofula', in Kiple, *op. cit.* (note 7), 998–1000: 998.

152. French points out that Queen Anne was the last British monarch to use the 'touch'; *ibid.*, 998.

153. Buchan, *op. cit.* (note 12), 507.

154. French, *op. cit.* (note 151), 999.

155. *Ibid.*; Buchan believed this disease to be infectious.

156. Wesley, *op. cit.* (note 3), 72.

157. Buchan, *op. cit.* (note 12), 505.

158. *Ibid.*, 507.

159. Wesley, *op. cit.* (note 3), 72.

160. Hill, *op. cit* (note 68), 111.

161. Wesley, *op. cit.* (note 3), 73.

162. *Ibid.*, 72, 90.

163. M.A. Screech, 'Good Madness in Christendom', in W.F. Bynum, R. Porter and M. Shepherd (eds), *The Anatomy of Madness: Essays in the History of Psychiatry*, 2 vols (London: Tavistock Publications, 1985), Vol. I, 25–39: 34.

164. J. Wesley, *Thoughts on Nervous Disorders* (1784), in T. Jackson (ed.), *The Works of the Rev. John Wesley, A.M.*, 14 vols (London: Wesleyan Methodist Book-Room, 1831), Vol. XI, 515.

165. *Ibid.*, 516.

166. P. Laffey, 'John Wesley on Insanity', *History of Psychiatry*, 12 (2001), 467–79: 469.

167. Wesley, *op. cit.* (note 133), Vol. V, 173.

168. Laffey, *op. cit.* (note 166), 472.

169. *Ibid.*, 472–3.

170. R. Porter, *Mind Forg'd Manacles: A History of Madness in England from the Restoration to the Regency* (London: Penguin, 1987), 48.

171. Wesley, *op. cit.* (note 3), 75, 79.

172. *Ibid.*, 75n *.

173. R. Mead, *Medical Precepts and Cautions*, T. Stack (trans.), 2nd edn (London, 1751). Cold-water therapy was recommended by Mead in his *A Mechanical Account of Poisons*. Mead accepted the traditional division between maniacs and melancholics: the outrageous behaviour of the former needed to be

conquered by authority, whilst the despondency of the latter was to be dissipated by raising their spirits; J. Andrews, 'A Respectable Mad-Doctor? Dr Richard Hale, FRS (1670–1728)', *Notes and Records of the Royal Society of London*, 44 (1990), 169–204.

174. T. Smollet, *An Essay on the External Use of Water,* 1st edn (London, 1752).

175. Porter, *op. cit.* (note 170), 221; A. Digby, *Madness, Morality and Medicine* (Cambridge: Cambridge University, 1985); K. Jones shows how the Manchester Lunatic Hospital practiced 'tender treatment of the insane', but that the standard remedies of bleeding, purging, blistering and vomits continued. The York Retreat, however, abandoned these methods after a period of experimentation and developed instead a system of moral treatment; See K. Jones, *Asylums and After: A Revised History of the Mental Health Services* (London: Athlone Press, 1993), 23.

176. Buchan, *op. cit.* (note 12), 538.

177. Wesley, *op. cit.* (note 164), Vol. XI, 517.

178. Wesley, *op. cit.* (note 3), 79.

179. Porter, *op. cit.* (note 100), 271.

180. Porter, *op. cit.* (note 170), 206.

181. *Ibid.,* 271.

182. J. Wesley, *The Nature of Enthusiasm*, in A.C. Outler (ed.), *The Bicentennial Edition of the Works of John Wesley* (Nashville: Abingdon Press, 1984-), *Sermons,* Vol. II, 44–60: 49; Laffey, *op. cit.* (note 166), 468.

183. Laffey has rightly identified the way in which historians have misrepresented Wesley's approach to madness. Laffey argues that Wesley did not attempt to break down those distinctions between spiritual malaise and madness, but 'observed a strict division' between the experiences. Laffey, *ibid.,* 478.

184. Wesley, *op. cit.* (note 133), Vol. I, 217; Laffey, *ibid.,* 474.

185. Laffey, *ibid.,* 475.

186. Wesley, *op. cit.* (note 133), Vol. IV, 541; Laffey, *ibid.,* 475. St Luke's was built to rival Bedlam and Dr William Battie, physician to this institution, published a pamphlet in 1758, *Treatise on Madness,* which outlined his new methods. See Jones, *op. cit.* (note 175), 23.

187. Laffey, *ibid.,* 475–7.

188. J. Wesley, *A Farther Appeal to Men of Reason and Religion*, in G.R. Cragg (ed.), *The Bicentennial Edition of the Works of John Wesley* (Nashville: Abingdon Press, 1989), *The Appeals,* Vol. XI, 198.

189. S. Stidstone Gronim, 'Imagining Inoculation: Smallpox, the Body, and Social Relations of Healing in the Eighteenth Century', *Bulletin for the History of Medicine,* 80 (2006), 247–68: 247.

190. *Ibid.,* 248–9.

191. C.J. Lawrence, 'William Buchan: Medicine Laid Open', *Medical History,* 19 (1975), 20–35: 30.

192. *Ibid.*, 31; Buchan, *op. cit.* (note 12), 287.

193. Lawrence, *op. cit.* (note 191), 31.

194. See J. Wesley, *The Letters of the Rev. John Wesley A.M.,* J. Telford (ed.), 8 vols. (London: Epworth Press, 1931), Vol. V, 30.

195. Lawrence, *op. cit.* (note 191), 30.

196. Buchan, *op. cit.* (note 12), 269.

197. Phyllis Hembry points out that from 1665 the *Philosophical Transactions* had numerous specialist essays on the subject, whilst the eighteenth century produced a large volume of literature on mineral waters and spas. P. Hembry, *The English Spa 1560–1815: A Social History* (London: The Athlone Press, 1990).

198. J. Ecklund, 'Of a Spirit in the Water: Some Early Ideas on the Aerial Dimension', *Isis*, 67 (1976), 527–50.

199. N.G. Coley, 'Physicians, chemists and the analysis of mineral waters: "The most difficult part of chemistry"', in R. Porter (ed.), *The Medical History of Waters and Spas* (London: Wellcome Institute for the History of Medicine, 1990), 56–66.

200. Wesley, *op. cit.* (note 3), 118.

201. *Ibid.*, 117.

202. *Ibid.*, 118.

203. *Ibid.*, 22. This general advice is given under the receipts given for 'A Tertian Ague'.

204. Two valuable scientific studies conducted fairly recently have shown how water immersion can promote urine, which in turn can expel lead, water, sodium and calcium. Eighteenth-century physicians noted profound alterations in the body after water immersion. See, A. Heywood, H.A. Waldron, P. O'Hare *et al.*, 'The Effect of Immersion on Urinary Lead Excretion', *British Journal of Industrial Medicine*, 43 (1986), 713–15; A. Heywood, 'A Trial of the Bath Waters: The Treatment of Lead Poisoning', in Porter (ed.), *op. cit.* (note 199), 82–101. In the latter study, Heywood argues that one cause of gout might have been lead intoxication.

205. Smollet, *op. cit.* (note 174), 15–16.

206. M. Jenner, 'Bathing and Baptism: Sir John Floyer and the Politics of Cold Bathing', in K. Sharpe and S.N. Zwicker (eds.), *Refiguring Revolutions: Aesthetics and Politics from the English Revolution to the Romantic Revolution* (Berkeley: University of California Press, 1998), 197–216.

207. *Ibid.*, 203.

208. J. Wesley, *Treatise on Baptism* (1756), in Jackson, *op. cit.* (note 164), Vol. X, 188–201: 188.

209. B. Franklin, *Experiments and Observations on Electricity* (repr. London, 1769); J. Priestley, *History and Present State of Electricity,* 2nd edn (London, 1769); R. Lovett, *The Subtil Medium Prov'd*, 1st edn (London, 1756 [Part 1],

London, 1759 [Part 2]); R. Lovett, *An Appendix on Electricity rendered Useful in Medical Intentions,* 1st edn (London, 1760); R. Lovett, *The Electrical Philosopher,* 1st edn (Worcester, 1774); Wesley, *op. cit.* (note 133), Vol. III, 320

210. See Jackson, *op. cit.* (note 164), Vol. II, 388; M. Rowbottom and C. Susskind, *Electricity and Medicine: A History of their Interaction* (San Francisco: San Francisco Press, 1984), 20.

211. Rowbottom and Susskind, *ibid.*

212. Wesley, *op. cit.* (note 3), xvii.

213. J. Priestley, *The History and Present State of Electricity, with Original Experiments,* 2nd edn (London, 1769), 412–15.

214. Rowbottom and Susskind, *op. cit.* (note 210), 23.

215. P. Bertucci, 'Revealing Sparks: John Wesley and the Religious Utility of Electrical Healing', *British Journal for the History of Science,* 39/3, (2006), 341–62: 353, 344.

216. Priestley, *op. cit.* (note 213), 419. Other works referring to Wesley's electrical experiments include Lovett's *Electrical Philosopher* and James Ferguson's *Introduction to Electricity* (1770).

217. J. Wesley, *The Desideratum: Or, Electricity Made Plain and Useful by a Lover of Mankind and of Common Sense* (London, 1759; repr. London, 1871), n.p. The scholar A. Wesley Hill objects to Priestley's assumption of Wesley's 'ignorance' here: 'This senseless assumption of Wesley's ignorance by Priestley and others is most provoking of indignation… Wesley was no ignorant, meddlesome fellow… wide reading and great practical experience made him quite capable of distinguishing with accuracy both the nature of disorder and the consequence of a seeming cure'. A.W. Hill, *John Wesley Among the Physicians: A Study of Eighteenth-Century Medicine* (London: Epworth Press, 1958), 92.

218. Wesley, quoted in Rowbottom and Susskind, *op. cit.* (note 210), 20.

219. S.J. Rogal, 'Electricity: John Wesley's "Curious and Important Subject"', *Eighteenth-Century Life,* 13 (1989), 79–90.

220. Bertucci, *op. cit.* (note 215), 341, 347, 350–1, 358.

221. *Ibid.,* 342. See ftn. 5 where Bertucci criticises a number of other scholars on the same basis.

222. *Ibid.,* 362.

223. *Ibid.,* 354.

224. *Ibid.,* 361.

225. Wesley quoted by *ibid.,* 357.

226. Bertucci, *ibid.,* 357,

227. Priestley, *op. cit.* (note 213), 410; Rowbottom and Susskind, *op. cit.* (note 210).

228. Priestley, *ibid.,* 418.

229. Wesley, *op. cit.* (note 3), 119.
230. Hill, *op. cit.* (note 217), 90–1.
231. Priestley, *op. cit.* (note 213), 413.
232. *Ibid.*, 417.
233. Rogal, *op. cit.* (note 219), 90.
234. Wesley, quoted by Outler, *op. cit.* (note 182), Vol. II, 573 n. 26.
235. This was Wesley's conclusion after reading Priestley's *The History and Present State of Electricity* – though he thought it was an 'ingenious book'. Wesley, *op. cit.* (note 133), Vol. III, 302–4 (January 1768).
236. Wesley, *op. cit* (note 217), i.
237. Wesley, *op. cit.* (note 194), Vol. IV, 123.
238. Rowbottom and Susskind, *op. cit.* (note 210).
239. Bertucci, *op. cit.* (note 215), 353.
240. G. Rousseau, 'John Wesley's "Primitive Physick" (1747)', *Harvard Library Bulletin,* 16 (1968), 242–56: 294.
241. Wesley, *op. cit.* (note 3), 74.

6

Conclusion:
The Search for Pristine Purity

There is, they say, (and I believe there is)
A spark within us of th' immortal fire,
That animates and moulds the grosser frame;
And when the body sinks escapes to heaven,
Its native seat, and mixes with the Gods.
Meanwhile this heavenly particle pervades
The mortal elements; in every nerve
It thrills with pleasure, or grows mad with pain,
And, in its secret conclave, as it feels
The body's woes and joys, this ruling power
Wields at its will the dull material world,
And is the body's health or malady.

Dr John Armstrong, *The Art of Preserving Health.*

Homo sum; humani nihil a me alienum puto.

John Wesley, Title page, *Primitive Physic.*[1]

Wesley's quotation from Terence – 'I am a man; therefore I deem nothing human to be outside my interest' – thoroughly epitomises his cast of mind, as summed up by J.C. Bowmer:

> He was interested in everything that pertained to life – not life as a biological study or theological abstraction, but life lived, gloriously or sordidly, by men and women of flesh and blood.[2]

Theological abstraction and biological study were of interest to Wesley in as much as they could be used to correct man's nature. *Primitive Physic* was a manual designed to remedy that mortal condition: ordinary people could mitigate everyday diseases of the flesh, but its spiritual component involved an implicit desire for readers to pursue pristine purity and achieve a common life in the body of Christ. For Wesley, theological abstraction and biological study were fused together in a dynamic and powerful way because he was fascinated by the full range of human existence; nowhere is this more

267

apparent than in his *Journal,* which offers the historian many picaresque insights into eighteenth-century life. Georgian existence, however, was frequently shattered by disease and death, and Wesley's journal entries are repeatedly shot-through with such themes:

> I went to Yarn. There I found a lovely young woman in the last stage of a consumption; but such a one as I never read of, nor heard any Physician speak of, but Dr. Wilson. The seat of the ulcers is not the lungs, but the windpipe. I never knew it cured…this young woman died in a few weeks.[3]

In such a context as this, where physic was of little use, Wesley attempted to reassure those dying that they would receive hope and salvation in the eternal realm of the afterlife.

Wesley made a direct and simple connection between science, health and life, but never confused medicine and religion. He firmly believed in the power of spiritual healing, though this belief was not expressed in the remedies set out in *Primitive Physic.* His separation of the medical and religious is evidenced by the way he treated diseases suffered by his friends and family. We have seen how Wesley took a pragmatic, orthodox approach when asked to provide medical advice to his brother Charles, but his journal entries and letters reveal the extent to which he accepted medical opinion when it came to treating his own ailments. The following long passage extracted from a journal entry for 4 January 1774 demonstrates this very well:

> Three or four years ago a stumbling horse threw me forward on the pummel of the saddle. I felt a good deal of pain, but it soon went off, and I thought of it no more. Some months after I observed, *testiculum alterum altero duplo majorem esse.* I consulted a physician. He told me it was a common case, and did not imply any disease at all. In May twelvemonth it was grown near as large as a hen's egg. Being then at Edinburgh, Dr. Hamilton insisted on my having the advice of Dr. Gregory and Munro. They immediately saw it was a hydrocele, and advised me, as soon as I came to London, to aim at a radical cure…When I came to London, I consulted Mr. Wathen. He advised me, 1. Not to think of a radical cure, which could not be hoped for, without my lying in one posture fifteen or sixteen days; and he did not know whether this might not give wound to my constitution, which I should never recover. 2. To do nothing while I continued easy. And this advice I was determined to take.

> Last month the swelling was often painful. So on this day Mr. Wathen performed the operation, and drew off something more than half a pint of thin, yellow, transparent water. With this came out (to his no small surprise)

a pearl of the size of a small shot; which he supposed might be the cause of the disorder, by occasioning a conflux of humours to the part.[4]

The next day, Wesley felt so 'easy' that it was as though no operation had been performed. In this instance, he had been suffering from a hydrocele: a 'dropsy', or abnormal accumulation of serous fluid in the testicle. What is striking about the above extract is the way in which Wesley defers to the judgement of qualified practitioners – despite the fact that the practical advice given by Wathen contradicted Gregory and Munro's prescription.

On those rare occasions Wesley was taken ill he bowed to qualified medical opinion and took his medicine, albeit reluctantly. Deference to orthodox medical practitioners can also be seen time and again in *Primitive Physic*, where many are cited with approval. It can be seen too in Wesley's reaction to the criticism made by Hawes, a physician who was well respected and professionally esteemed. In terms of medical practice, Hawes clearly demonstrated shortcomings of his own, yet Wesley took much of the criticism levelled at *Primitive Physic* on board by gradually integrating some of the amendments into subsequent editions. Despite Wesley's sharply focused rhetoric in 'The Preface', which aimed its fire at 'professional' physicians, it is true to say that he generally respected them and conceded to their better judgement when it was appropriate.

Here, Wesley's lack of formal training led him to tread carefully, and perhaps the most impressive aspect of *Primitive Physic* is the way in which he amended and omitted various articles in the light of new medical discoveries. Wesley was not afraid to alter his position radically on a point of physic when presented with better techniques or more advanced medical evidence. His about-turn on the issue of fluid intake when treating the dropsy or bleeding of a fever adequately attests to an approach that was carefully considered. These were not the actions of an arrogant or unthinking empiricist, disrespectful of orthodox medical opinion.

Primitive Physic is a text that is of vital interest because it brings to light so many points of contact and difference between Wesley's medical practice and that of established physicians. It is precisely those areas of contact and difference which can illuminate how 'orthodox' *Primitive Physic* really was. Yet the adoption of orthodox methods did not prevent Wesley from entering into a critical dialogue with the medical profession in a way that could be extremely forthright. On the issue of abstruse, speculative medical theories, which he believed threatened to hinder medical progress altogether, Wesley made his feelings perfectly plain. Experience counted for more than theory, and although this stance contained its own theoretical traditions, of which Wesley was undoubtedly aware, its privileging of theory over fact was why he felt particularly aggrieved at the Faculty's lack of interest in electrical therapy. Experience had shown Wesley that electricity worked very well on a range of illnesses, but specifically on those nervous disorders.

Undoubtedly, Wesley's interest in medicine must have been partly informed by his own health considerations. Though Wesley was rarely ill, he was not completely immune from those diseases that dominated the eighteenth-century; over the period of his long life, Wesley suffered from diabetes, smallpox, the ague, consumption and gout – consumption had nearly killed Wesley in 1753. His mother suffered from gout and he came from a family where many of his siblings failed to reach adulthood. For Wesley finding the golden mean, physically and spiritually, was the goal of all self-aware Christians. Motivated by Christian ideals of pristine purity and practical piety, *Primitive Physic* represents, quite literally, what he tried to achieve: a belief, which he committed to paper, so that the poor could regulate their lifestyle and mitigate disease.

Primitive Physic was Wesley's way of making sure the poor had a physician in their home – one that could be called upon at any time and who would not charge exorbitant fees. Healing was central to his theology and so it followed that *Primitive Physic* became an essential text, which was distributed amongst the Methodist societies. Hence, it was made clear in every edition of *Primitive Physic* that this text was on sale 'at the Chapel, City Road, and at all the Methodist Preaching-Houses in Town and Country'.[5] In addition to this, Wesley penned numerous anxious letters to Methodist preachers stressing the importance of distributing *Primitive Physic*, amongst other valuable works:

> Dear Richard,
>
> You should take particular care that your circuit be never without an assortment of all the valuable books, especially the *Appeals*, the *Sermons*, Kempis, and the *Primitive Physic*, which no family should be without.[6]

Interesting to note here is how Wesley's selection of the 'valuable books' involved looking after the mind (*Appeals*), spirit (*Sermons*) and body (*Primitive Physic*). *Primitive Physic* provided an extensive range of remedies for individuals to select, and through regimen it encouraged them to be proactive in their physical wellbeing.

In this sense, although physic was to be mediated to some extent through Methodist preachers, the general populace was not merely regarded as being a passive receptacle. *Primitive Physic* could complement other forms of 'popular' healing and kitchen–physic. Wesley thus asked his preachers to keep their eyes open for any efficacious remedy they might pick up when visiting their flock so that it could be added to subsequent editions of his manual.[7] But although *Primitive Physic* sometimes enjoyed a dialogical relationship with its readers and mediators, Wesley continued to exercise tight editorial control. To his Book Steward, John Atlay, he gave the following instructions regarding the 20th edition in 1781:

> My Dear Brother,
>
> I prepared the new edition of the *Primitive Physic* for the press before I left London. It lies in the corner of the upper drawer of my bureau. I have placed all the additions exactly. See that they be not displaced.[8]

Wesley's instruction here probably has an additional frisson to it because his editorial skills had been so severely scrutinised by Hawes and 'ANTIDOTE' in the public press. Even though every addition or omission had always been subject to Wesley's critical judgement, after the 16th edition this process became more rigorous and was backed up by orthodox medical practice. The plain style and apparent simplicity of *Primitive Physic* was authoritatively sourced and underwritten by contemporary theory and practice as espoused by leading physicians. Following Wesley's reading of Hawes's *An Examination*, these leading physicians were actually cited.

Wesley was no peddler or dilettante in the area of medicine. Nor was he just a collector of 'popular' kitchen–physic recipes. On the contrary, he was an active exponent of English enlightened medicine. Like Boyle, Locke and Sydenham, Wesley was an empiricist and medical pragmatist who utilised this approach to encourage men and women to relieve and improve physical conditions. This he did primarily through *Primitive Physic*, but his thoroughly medical cast-of-mind meant that he could not resist giving physic in whatever context he found himself. We have seen how Wesley's sermons consistently sought recourse to medical terminology and language, and how he constantly observed and commented on the various medical issues of his day in the *Journal*. This tendency, however, was echoed in his letters, where Wesley provided post-bag medical advice and commentary with great enthusiasm:

> My Dear Brother,
>
> Use the decoction of burdock largely, and I think it will have a good effect. And certainly the *Primitive Physic* will teach you a remedy either for the outward or inward piles.[9]

> Dear Charles, [Atmore]
>
> Agues this year spread all over the kingdom, and they are far more stubborn than usual. If you have not tried Dr. Sander's pills, you should (after taking a little vomit). They are entirely safe, as has been proved in a thousand

instances. Take, - Castile soap, two scruples; *arsenicum album*, two grains. Mix thoroughly, and make into eight pills. Take one every four hours between the fits. It seldom fails.[10]

My Dear Sister,

It pleases God to lead you in a rough path for the present; but it is enough that all will end well. I never knew any disorder in the bowels which might not be speedily cured by drinking plentifully of lemonade; unless in a few peculiar constitutions, which could not bear lemons. And the drinking of nettle-tea (instead of common tea) will commonly perfect the cure.[11]

These are three letters out of a range of possible choices that cover the full medical spectrum. Common to all of the letters though, and a feature of those cited above, is Wesley's compassionate regard for the necessity of reassurance and hope. Hence his repeated use of phrases such as 'I think it will have a good effect', 'it seldom fails' and 'will commonly perfect the cure'.

Healing was central to Wesley's theology but hope was pivotal to both medical and spiritual holism. Wesley refused to believe that even the most entrenched disease was incurable and the remedies set out in *Primitive Physic* for cancer, consumption and gout defied those physicians who inclined towards pessimism. Wesley's assurances on this score were not merely deluded; hope, he argued, could strengthen mind and body against even the most inveterate condition – whether it was physical, psychological or spiritual. This stance was mirrored theologically in his adamant refusal to concede to the Calvinist doctrine of Predestination, insisting instead that man could work towards his own salvation: pristine purity and eschatological hope was God's gift to everyone.

Wesley's emphasis on the doctrine of Christian Perfection, and of what Primitive Christianity really meant, embroiled him in theological controversy with Anglicans and Calvinists alike. Yet he detested division between Christians and loathed religious sectarianism. He sought instead to achieve a general Christian alliance that recognised difference of opinion but which was based on a union of affection and practical piety. In this sense, he wished to revive all that was best about those reforming Anglican societies characteristic of the Restoration period. In this vein, the Methodist movement took an eirenic stance and strove to promote social projects, which included welfare provision, lending services, schools, bookshops and medical dispensaries. This project also involved prison work, hygiene movements and anti-slavery campaigns. Wesley's philanthropic endeavours were an attempt to replicate those acts of charity undertaken by Primitive Christians, but fitted well with the values of English enlightened thought.

Primitive Physic puts an active religion and an empiricist, experimental philosophy to useful effect. In writing this text Wesley sought to address those very real problems faced by the labouring poor in eighteenth-century England – problems that revolved around health, hygiene and nutrition. Attendant to these, were the interrelated issues of the cost and accessibility of healthcare. When dispensing physic, Wesley also needed to think carefully about the burden of responsibility attached to safeguarding his reading public from the danger of 'quack' methods and polypharmacy, both of which profited from the use of lethal nostrums and chemical compounds. That Wesley managed to address each of these crucial issues, while simultaneously negotiating his way through a maze of complex disease-related theory, is a testament to his success as a 'non-professional' physician.

By compiling that list of receipts which made up *Primitive Physic*, Wesley placed into the hands of the poor a remedy for their physical ills. *Primitive Physic* concentrates its focus on treating the purely physical symptoms of disease, as opposed to specifying ways in which to combat the spiritual disorder of *dis-ease*, that marker of original sin. Yet Wesley's motivation in the opening paragraphs of 'The Preface' to *Primitive Physic* was to show that the alleviation of bodily disorder was inextricably linked to man recovering his pristine state. Perfect bodily and spiritual health involved using 'all the means which reason and experience can dictate...'[12] Wesley adopted this injunction as his guide and method in everything, but in *Primitive Physic* it was used to identify a standard set down in physic by tradition, while pointing also to those new, progressive and enlightened discoveries that were beginning to re-configure Georgian medical practice. In this sense, *Primitive Physic* was at the very heart of discontinuity and change in eighteenth-century England.

Notes

1. J. Armstrong, *The Art of Preserving Health* (London, 1744), in *English Poetry Full-Text Database* [Windows CD-ROM] (Cambridge: Chadwyck-Healey, 1993); J. Wesley, *Primitive Physic,* 1st edn (London, 1747) n.p.
2. J.C. Bowmer, 'John Wesley's Philosophy of Suffering', *London Quarterly and Holburn Review,* 184 (1959), 60–6: 60.
3. J. Wesley, *The Journal of the Rev. John Wesley, A.M.,* 4 vols (London: J. Kershaw, 1827), Vol IV, 94 (Thursday, 8 May 1777).
4. *Ibid.,* 6. Dr Hamilton was a Scots physician who joined the Methodists and also became a preacher. He was elected physician to the London Dispensary and became eminent within the medical profession.
5. See the title page of *Primitive Physic* (any edition).
6. Letter from Wesley to Richard Rodda, preacher on the Oxfordshire circuit, in J. Telford (ed.), *The Letters of the Rev. John Wesley A.M.,* 8 vols (London:

Epworth Press, 1931), Vol. VIII, 138 (9 September 1782).

7. This can be seen in several of Wesley's letters to local preachers. I have deliberately refrained from using material or data that can cast light on the reception of Wesley's medical manual amongst the general populace. This topic lies outside the purview of concerns set down here and will form the basis of a forthcoming volume, *Medicine on Demand: The Reception of John Wesley's 'Primitive Physic'*.

8. Wesley, *op. cit.* (note 6), Vol. VIII, 63 (8 May 1781).

9. Letter from Wesley to John Bredin, preacher in Bandon (Cork), *op. cit.* (note 5), Vol. VIII, 24 (19 June 1780).

10. Letter from Wesley to Charles Atmore, Methodist itinerant, appointed to Scarborough, *op. cit.* (note 6), Vol. VII, 124 (28 May 1782).

11. Letter from Wesley to Ellen Gretton, Methodist member, *op. cit.* (note 6), Vol. VII, 13 (9 September 1782).

12. J. Wesley, *Advice with Respect to Health,* 4th edn (London, 1789), viii.

Bibliography

Primary Texts

Anonymous, *The Family Guide to Health: Or, A Practice of Physic: In a Familiar Way* (1st edn, London, 1767).

Anonymous, *A Cheap, Sure and Ready Guide to Health: Or, A Cure for a Disease Call'd the Doctor* (1742; 2nd edn, London, 1742).

Arbuthnot, J., *An Essay Concerning the Effects of Air in Human Bodies* (1st edn, London, 1733).

——, *An Essay Concerning the Nature of Aliments, and the Choice of Them, According to the Different Constitutions of Human Bodies* (1731; 4th edn, London, 1756).

Armstrong, John, *The Art of Preserving Health* (London, 1744), in *English Poetry Full-Text Database*.

Baxter, R., *The Reformed Pastor* (1656; repr. London, 1841).

Blackmore, Sir Richard, *Dissertations on a Dropsy, a Tympany, the Jaundice, the Stone, and a Diabetes* (1st edn, London, 1727).

——, *A Treatise of Consumptions and other Distempers belonging to the Breast and Lungs* (1724; 2nd edn, London, 1725).

Boerhaave, Herman, *Boerhaave's Aphorisms: Concerning the Knowledge and Cure of Diseases,* tr. Anonymous (London, 1742); orig. pub. as *Aphorismi de cognoscendis et curandis morbis in usum doctrinae domesticae digesti* (1722; Leyden, 1728).

Boyle, Robert, *The Works of Robert Boyle*, Michael Hunter and Edward B. Davis (eds), 14 vols (London: Pickering & Chatto, 2000).

——, *General History of the Air* (London, 1692).

——, *Medicinal Experiments: Or, A Collection of Choice and Safe Remedies For the Most Part Simple and Easily Prepared* (1692; 4th edn, London, 1703).

Buchan, William, *Domestic Medicine: Or, A Treatise on the Prevention and Cure of Diseases by Regimen and Simple Medicines* (1769; 2nd edn, London, 1772).

Burton, Robert, *The Anatomy of Melancholy*, Holbrook Jackson (ed.), 3 vols (London: Dent, 1968).

Cadogan, W., *A Dissertation on the Gout, and All Chronic Diseases, Jointly Considered as Proceeding from the Same Causes* (1771; 9th edn, London, 1771).

Casaubon, Meric, *Treatise Concerning Enthusiasm: As it is an Effect of Nature* (London, 1655), *see* Korshin.

Cave, William, *Primitive Christianity: Or, the Religion of the Ancient Christians in the First Ages of the Gospel* (1673; 6th edn, London, 1702).

Cheyne, G., *A New Theory of Continual Fevers: Wherein, Besides the Appearances of Such Fevers, and the Method of Their Cure, Occasionally, the Structure of the Glands, and the Manner and Laws of Secretion, the Operation of Purgative, Vomitive, and Mecurial Medicines, are Mechanically Explain'd* (1st edn, London, 1701).

——, *A New Theory of Continu'd Fevers* (1702; 2nd edn, London, 1722).

——, *An Essay of Health and Long Life* (1st edn, London, 1724).

——, *An Essay of Health and Long Life* (6th edn, London 1725).

——, *An Essay on the True Nature and Due Method of Treating the Gout* (1722; 5th edn, London, 1723).

——, *An Essay on the True Nature and Due Method of Treating the Gout* (1722; 6th edn, London, 1724).

——, *The English Malady* (London, 1733), *see* Porter.

——, *An Essay on Regimen: Together with Five Discourses, Medical, Moral, and Philosophical: Serving to Illustrate the Principles and Theory of Philosophical Medicine, and Point Out Some of its Moral Consequences* (1st edn, London, 1740).

——, *The Natural Method of Curing the Diseases of the Body, and the Disorders of the Mind Depending on the Body* (1st edn, London, 1742).

Cyprian, *Epistles,* tr. C.H. Collyns (Oxford: Library of the Fathers of the Holy Catholic Church, 1844).

Derham, William, *Astro-Theology: Or, A Demonstration of the Being and Attributes of God, from a Survey of the Heavens* (1713; 4th edn, London, 1715).

Dover, Thomas, *The Ancient Physician's Legacy to his Country* (1732; 6th edn, London, 1742).

Elliot, John (ed.), *A Complete Collection of the Medical and Philosophical Works of John Fothergill* (London, 1781).

English Poetry Full-Text Database [Windows CD-ROM], (Cambridge: Chadwyck-Healey, 1993).

Eusibius of Caesarea, *The History of the Church*, tr. G.A. Williamson (London: Penguin, 1989).

Evans, Theophilus, *The History of Modern Enthusiasm from the Reformation to the Present Times* (1st edn, London, 1752).

Falconer, William, *A Dissertation on the Influence of the Passions upon the Disorders of the Body* (1772; 2nd edn, London, 1791).

Fleury, Claude, *The Manners of the Antient Christians, Extracted from a French Author,* ed. John Wesley (1st edn, Bristol, 1749).

Floyer, John and Baynard, Edward, *Psychroloysia: Or, The History of Cold-Bathing, Both Ancient and Modern: In Two Parts: The First Written by Sir John Floyer of Litchfield, kt.: The Second, Treating of the Genuine Use of Hot and Cold Baths...by Dr. Edward Baynard* (1707; 5th edn, London, 1722).

Franklin, B., *Experiments and Observations on Electricity* (1751; repr. London, 1769).

Hales, Stephen, *A Sermon Preached Before the Royal College of Physicians* (1st edn, London, 1751).

——, *A Description of Ventilators* (1st edn, London, 1743).

——, *A Treatise on Ventilators* (1st edn, London, 1758).

Hartley, David, *Observations on Man, His Frame, His Duty, and His Expectations,* 2 vols (1st edn, London, 1749).

Hawes, William, *An Account of the Late Dr Goldsmith's Illness, so far as it relates to Dr James's Powders* (1780; 4th edn, London, 1780).

——, *An Examination of the Rev. Mr John Wesley's Primitive Physic* (1780; 2nd edn, London, 1780).

Herbert, G., *The Country Parson* (1st edn, London, 1671).

——, *The Temple: Sacred Poems and Private Ejaculations* (1633) (London: Nonesuch Press, 1927).

Hill, John, *The Virtues of Honey in Preventing the Worst Disorders* (1st edn, London, 1760).

——, *The Virtues of Sage in Lengthening Life* (1st edn, London, 1763).

——, *The Family Herbal: Or, An Account of all those English Plants, which are Remarkable for their Virtues* (1st edn, London, 1755).

Horneck, A., *The Happy Ascetick: or the Best Exercise... to which is added, A Letter to a Person of Quality, concerning the holy lives of the Primitive Christians* (1681; 2nd edn, London, 1685).

Huxham, John, *An Essay on Fevers and their Various Kinds* (1st edn, London,1750).

James, Robert, *A Medicinal Dictionary: Including Physic, Surgery, Anatomy, Chymistry and Botany... together with a History of Drugs* (1st edn, London, 1743).

Jones, John, *Mysteries of Opium Reveal'd* (1701; 2nd edn, London, 1701).

Kant, Immanuel, 'An Answer to the Question: "What is Enlightenment"', in *Kant's Political Writings,* ed. Hans Reiss (Cambridge: Cambridge University Press, 1970), 54–60.

Korshin, P.J. (ed.), *Casaubon's Treatise* (Florida: Scholars Facsimiles and Reprints, 1970), *see* Casaubon.

Lavington, G., *The Enthusiasm of Methodists and Papists Compared* (1749–54; 2nd edn, London, 1754).

Law, William, *A Serious Call to a Devout and Holy Life: The Spirit of Love,* Paul G. Stanwood (ed.), (1729; London: SPCK, 1978).

Locke, J., *An Essay Concerning Human Understanding,* John Yolton (ed.), (1690; London: Everyman, 1994).

——, *The Reasonableness of Christianity: As Delivered in the Scriptures,* J.C. Higgins Biddle (ed.), (1695; Cambridge: Cambridge University Press, 1999).

——, *Some Familiar Letters between Mr Locke, and Several of his Friends* (1742; 4th edn, London, 1742).

Lovett, Richard, *The Subtil Medium Prov'd* (1st edn, London, 1756 [Part 1], London, 1759 [Part 2]).

——, *An Appendix on Electricity rendered Useful in Medical Intentions* (1st edn, London, 1760).

——, *The Electrical Philosopher* (1st edn, Worcester, 1774).

Macarius (Pseudo-), *The Fifty Spiritual Homilies*, George A. Maloney (ed.), (New York: Paulist Press, 1992).

Mandeville, B., *The Fable of the Bees: Or, Private Vices, Publick Benefits,* with a commentary by F.B. Kaye, 2 vols (1723, 1728; Oxford: Oxford University Press, 1924; repr., Indianapolis: Liberty Fund, 1988).

——, *An Essay on Charity and Charity Schools* (1724; 4th edn, London, 1725).

Mead, Richard, *A Mechanical Account of Poisons in Several Essays* (1st edn, London, 1702).

——, *Of the Influence of the Sun and Moon on Humane Bodies* (1st edn, London, 1704).

——, *Medical Precepts and Cautions,* tr. Thomas Stack (2nd edn, London, 1751).

More, H, *Enthusiasmus Triumphatus,* with an introduction by M.V. Deporte (1656; repr. California: University of California Press, 1966).

Nelson, Robert, *A Companion for the Festivals and Fasts of the Church of England* (London: W. B. for A. and J. Churchil [*sic*], 1704).

Porter, Roy (ed.), *George Cheyne: The English Malady: Or, A Treatise of Nervous Diseases of all Kinds (1733)* (Tavistock Classics in the History of Psychiatry; London: Routledge, 1991), *see* Cheyne.

Priestley, J., *The History and Present State of Electricity, with Original Experiments.* (1767; 2nd edn, London, 1769).

Radcliffe, John, *Pharmacopaeia Radcliffeana: Or, Dr Radcliffe's Prescriptions, Faithfully Gathered from his Original Recipes* (1715; 3rd edn, London, 1718).

Ray, John, *The Wisdom of God Manifested in the Works of the Creation* (1691; 10th edn, London, 1735).

Smollet, Tobias, *An Essay on the External Use of Water* (1st edn, London, 1752).

St Ignatius of Antioch, *The Epistles of St Clement of Rome and St Ignatius of Antioch,* J.A. Kleist (ed.), (London: Newman Press, 1946).

Stephen, L., *History of English Thought in the Eighteenth Century* (1876; 3rd edn, London, 1902).

Stevens, George Alexander, *The Specifick* (London, 1788), in *English Poetry Full-Text Database.*

Stukley, William, *Of the Gout* (1st edn, London, 1735).

Sydenham, Thomas, *The Works of Thomas Sydenham M.D.,* tr. R.G. Latham, 2 vols (London: Sydenham Society, 1868).

Taylor, Jeremy, *The Rule and Exercises of Holy Living* (1650; 22nd edn, London, 1715).

Thomas à Kempis, *Imitatio Christi* (London: Penguin, 1952).

Tissot, Samuel August Andre, *L'Avis au Peuple sur sa Santé,* tr. J. Kirkpatrick (1762; 2nd edn, London, 1765).

——, *An Essay on the Disorders of People of Fashion,* tr. Francis Bacon Lee (1768; London, 1771).

Tyerman, Luke, *The Life and Times of the Rev. Samuel Wesley, M.A.,* 3 vols (London, 1866).

——, *The Life and Times of the Rev. John Wesley, MA.,* 3 vols (London, 1870–2).

Wainewright, Jeremiah, *A Mechanical Account of the Non-Naturals: Being a Brief Explication of the Changes Made in Humane Bodies by Air, Diet, together with an Enquiry into the Nature and Use of the Baths* (1st edn, London, 1708).

Warburton, W., *The Doctrine of Grace: Or, The Office and Operations of the Holy Spirit Vindicated from the Insults of Infidelity and the Abuses of Fanaticism* (1st edn, London, 1763).

Wesley, John, *Primitive Physic: or, An Easy and Natural Method of Curing Most Diseases* (1st edn, London, 1747).

——, *Primitive Physic* (5th edn, Bristol, 1755).

——, *Primitive Physic* (8th edn, Bristol, 1759).

——, *Primitive Physic* (15th edn, London, 1772).

——, *Primitive Physic* (16th edn, London, 1774).

——, *Primitive Physic,* A. Wesley Hill (ed.), (23rd edn, London, 1791; repr. London: Epworth Press, 1960).

——, *Primitive Physic* (24th edn, London, 1792).

——, *The Christian Pattern; Or, A Treatise of the Imitation of Christ* (London, 1735).

——, *The Character of a Methodist* (3rd edn, Bristol, 1743).

——, *A Plain Account of the People Call'd Methodists* (London, 1748).

—— (ed.), *A Christian Library: Consisting of Extracts from and Abridgements of the Choicest Pieces of Practical Divinity which have been published in the English Language,* 50 vols (1st edn, Bristol, 1749–55).

——, *An Address to the Clergy* (London, 1756).

——, *The Desideratum: Or, Electricity Made Plain and Useful by a Lover of Mankind and of Common Sense* (London, 1759; repr. London, 1871).

——, *A Survey of the Wisdom of God in the Creation: Or, A Compendium of Natural Philosophy,* 5 vols (3rd edn, London, 1763).

——, *An Extract from Dr Cadogan's Dissertation on the Gout and all chronic Diseases* (1st edn, London, 1774).

—— (ed.), *Advice with Respect to Health* (4th edn, London, 1789)

—— (ed.), *The Family Physician: or, Advice with Respect to Health, including Directions for the Prevention and Cure of Acute Diseases, extracted from Dr Tissot* (6th edn, London, 1797).

——, *The Journal of the Rev. John Wesley, A.M.,* 4 vols (London: J. Kershaw, 1827).

——, *The Works of the Rev. John Wesley, A.M.,* Thomas Jackson (ed.), 14 vols (London: Wesleyan Methodist Book-Room, 1831).

——, *Thoughts Upon Self Denial* (repr. London, 1857).

——, *The Journal of the Revd John Wesley, A.M.,* N. Curnock (ed.), 8 vols (London: n.p., 1909–16).

——, *The Letters of the Rev. John Wesley A.M.,* J. Telford (ed.), 8 vols (London: Epworth Press, 1931).

——, *The Bicentennial Edition of the Works of John Wesley,* vols i–iv: *Sermons,* Albert C. Outler (ed.), (Nashville: Abingdon Press, 1985).

Wesley, John [*cont...*], *An Earnest Appeal to Men of Reason and Religion* (1743), in *The Bicentennial Edition of the Works of John Wesley,* Vol. XI, *The Appeals,* G.R. Cragg (ed.), (Nashville: Abingdon Press, 1989), 37–94.

Wesley, Samuel, *Sermon Preached before the Society for the Reformation of Manners* (1698), repr. *Methodist Magazine,* 1841, 648–65, 727–36.

——, *Advice to a Young Clergyman* (London, 1735).

Young, George, *Treatise on Opium, Founded Upon Practical Observations* (1st edn, London, 1753).

Secondary Texts

Aarsleff, Hans, *From Locke to Saussure: Essays on the Study of Language and Intellectual History* (London: Athlone, 1982).

Andrews, Jonathan, 'A Respectable Mad Doctor? Dr Richard Hale, FRS (1670–1728)', *Notes and Records of the Royal Society,* 44 (1990), 169–201.

—— and Scull, Andrew, *Undertaker of the Mind: John Monro and Mad-Doctoring in Eighteenth-Century England* (California: University of California Press, 2001).

Armstrong, G. Kelly, 'Irrationalism and Politics in the Eighteenth Century', *Studies in Eighteenth-Century Culture,* 2 (1972), 239–53.

Baragar, C.A., 'John Wesley and Medicine', *Annals of Medical History,* 10 (1928), 59–65.

Bardell, E.B., 'Primitive Physick: John Wesley's Receipts', *Pharmacy in History,* 21 (1979), 111–21.

Barker, G.F.R., 'Hill, John…', in *Dictionary of National Biography.*

Barry, J, 'Piety and Patient: Medicine and Religion in Eighteenth-Century Bristol', in Porter (ed.), *Patients and Practitioners,* 145–75.

—— and Jones, C. (eds), *Medicine and Charity before the Welfare State* (London: Routledge, 1991).

Beckwith, S., *Christ's Body: Identity, Culture and Society in Late Medieval Writings* (London: Routledge, 1993).

Benjamin, M., 'Medicine, Morality and the Politics of Berkeley's Tar-water', in Cunningham and French (eds), *The Medical Enlightenment of the Eighteenth Century*, 165–93.

Bennett, G.V., 'Patristic Tradition in Anglican Thought, 1660–1900', *Oecumenica* (Minneapolis 1966–72), 1971–2 63–85.

Bennett, J.M., 'Conviviality and Charity in Medieval and Early Modern England', *Past and Present*, 134 (1992), 19–41.

Bertucci, Paola, 'Revealing Sparks: John Wesley and the Religious Utility of Electrical Healing', *British Journal for the History of Science*, 39/3, (2006), 341–62.

Bono, James, 'Science, Discourse, and Literature: The Role/Rule of Metaphor in Science', in Stuart Peterfreund (ed.), *Literature and Science: Theory and Practice* (Boston: Northeastern University Press, 1990), 59–89.

Bowmer, J.C., 'John Wesley's Philosophy of Suffering', *London Quarterly and Holburn Review*, 184 (1959), 60–6.

Brantley, Richard E., *Locke, Wesley, and the Method of English Romanticism* (Gainesville: University of Florida Press, 1984).

Brewer, J. and Porter, Roy (eds), *Consumption and the World of Goods* (London: Routledge, 1993).

Brooke, John Hedley, *Science and Religion: Some Historical Perspectives* (Cambridge: Cambridge University Press, 1991).

Brown, Peter, *The Body and Society: Men, Women, and Sexual Renunciation in Early Christianity* (New York: Columbia University Press, 1988).

Bynum, W.F., 'Health, Disease and Medical Care', in Rousseau and Porter (eds), *The Ferment of Knowledge: Studies in the Historiography of Eighteenth-Century Science*, 211–54.

—— and Porter, Roy (eds), *Companion Encyclopedia of the History of Medicine*, 2 vols (London: Routledge, 1993).

Campbell, T., *John Wesley and Christian Antiquity: Religious Vision and Cultural Change* (Nashville: Kingswood Books, 1991).

Carmichael, Ann G., 'St Anthony's Fire', in Kiple (ed.), *The Cambridge World of Human Disease*, 989–90.

Cassirer, E., *The Philosophy of the Enlightenment*, tr. Fritz C.A. Koelln and James P. Pettegrove (Princeton: Princeton University Press, 1979).

Chadwick, Henry, *The Early Church* (London: Penguin, 1967, rev. ed. 1993).

Champion, J., 'Toleration and Citizenship in Enlightenment England: John Toland and the Naturalisation of the Jews, 1714–1753', in Grell and Porter (eds), *Toleration in Enlightenment Europe*, 133–56.

Clark, J.C.D., *English Society 1688-1832* (Cambridge: Cambridge University Press, 1985).

Clark, William; Golinski, Jan and Schaffer, Simon, 'Introduction', in Clark, Golinski and Schaffer (eds), *The Sciences in Enlightened Europe*, 3–31.

—— —— —— (eds), *The Sciences in Enlightened Europe* (Chicago: University of Chicago Press, 1999).

Coley, Noel G., 'Physicians, Chemists and the Analysis of Mineral Waters: "The Most Difficult Part of Chemistry"', in Porter (ed.), *The Medical History of Waters and Spas*, 56–66.

Collier, F.W., *John Wesley Among the Scientists* (New York: Abingdon Press, 1928).

Concise Oxford English Dictionary (10th edn, Oxford: Oxford University Press, 1999).

Conrad, L., *et al.* (eds), *The Western Medical Tradition* (Cambridge: Cambridge University Press, 1995).

Cragg, G.R., *Freedom and Authority: A Study of English Thought in the Early Seventeenth Century* (Philadelphia: Westminster Press, 1975).

Croxson, Bronwyn, 'The Public and Private Faces of Eighteenth-Century London Dispensary Charity', *Medical History*, 41 (1997), 127–49.

Cule, J., 'The Rev. John Wesley, M.A. (Oxon), 1703–1791: "The Naked Empiricist" and Orthodox Medicine', *The Journal of the History of Medicine,* 45 (1990), 41–63.

Cunningham, A. and French, R. (eds), *The Medical Enlightenment of the Eighteenth Century* (Cambridge: Cambridge University Press, 1990).

Cunningham, A., 'How the *Principia* Got Its Name; Or, Taking Natural Philosophy Seriously', *History of Science*, 29 (1991), 377–92.

Darwin, Frances, 'Hales, Stephen 1677–1761', in *Dictionary of National Biography*.

Davison, L., *et al.* (eds), *Stilling the Grumbling Hive: The Response to Social and Economic Problems in England, 1689–1750* (New York: St Martin's Press, 1992)

DeLacy, Margaret, 'The Conceptualization of Influenza in Eighteenth-Century Britain: Specificity and Contagion', *Bulletin of the History of Medicine*, 67 (1993), 74–118.

De Porte, M., *Nightmares and Hobbyhorses: Swift, Sterne and Augustan Ideas of Madness* (San Marino, CA: The Huntingdon Library, 1974).

Dewhurst, Kenneth, *The Quicksilver Doctor: The Life and Times of Thomas Dover. Physician and Adventurer* (Bristol: John Wright & Sons, 1957).

——, 'An Oxford Medical Student's Notebook (1652–1659)', *Oxford Medical School Gazette*, 2 (1959), 141–6.

——, *Locke's Contribution to Boyle's Researches on the Air and on Human Blood* (London: Royal Society of London, 1962).

——, 'A Review of John Locke's Research into Social and Preventive Medicine', *Bulletin of the History of Medicine*, 36 (1962), 317–40.

——, *John Locke (1632–1704), Physician and Philosopher: A Medical Biography with an Edition of the Medical Notes in his Journals* (London: Wellcome Historical Medical Library, 1963).

——, 'An Oxford Medical Quartet: Sydenham, Willis, Locke and Lower', in *Oxford Medicine: Essays on the Evolution of the Oxford Clinical School to Commemorate the Bicentenary of the Radcliffe Infimary, 1770–1970* (Oxford: Sandford Publications, 1970), 23–31.

——, *Thomas Willis as a Physician* (Los Angeles: William Andrews Clark Memorial Library, 1964).

——, *Dr. Thomas Sydenham (1624–1689): His Life and Original Writings* (London: Wellcome Historical Medical Library, 1966).

Dictionary of National Biography [Windows CD-ROM], (1890; Oxford: Oxford University Press, 1995).

Digby, Anne, *Madness, Morality and Medicine* (Cambridge: Cambridge University Press, 1985).

Dock, G., 'The *Primitive Physick* of Revd John Wesley: A Picture of Eighteenth-Century Medicine', *Journal of the American Medical Association,* 64 (1915), 629–38.

Dreyer, Frederick, 'Faith and Experience in the Thought of John Wesley', *The American Historical Review,* 88 (1983), 12–30.

Duffy, Eamon, 'Primitive Christianity Revived: Religious Renewal in Augustan England', in D. Baker (ed.), *Renaissance and Renewal in Christian History* (Studies in Church History, 14), (Oxford: Blackwell, 1977), 287–300.

Dunn, J.D.G., *The Acts of the Apostles* (Peterborough: Epworth Press, 1996).

Eklund, J., 'Of a Spirit in the Water: Some Early Ideas on the Aerial Dimension', *Isis,* 67 (1976), 527–50.

Emch-Dériaz, Antoinette, 'The Non-Naturals Made Easy', in Porter (ed.), *The Popularization of Medicine, 1650–1850* (London: Routledge, 1992), 134–59.

English, J.C., 'John Wesley and the Anglican Moderates of the Seventeenth Century', *Anglican Theological Review,* 51 (1969), 203–20.

——, 'John Wesley and Isaac Newton's "System of the World"', *Proceedings of the Wesley Historical Society,* 48/3 (1991), 69–86.

Estes, J. Worth, 'Dropsy', in Kiple (ed.), *The Cambridge World of Human Disease,* 689–96.

Felleman Bartels, Laura, 'John Wesley's *Survey of the Wisdom of God in Creation:* A Methodological Inquiry', *Perspectives on Science and Christian Faith,* 58/1 (2006), 1–6.

——, 'John Wesley and Dr George Cheyne on the Spiritual Senses', *Wesleyan Theological Journal,* (2004), 163–72.

Ferguson, P., 'Me and My Shadows: On the Accumulation of Body-Images in Western Society. Part One – The Image and the Image of Body in Pre-Modern Society', *Body and Society,* 3 (September 1997), 1–31.

Fissell, M.E., 'Charity Universal? Institutions and Moral Reform in Eighteenth-Century Bristol', in Davison, *et al.* (eds), *Stilling the Grumbling Hive: The Response to Social and Economic Problems in England, 1689–1750* (New York: St Martin's Press, 1992), 121–44.

Fox, R. Hingston, *Dr John Fothergill and his Friends: Chapters in Eighteenth-Century Life* (Macmillan: London, 1919).

French, R., 'Scrofula', in Kiple (ed.), *The Cambridge World History of Human Disease*, 998–1000.

Furnish, Victor Paul, *II Corinthians* (New York: Doubleday, 1984).

Garnett, Jane and Colin, Matthew (eds), *Revival and Religion since 1700: Essays for John Walsh* (London: The Hambledon Press, 1993).

Green, Richard, *Anti-Methodist Publications Issued during the Eighteenth Century* (London: C. H. Kelly, 1902).

Green, V.H.H., *The Young Mr Wesley: A Study of John Wesley and Oxford* (London: Epworth Press, 1963).

Grell, Ole Peter, and Cunningham, A. (eds), *Health Care and Poor Relief in Protestant Europe, 1500–1700* (London: Routledge, 1997).

——, Israel, J.I., Tyacke, N. (eds), *From Persecution to Toleration: The Glorious Revolution and Religion in England* (Oxford: Oxford University Press, 1991).

—— and Porter, Roy, 'Introduction', in *idem* (eds), *Toleration in Enlightenment Europe*, 1–22.

—— and Porter, Roy (eds), *Toleration in Enlightenment Europe* (Cambridge: Cambridge University Press, 2000).

Gronim Stidstone, Sara, 'Imagining Inoculation: Smallpox, the Body, and Social Relations of Healing in the Eighteenth Century', *Bulletin for the History of Medicine*, 80, (2006), 247–68.

Guerrini, A., '"A Club of Little Villains": Rhetoric, Professional Identity, and Medical Pamphlet Wars', in Porter and Roberts (eds), *Literature and Medicine during the Eighteenth Century*, 226–44.

——, 'Ether Madness: Newtonianism, Religion, and Insanity', in Adele Seef and Paul Theerman (eds), *Action and Reaction* (Newark: University of Delaware Press, 1993), 232–54.

——, *Obesity and Depression in the Enlightenment: The Life and Times of George Cheyne* (Oklahoma: University of Oklahoma Press, 2000).

Haakonssen, Lisbeth (ed.), *Medicine and Morals in The Enlightenment: John Gregory, Thomas Percival and Benjamin Rush* (Amsterdam: Clio Medica, 1997).

Haas, J.W., 'John Wesley's Views on Science and Christianity: An Examination of the Charge of Anti-Science', *American Society of Church History,* 63 (1994), 378–92.

Habermas, J., *The Structural Transformation of the Public Sphere: An Enquiry into a Category of Bourgeois Society*, tr. Thomas Burger (Cambridge, MA: MIT Press, 1989).

Hagner, M., 'Enlightened Monsters', in Clark, Golinski, Schaffer (eds), *The Sciences in Enlightened Europe*, 175–217.

Hannaway, Caroline, 'Environment and Miasmata', in Bynum and Porter (eds), *Companion Encyclopedia of the History of Medicine*, (London: Routledge, 1993), Vol. I, 292–308.

Harré, Rom, 'Knowledge', in Rousseau and Porter (eds), *The Ferment of Knowledge: Studies in the Historiography of Eighteenth-Century Science*, 11–54.

Harrison, P., *'Religion' and the Religions in the English Enlightenment* (Cambridge: Cambridge University Press, 1990).

Heal, F., *Hospitality in Early Modern England* (Oxford: Oxford University Press, 1990).

Heller, R., 'Priest-Doctors as a Rural Health Service in the Age of Enlightenment', *Medical History,* 20 (1976), 361–83.

Hembry, Phyllis, *The English Spa, 1560–1815: A Social History* (London: Athlone Press, 1990).

Heyd, Michael, *'Be Sober and Reasonable': The Critique of Enthusiasm in the Seventeenth and Early Eighteenth Centuries* (New York: E.J. Brill, 1995).

Heywood, Audrey, 'A Trial of the Bath Waters: The Treatment of Lead Poisoning', in Porter (ed.), *The Medical History of Waters and Spas*, 82–101.

——, Waldron, H.A., *et al.,* 'The Effect of Immersion on Urinary Lead Excretion', *British Journal of Industrial Medicine*, 43 (1986), 713–715.

Hill, Wesley A., *John Wesley Among the Physicians: A Study of Eighteenth-Century Medicine* (London: Epworth Press, 1958).

Hitchcock, T., 'Paupers and Preachers: The SPCK and the Parochial Workhouse Movement', in Davison, *et al.* (eds), *Stilling the Grumbling Hive*, 145–66.

Holifield, Brookes, E., *Health and Medicine in the Methodist Tradition.* (New York: Crossroad, 1986).

Holmes, Geoffrey, *Augustan England: Professions, State and Society, 1680–1730* (London: George Allen & Unwin, 1982).

Horkheimer, Max and Adorno, Theodor, *Dialectic of Enlightenment*, tr. John Cumming (London: Allen Lane, 1973).

Houlbrooke, R. (ed.), *Death, Ritual and Bereavement* (London: Routledge, 1989).

——, 'Introduction', in *idem* (ed.), *Death, Ritual and Bereavement*, 1–24.

Humble, J.G., and Hansell, P. (eds), *The Westminster Hospital, 1716–1966* (London: Pitman Medical Publishing, 1966).

Hundert, E.J., 'Sociability and Self-Love in the Theatre of Moral Sentiments: Mandeville to Adam Smith', in Stefan Collini, Richard Whatmore, Brian Young (eds), *Economy, Polity, and Society: British Intellectual History, 1750–1950* (Cambridge: Cambridge University Press, 2000), 31–47.

Jacob, Margaret, 'Christianity and the Newtonian Worldview', in David C. Lindberg and Ronald L. Numbers (eds), *God and Nature: Historical Essays on the Encounter between Christianity and Science* (Los Angeles: University of California Press, 1986), 238–55.

Jenner, Mark, 'Bathing and Baptism: Sir John Floyer and the Politics of Cold Bathing', in Kevin Sharpe and Steven N. Zwicker (eds), *Refiguring Revolutions: Aesthetics and Politics from the English Revolution to the Romantic Revolution* (Berkeley: University of California Press, 1998), 197–216.

Jewson, N.D., 'Medical Knowledge and the Patronage System in Eighteenth-Century England', *Sociology*, 8 (1974), 369–85.

Jones, K., *Asylums and After: A Revised History of the Mental Health Services* (London: Athlone Press, 1993).

Jordanova, L., *The Sense of a Past in Eighteenth-Century Medicine* (Reading: University of Reading, 1999).

Juster, S., 'Mystical Pregnancy and Holy Bleeding: Visionary Experience in Early Modern Britain and America', *William and Mary Quarterly*, 57 (2000), 249–88.

Kaplan, Barbara Beigun, *"Divulging of Useful Truths in Physic": The Medical Agenda of Robert Boyle* (Baltimore and London: John Hopkins Press, 1993).

Kasting, N., 'A Rationale for Centuries of Therapeutic Bloodletting: Antipyretic Therapy for Febrile Diseases', *Perspectives in Biology and Medicine,* 33 (1990), 509–16.

Keefer, L.L., 'John Wesley: Disciple of Early Christianity', *Wesleyan Theological Journal,* 19 (1984), 23–32.

King, Lester. S., *The Medical World of the Eighteenth Century* (Chicago: University of Chicago Press, 1958).

Kiple, Kenneth F. (ed.), *The Cambridge World of Human Disease* (Cambridge: Cambridge University Press, 1993).

Knox, R. A., *Enthusiasm: A Chapter in the History of Religion, with Special Reference to the Seventeenth and Eighteenth Centuries* (Oxford: Clarendon Press, 1950).

Kramer, John C., 'Opium Rampant: Medical Use, Misuse, and Abuse in Britain and the West in the Seventeenth and Eighteenth Centuries', *British Journal of Addiction to Alcohol and Other Drugs,* 74 (1979), 377–89.

Laffey, Paul, 'John Wesley on Insanity', *History of Psychiatry,* 12 (2001), 467–79.

Lane, Joan, *A Social History of Medicine: Health, Healing and Disease in England, 1750–1950* (London: Routledge, 2001).

Lawlor, Clark and Suzuki, Akihito, 'The Disease of the Self: Representing Consumption, 1700–1830, *Bulletin of the History of Medicine,* 74, (2000), 458–494.

Lawrence, C.J., 'William Buchan: Medicine Laid Open', *Medical History,* 19 (1975), 20–35.

——, *Medicine in the Making of Modern Britain, 1700–1920* (London: Routledge, 1994).

Lawrence, S.C., 'Anatomy and Address: Creating Medical Gentlemen in Eighteenth-Century London', in Nutton and Porter (eds), *The History of Medical Education in Britain,* 199–228.

——, *Charitable Knowledge: Hospital Pupils and Practitioners in Eighteenth-Century London* (Cambridge: Cambridge University Press, 1996).

Lawton, George, *John Wesley's English: A Study of his Literary Style* (London: George Allen & Unwin, 1962).

Lindeboom, G. A., *Herman Boerhaave: The Man and His Work* (London: Methuen, 1968).

Louden, Irvine, *Medical Care and the General Practitioner, 1750–1850* (Oxford: Clarendon Press, 1986).

Lund, R.D. (ed.), *The Margins of Orthodoxy: Heterodox Writing and Cultural Response* (Cambridge: Cambridge University Press, 1995).

Lyles, A.M., *Methodism Mocked: The Satiric Reaction to Methodism in the Eighteenth Century* (London: Epworth Press, 1960).

MacDonald, M., *Mystical Bedlam: Madness, Anxiety and Healing in Seventeenth-Century England* (Cambridge: Cambridge University Press, 1981).

——, 'Religion, Social Change and Psychological Healing in England 1600–1800', in Sheils (ed.), *The Church and Healing*, 101–25.

Mack, P., 'Religious Dissenters in Enlightenment England', *History Workshop Journal,* 49 (2000), 1–23.

Madden, D., review of Grell and Porter (eds), *Toleration in Enlightenment Europe,* in *History of European Ideas,* 26 (2000), 74–7.

—— and Towsey, D., 'Derrida, Faith and St Paul', *Literature and Theology,* 16 (2002), 396–409.

——, 'Experience and the Common Interest of Mankind: The Enlightened Empiricism of John Wesley's *Primitive Physic*', *British Journal for Eighteenth-Century Studies,* 26/1 (2003), 41–53.

——, 'Pristine Purity: Primitivism and Practical Piety in the Art of John Wesley's Physic', Ph.D. thesis (Oxford University, 2003), 1–360.

——, 'Contemporary Reaction to John Wesley's *Primitive Physic:* Or, The case of William Hawes Examined', *Social History of Medicine* 17/3 (2004), 365–78.

——, 'Medicine and Moral Reform: The Place of Practical Piety in John Wesley's Art of Physic', *Church History* 73/4 (2004), 741–758.

——, 'The Limitation of Human Knowledge: Faith and the Empirical Method in John Wesley's Medical Holism', *History of European Ideas* 32 (2006), 162–72.

Maddox, R., 'A Heritage Reclaimed: John Wesley on Holistic Health and Healing', in Mary Elizabeth Mullino Moore (ed.), *A Living Tradition* (Nashville, TN: Kingswood Books, forthcoming).

Maehle, Andreas-Holger, 'Pharmacological Experimentation with Opium in the Eighteenth Century', in Porter and Teich (eds), *Drugs and Narcotics in History*, 52–76.

Matthee, Rudi, 'Exotic Substances: the Introduction and Global Spread of Tobacco, Coffee, Cocoa, Tea and Distilled Liquor, Sixteenth to Eighteenth Centuries', in Porter and Teich (eds), *Drugs and Narcotics in History*, 24–53.

Matthews, Rex D., 'Religion and Reason Joined', PhD thesis (Harvard University, 1986), 1–269.

——,'"With the Eyes of Faith': Spiritual Experience and the Knowledge of God in the Theology of John Wesley' in Theodore Runyon (ed.), *Wesleyan Theology Today: A Bicentennial Theological Consultation*, (Nashville, TN: Kingswood Books, 1985), 409–26.

Melling, D.J., 'Suffering and Sanctification in Christianity', in J.R. Hinnells and Roy Porter (eds), *Religion, Health and Suffering* (London: Kegan Paul, 1999), 46–64.

Mendus, S., *Justifying Toleration: Conceptual and Historical Perspectives* (Cambridge: Cambridge University Press, 1988).

Mitsuo, Shimizu, 'Epistemology in the Thought of John Wesley', PhD thesis (Drew University, 1980).

Morgan, R., *Romans* (Sheffield: Sheffield Academic Press, 1995).

Nutton, V. and Porter, Roy (eds), *The History of Medical Education in Britain* (Amsterdam: Clio Medica, 1995).

Ott, P.W., 'John Wesley on Health: A Word for Sensible Regimen', *Methodist History*, 18 (1979–80), 193–204.

——, 'John Wesley on Health as Wholeness', *Journal of Religion and Health*, 30 (1991), 43–57.

——, 'Medicine as Metaphor: John Wesley on Therapy of the Soul', *Methodist History*, 33 (1995), 178–91.

Outler, Albert C., 'Introduction', in *The Bicentennial Edition of the Works of John Wesley*, Vol. I, 1–100.

Outram, Dorinda, 'The Enlightenment Our Contemporary', in Clark, Golinski, Schaffer (eds), *The Sciences in Enlightened Europe,* 32–40.

Pagels, E., *Adam, Eve and the Serpent* (London: Penguin, 1988).

Pelling, M., 'Medical Practice in Early Modern England: Trade or Profession?', in Wilfred Prest (ed.), *The Professions in Early Modern England* (London: Croom Helm, 1987), 90–128.

——, 'Knowledge Common and Acquired: The Education of Unlicensed Medical Practitioners in Early Modern London', in Nutton and Porter (eds), *The History of Medical Education in Britain,* 250–79.

Plaut, G.S., 'Dr Fothergill and Eighteenth-Century Medicine', *Journal of Medical Biography,* 7 (1999), 192–6.

Plumb, J.H., *England in the Eighteenth Century* (London: Penguin, 1950).

Pocock, J., 'Enthusiasm: The Antiself of Enlightenment', in Lawrence E. Klein and Anthony La Vopa (eds), *Enthusiasm and Enlightenment in Europe: 1650–1850* (San Marino, CA: Huntingdon Library, 1998), 7–28.

Porter, Dorothy, 'Public Health', in Bynum and Porter (eds), *Companion Encyclopedia of the History of Medicine,* Vol. II, 1231–61.

Porter, Roy, (ed.), *The Enlightenment in National Context* (Cambridge: Cambridge University Press, 1981).

—— (ed.), *Patients and Practitioners* (Cambridge: Cambridge University Press, 1985).

——, *Mind Forg'd Manacles: A History of Madness in England from the Restoration to the Regency* (London: Penguin, 1987).

—— and Porter, Dorothy, *In Sickness and in Health* (New York: Blackwell, 1989).

——, *Health For Sale: Quackery in England 1660–1850* (Manchester: Manchester University Press, 1989).

——, 'Death and the Doctors in Georgian England', in Houlbrooke (ed.), *Death, Ritual and Bereavement,* 77–94.

——, 'The Gift Relation: Philanthropy and Provincial Hospitals in Eighteenth-Century England', in L. Granshaw and Roy Porter (eds), *The Hospital in History* (London: Routledge, 1989), 149–78.

Porter, Roy [*cont...*] (ed.), *The Medical History of Waters and Spas* (London: Wellcome Institute for the History of Medicine, 1990).

——, 'Barely Touching: A Social Perspective on Mind and Body', in G. S. Rousseau (ed.), *The Languages of Psyche: Mind and Body in Enlightenment Thought* (Berkeley: University of California Press, 1990), 45–80.

——, 'Introduction', in Porter (ed.), *George Cheyne: The English Malady: Or, A Treatise of Nervous Diseases of all Kinds (1733)*, ix–xlix.

——, 'The Patient in England, *c.*1660–*c.*1800', in Wear (ed.), *Medicine in Society: Historical Essays*, 91–118.

—— (ed.), *The Popularization of Medicine, 1650–1850* (London: Routledge, 1992).

——, *Doctor of Society: Thomas Beddoes and the Sick Trade in Late-Enlightenment England* (London: Routledge, 1992).

——, 'Spreading Medical Enlightenment: The Popularization of Medicine in Georgian England, and its Paradoxes', in *idem* (ed.), *The Popularization of Medicine*, 215–31.

—— and Roberts, Marie (eds), *Literature and Medicine during the Eighteenth Century* (London: Routledge, 1993).

——, 'The Rise of Physical Examination', in W. F. Bynum and *idem* (eds), *Medicine and the Five Senses* (Cambridge: Cambridge University Press, 1993), 179–97.

——, 'Consumption: Disease of the Consumer Society?' in Brewer and Porter (eds), *Consumption and the World of Goods*, 58–81.

——, 'The Eighteenth Century', in Conrad, *et al.* (eds), *The Western Medical Tradition* (Cambridge: Cambridge University Press, 1995), 371–475.

—— and Teich, Mikuláš (eds), *Drugs and Narcotics in History* (Cambridge: Cambridge University Press, 1995).

—— (ed.), *Medicine in the Enlightenment* (Amsterdam: Clio Medica, 1995).

——, *The Greatest Benefit to Mankind: A Medical History of Humanity from Antiquity to the Present* (London: Harper Collins, 1997).

—— and Rousseau, G. S., *Gout: The Patrician Malady* (London: Yale University Press, 2000).

——, *Enlightenment: Britain and the Creation of the Modern World* (London: Penguin, 2000).

Príhoda, Antonín, *The Healing Powers of Nature* (Leicester: Blitz Editions, 1998).

Rack, Henry D., 'Doctors, Demons and Early Methodist Healing', in Sheils (ed.), *The Church and Healing*, 137–52.

——, *Reasonable Enthusiast: John Wesley and the Rise of Methodism* (London: Epworth Press, 1992).

Redwood, John, *Reason, Ridicule and Religion: The Age of Enlightenment in England, 1660–1750* (London: Thames and Hudson, 1976).

Rey, R., 'Vitalism, Disease and Society', in Porter (ed.), *Medicine in the Enlightenment*, 274–88.

Riddell, W.R., 'Wesley's System of Medicine', *New York Medical Journal*, 99 (1914), 64–8.

Riley, James C., *The Eighteenth-Century Campaign to Avoid Disease* (London: Macmillan, 1987).

Risse, Guenter B., 'Medicine in the Age of Enlightenment', in Wear (ed.), *Medicine in Society*, 149–95.

Rivers, I., *Reason, Grace and Sentiment: A Study of the Language of Religion and Ethics in England, 1660–1780*, 2 vols (Cambridge: Cambridge University Press, 1991).

Roberts, Marie, '"A physic against death": Eternal Life and the Enlightenment – Gender and Gerontology', in Porter and *idem* (eds), *Literature and Medicine during the Eighteenth Century*, 151–67.

Rogal, S.J., 'Pills for the Poor: John Wesley's "Primitive Physick"', *Yale Journal of Biology and Medicine*, 51 (1978), 81–90.

——, 'Electricity: John Wesley's "Curious and Important Subject"', *Eighteenth-Century Life*, 13 (1989), 79–90.

Root-Bernstein, R. and Root-Bernstein, M., *Honey, Mud, Maggots and other Medical Marvels: The Science behind Folk Remedies and Old Wives' Tales* (London: Pan Books, 2000).

Rose, C., 'Evangelical Philanthropy and Anglican Revival: The Charity Schools in Augustan London, 1698–1740', *London Review*, 16 (1991), 35–65.

Rose, C. [*cont...*], 'The Origins and Ideals of the SPCK 1699–1716', in Walsh, Haydon, Taylor (eds), *The Church of England c.1689–c.1833: From Toleration to Tractarianism*, 172–90.

Rosner, Lisa, *Medical Education in the Age of Improvement* (Edinburgh: Edinburgh University Press, 1991).

Rousseau, G.S., 'John Wesley's "Primitive Physick" (1747)', *Harvard Library Bulletin*, 16 (1968), 242–56.

—— and Porter, Roy (eds), *The Ferment of Knowledge: Studies in the Historiography of Eighteenth-Century Science* (Cambridge: Cambridge University Press, 1980).

Rowbottom, M. and Susskind, C., *Electricity and Medicine: A History of their Interaction* (San Francisco: San Francisco Press, 1984).

Rowe, K.E (ed.), *The Place of Wesley in the Christian Tradition* (Metuchen, NJ: Scarecrow Press, 1976).

Rupp, G. and Davies, R. (eds), *A History of the Methodist Church in Great Britain* (London: Epworth Press,1965).

Ryder, M.R., 'Avoiding the "Many-Headed Monster": Wesley and Johnson on Enthusiasm', *Methodist History*, 23 (1984–85), 214–22.

Schaffer, S., 'Measuring Virtue: Eudiometry, Enlightenment and Pneumatic Medicine'. in Cunningham and French (eds), *The Medical Enlightenment of the Eighteenth Century*, 281–318.

——, '"The Consuming Flame": Electric Showmen and Tory Mystics in the World of Goods', in Brewer and Porter (eds), *Consumption and the World of Goods*, 489–526.

Schmidt, M., *John Wesley: A Theological Biography*, tr. N. P. Goldhawk, 2 vols (London: Epworth Press, 1985).

——, 'John Wesley's Place in Church History', in Rowe (ed.), *The Place of Wesley in the Christian Tradition*, 67–93

Schofield, R.E., 'John Wesley and Science in 18th Century England', *Isis,* 44 (1953), 331–40.

Screech, M.A., 'Good Madness in Christendom', in W. F. Bynum, Roy Porter, Michael Shepherd (eds), *The Anatomy of Madness: Essays in the History of Psychiatry*, 2 vols (London: Tavistock Publications, 1985), Vol. I, 25–39.

Semmel, B., *The Methodist Revolution* (London: Heinemann, 1973).

Shapin, Steven, 'Trusting George Cheyne: Scientific Expertise, Common Sense and Moral Authority in Early Eighteenth-Century Dietetic Medicine', *Bulletin of the History of Medicine*, 77, (2003), 263–97.

Sheils, W.J. (ed.), *The Church and Healing* (Studies in Church History, 19), (Oxford: Oxford University Press, 1982).

Shuttleton, David, 'Methodism and Dr Cheyne's "More Enlightening Principles"', in Porter (ed.), *Medicine in the Enlightenment*, 316–35.

Smith, G., 'Prescribing the Rules of Health: Self-Help and Advice in the Late Eighteenth Century', in Porter (ed.), *Patients and Practitioners,* 249–82.

Stewart, Larry, 'Seeing Through the Scholium: Religion and Reading Newton in the Eighteenth Century', *History of Science*, 36 (1996), 123–65.

Ronald H. Stone, *John Wesley's Life and Ethics* (Nashville: Abingdon Press, 2001)

Suzuki, A., 'Anti-Lockean Enlightenment: Mind and Body in Early Eighteenth-Century English Medicine', in Porter (ed.), *Medicine in the Enlightenment*, 336–59.

Thomas, B.G., 'John Wesley and the Art of Healing', *American Physician*, 32 (1906), 295–98.

Thompson, E.P., *The Making of the English Working Class* (Harmondsworth: Penguin, 1963).

——, *Customs in Common* (London: Penguin, 1993).

Tucker, S., *Enthusiasm: A Study in Semantic Change* (Cambridge: Cambridge University Press, 1972).

Turrell, W. J., *John Wesley: Physician and Electrotherapist* (Oxford: Blackwell, 1938).

Valenze, D., *Prophetic Sons and Daughters* (Princeton, NJ: Princeton University Press, 1985).

——, 'Charity, Custom, and Humanity: Changing Attitudes Towards the Poor in Eighteenth-Century England', in Garnett and Matthew (eds), *Revival and Religion since 1700: Essays for John Walsh*, 59–78.

Walsh, John, 'Origins of the Evangelical Revival', in G. V. Bennett and J. D. Walsh (eds), *Essays in Modern Church History in Memory of Norman Sykes* (Oxford: Oxford University Press, 1966), 132–62.

——, 'John Wesley and the Community of Goods', in K. Robbins (ed.), *Protestant Evangelicalism: Britain, Ireland, Germany and America, c.1750–c.1950. Essays in Honour of W.R. Ward* (Oxford: Oxford University Press, 1990), 22–50.

——, Haydon, C., Taylor, S. (eds), *The Church of England c.1689–c.1833: From Toleration to Tractarianism* (Cambridge: Cambridge University Press, 1993).

Ware, Kallistos, 'Preface', in Macarius (Pseudo-), *The Fifty Spiritual Homilies*, xi-xviii.

Wear, Andrew, 'Puritan Perceptions of Illness in Seventeenth-Century England', in Porter (ed.), *Patients and Practitioners*, 55–99.

—— (ed.), 'Early Modern Europe: 1500–1700', in Conrad, *et al.* (eds), *The Western Medical Tradition*, 215–361.

—— (ed.), *Medicine in Society: Historical Essays* (Cambridge: Cambridge University Press, 1992).

Weinberg, Bennet Alan and Bealer, Bonnie K., *The World of Caffeine: The Science and Culture of the World's Most Popular Drug* (London: Routledge, 2001).

White, Andrew Dixon, *History of the Warfare of Science with Theology in Christendom,* 2 vols (New York, 1895).

Wilson, A., 'The Politics of Medical Improvement in Early Hanoverian London', in Cunningham and French (eds), *The Medical Enlightenment of the Eighteenth Century,* 4–39.

Wilson, K., 'Urban Culture and Political Activism in Hanoverian England', in E. Hellmuth (ed.), *The Transformation of Political Culture: England and Germany in Late Eighteenth Century* (Oxford: Oxford University Press, 1990), 165–84.

Young, B.W., *Religion and Enlightenment in Eighteenth-Century England* (Oxford: Clarendon Press, 1998).

Index